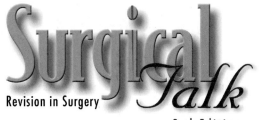

Revision in Surgery

2nd Edition

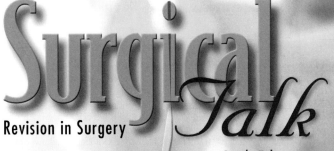

Revision in Surgery

2nd Edition

Andrew Goldberg
Stanmore Royal National Orthopaedic Hospital
Middlesex, UK

Gerard Stansby
University of Newcastle and Freeman Hospital
Newcastle Hospitals NHS Trust
UK

Imperial College Press

Published by

Imperial College Press
57 Shelton Street
Covent Garden
London WC2H 9HE

Distributed by

World Scientific Publishing Co. Pte. Ltd.
5 Toh Tuck Link, Singapore 596224
USA office: 27 Warren Street, Suite 401-402, Hackensack, NJ 07601
UK office: 57 Shelton Street, Covent Garden, London WC2H 9HE

Library of Congress Cataloging-in-Publication Data
Surgical talk : revision in surgery / edited by Andrew Goldberg, Gerard Stansby.-- 2nd ed.
   p. ; cm.
   Includes index.
   Rev. ed. of: Surgical talk / Andrew Goldberg, Gerard Stansby. c1999.
   ISBN-13 978-1-86094-494-9 (pbk) -- ISBN-10 1-86094-494-9 (pbk. : alk. paper)
   1. Surgery. I. Goldberg, Andrew. II. Stansby, Gerard. III. Goldberg, Andrew. Surgical
talk.
   [DNLM: 1. Surgical Procedures, Operative. WO 500 S961867 2005]
   RD31.S9265 2005
   617--dc22

                                                2004065844

British Library Cataloguing-in-Publication Data
A catalogue record for this book is available from the British Library.

First published 2005
Reprinted 2006, 2007, 2008, 2009, 2010

Typeset by Stallion Press
Email: enquiries@stallionpress.com

Printed in Singapore by World Scientific Printers

CONTENTS

Contributors   vii

Foreword   ix
(*by Prof. Averil Mansfield*)

Preface to First Edition   xi

Preface to Second Edition   xiii

Acknowledgements   xv

1. Surgical Talk   1

2. Fluid Balance and Parenteral Nutrition   13

3. Pre- and Postoperative Management   25

4. Trauma, Shock, Head Injuries and Burns   43

5. Liver, Biliary Tract and Pancreas   79

6. Disorders of the Oesophagus, Stomach and Duodenum   105

7. Small Intestine and Colon   127

8. Rectum and Anus   157

9. The Acute Abdomen   165

10. Breast Surgery   175

11. Lumps in the Head, Neck and Skin   197

12. Hernias   217

13. Vascular Disease   229

14. Urology   255

15. Orthopaedics   279

16. Ear, Nose and Throat   361

17. The Exam   379

Index   393

CONTRIBUTORS

Mr. Ben Bannerjee MD, FRCS. Consultant Surgeon and Honorary Senior Lecturer, Sunderland Royal Hospitals, Sunderland, UK.

Mr. Richard M Charnley DM, FRCS. Consultant Hepato-pancreato-biliary Surgeon, Freeman Hospital, Newcastle upon Tyne, UK.

Mr. Jonathan Glass MBBS, BSc, FRCS (Urol). Consultant Urologist, Guys & St. Thomas's Hospital NHS Trust, London, UK.

Prof. S Michael Griffin MD, FRCS. Professor of Gastrointestinal Surgery, Northern Oesophagogastric Unit, Royal Victoria Infirmary, Newcastle upon Tyne, UK.

Mr. Andrew Hilton MBBS, BSc(Hons), FRCS(Orth), Specialist Registrar in Trauma & Orthopaedics, South East Thames, UK.

Mr. Alan F Horgan MD, FRCS. Consultant Colorectal Surgeon, Freeman Hospital, Newcastle upon Tyne, UK.

Mr. Nigel Jones MS, FRCS. Consultant Surgeon, Freeman Hospital, Newcastle upon Tyne, UK.

Dr. Ian Nesbitt FRCA, Dip. ICM. Consultant Anaesthetist, Freeman Hospital, Newcastle upon Tyne, UK.

Mr. Michael Oko FRCS. Higher Surgical Trainee (ENT), Glasgow, UK.

Ms. Sarah Robinson FRCS. Research Registrar, Northern Oesophagogastric Unit, Royal Victoria Infirmary, Newcastle upon Tyne, UK.

Mr. Alan Wilson MSc, MD, FRCS. Consultant Surgeon, Whittington Hospital, London, UK.

FOREWORD

The authors are to be congratulated on a clearly written and presented text. Using this book the student can build up a firm foundation of both knowledge and skills, which will not only enable the hurdle of finals to be negotiated with confidence, but will also be of everyday value in clinical practice.

Visually attractive, readable and scientifically sound, the book makes relatively light work of the large volume of information contained within. It seems likely to me that this book will appeal not only to students with final examinations in mind, but also to house surgeons and senior house officers with patients to diagnose and treat and, perhaps, with the MRCS on the horizon.

Professor Averil Mansfield, CBE, ChM, FRCS

PREFACE TO FIRST EDITION

When you are a medical student, finals seem a daunting prospect. However, the truth is that most candidates pass the exam easily and most junior doctors look back at finals as being relatively straightforward. The reason for this is that this exam is simply the last hurdle in a long and draining race and by the time you have reached this point, the odds are with you to finish the course. The examiners are not there to fail candidates per se; in fact, the opposite is true and they are really trying to help you pass. However, they must ensure that a safe junior doctor is unleashed on the public. Because of this fact you must know the basics of all the common emergency situations. Luck plays only a small part in finals for most students and, as someone once said, "The harder you work, the luckier you get."

The philosophy of this book is to focus on the level of knowledge and the approach that would be expected of the better students arriving at finals. We have tried to include as much as possible without making the book too cumbersome. No book of this scope can include every possible topic, but we hope that we have included all that could legitimately be expected of you for the final exam. The book also contains comprehensive sections on trauma, orthopaedics and urology, which so often get left out of other texts, and a section on fluid balance that may continue to be of use when you are a junior house officer.

The text has been deliberately written in a tutorial-like story format as opposed to a set of lists, since this makes it easier to understand and remember. Everyone loves a list but we must assure you that you are much more likely to remember a list if you have written it yourself. Therefore, space has been left adjacent to the text for you to pick out important details from the text and jot down your own lists. If you do this as you go along, you will effectively produce your own textbook which will become an invaluable tool, with all you need for success at your fingertips.

Good luck with your revision and the exam, and we hope this book will help.

Andrew Goldberg
Gerard Stansby

PREFACE TO SECOND EDITION

We were delighted with the positive feedback that the first edition received from medical students as well as many junior doctors who had long passed their final examinations yet still found the book useful in their working lives.

Over the last few years, the world of medicine has moved on with advances in almost every field. With this in mind, we decided to bring the text up to date and to bring in expertise to co-author many of the chapters, especially those in which we were no longer experts! Each chapter has been reviewed and updated by the co-author whose name is listed at the beginning of the chapter. In addition, we have added an entirely new chapter on ENT, making *Surgical Talk* one of the only texts which comprehensively reviews all of the surgical specialities required for final surgical examinations.

We hope that those of you at that scary point in your career, namely just before you start a job in a new specialty, will also find this book a great overview of the subjects you need to know.

The teaching focus of the text remains. It is still full of 'top tips' to keep the reader one step ahead of the examiner. Exams are a mechanism to sell books. So consider this book a mechanism to pass exams. All feedback is welcome and we look forward to hearing from you.

Andrew Goldberg
Gerard Stansby

ACKNOWLEDGEMENTS

To our *parents* and *wives* who are always there for us and always a forethought.

Marie Stansby, for her help with the illustrations.

The *American College of Surgeons* Committee on Trauma, for their kind permission to use the ATLS® principles.

All the *medical students*, for their suggestions before, whilst and after the first book was written.

1

SURGICAL TALK

There is no doubt that the best performers in finals are those candidates who think logically, express themselves clearly and avoid putting their foot in their mouth by saying something stupid. Their depth of knowledge is not necessarily greater than that of their fellow candidates, but they do well in every part of the exam — writtens, clinicals and the viva. The message is clear: you must start early, practising a systematic approach to the subject. In this chapter several examples of such approaches are given. You may not like all of them, so choose a method that you can use and spend a great deal of time perfecting it. Also, note that a short pause before answering does not detract from the answer and may avoid a dreadful mistake.

Remember also that in finals the examiners are looking for a minimum standard across the breadth of medicine and surgery. Effectively, they wish to assess whether you will be safe as a house officer subsequently. They will not be impressed by superb knowledge in one area if there is ignorance about basic facts in another. You will not be expected to know the technical details of any particular operation but should have an understanding of the broad principles and common complications that would be explained to the patient. An example question might be, 'What would you say to the patient when consenting him for this operation?' If you did not know that there were two incisions or that there was a high chance of needing a colostomy, then how could you be expected to inform the patient correctly?

It follows that it is in your best interest to make sure that you know the essential basics about all relevant topics before attempting to learn some topics in greater detail. It is also a basic fact of human psychology that, when revising, students tend to revise more often the areas they feel comfortable about. In fact it is the areas you feel uncomfortable about that you need to spend time on. To avoid leaving gaps in your revision take the chapter headings of your surgical textbook and make sure that you feel you could give a short summary of the basic points in each chapter. If you cannot say much about a particular subject (and would dread being asked about it in finals), then that is your most urgent revision priority — do not leave it to chance.

SURGICAL SIEVES

Sometimes you are asked an obscure question, which throws you. Your mind goes blank, you blurt out the first thing that comes into your head, and you end up in a deep hole. Afterwards you often realise that you did know the answer, or at least some of it. A sieve allows you to gather your thoughts, working from first principles, and come up with at least some sensible statements. When you answer a question, you should really talk about the most common things first and the rarities at the end, and one disadvantage of using a sieve is that you may not be able to rapidly reorganise your thoughts in this way, but still it is useful when all else fails and is invaluable in essay writing.

The Aetiological Sieve

- Congenital
- Acquired
  - Traumatic
  - Inflammatory (physical, chemical, infective)
  - Neoplastic (benign or malignant, primary or secondary)
  - Circulatory
  - Autoimmune
  - Nutritional
  - Metabolic
  - Endocrine

- Drugs
- Degenerative
- Iatrogenic
- Psychosomatic

TIN CAN MED DIP is one way of remembering it, but you probably have your own method.

The Anatomical Sieve

This can apply to anatomical sites, structures or tissue types. If asked 'What are the causes of mechanical bowel obstruction?', you could say 'Adhesions.' This is a correct answer but an incorrect way of saying it. Start by saying that the bowel is a structure consisting of several anatomical regions and hence obstruction can occur anywhere along its length, for example, stomach outflow obstruction, small bowel obstruction and large bowel obstruction. The examiner will then usually pick one route and lead you along it. If writing an essay, you obviously need to discuss all three. Then, add that the bowel is a hollow tube, and like any hollow tube (cf. ureters) it can become blocked at three sites: from outside the tube pressing in (extramural), within the wall of the tube (intramural) and within the lumen of the tube (luminal). Where appropriate, answers should be structured in this way.

Causes of Mechanical Bowel Obstruction

Extramural	*Intramural*	*Luminal*
Adhesions	Tumours	Impacted faeces
Strangulated hernia	Infarction	Foreign body
Volvulus	Strictures	Large polyps
Extrinsic	Inflammation	Intussusception
compression	(e.g. Crohn's)	

Do not forget that there are other structures such as muscle, bone, joints and nerves in the region, but in this case these would rarely be the cause.

If possible, when listing differential diagnoses try to do so in the order of their likelihood (i.e. do not mention vanishingly rare things before common things).

General and Specific

'Tell me about postoperative complications.' When asked such a question it is difficult to know where to start. As before, you must avoid saying the first thing that comes into your head, as this may not be the most relevant. Here, we can use two types of classification: one applies to the type of complication, and the other gives a time scale.

Postoperative complications can be *generalized*, i.e. applying to any operation (such as the effects of anaesthesia), or *specific*, i.e. applying to a particular operation (such as damage to the recurrent laryngeal nerve in thyroidectomy).

Once classified into general and specific the complications can be broken down further into time scales. These complications can be *immediate*, *early* or *late* (see chapter on pre- and postoperative complications for further details).

Once you use these principles, it becomes easy to answer most questions logically. For example: 'What are the causes of haematuria?' The causes can be *generalized* (e.g. a bleeding disorder or use of anticoagulants) or *specific*, relating to any of the *anatomical structures* in the region. The following structures (starting from the top) are part of the urinary tract:

Structure	Causes
Kidney	Stones, trauma, carcinoma (use the aetiological sieve)
Ureter	Tumours, stones, infection
Bladder	Infection, tumour, stones
Prostate	Benign hypertrophy, tumour, infection
Urethra	Stone, infection, trauma, etc.

NB. Confirm true haematuria, since the appearance of red urine can occur following beetroot ingestion or with certain drugs such as rifampicin. Also, exclude bleeding from the vagina or anus.

Tissue Types

Try to list the causes of a lump in the groin. It is difficult to be exhaustive is it not? A good method is to use tissue types, i.e. say that this lump can arise from any of the tissue types in this region. For example:

Tissue type	Example
Skin	Sebaceous cyst
Adipose tissue	Lipoma
Connective tissue	Fibroma
Lymphatics	Enlarged lymph node
Blood vessels	Saphena varix, femoral artery aneurysm
Inguinal canal	Inguinal hernia, hydrocoele of the cord
Femoral canal	Femoral hernia
Testes	Undescended testes

Investigations

Always break down investigations in the following manner:

1. *Simple urine and faecal tests* (e.g. urine dipstix, microscopy and culture, pregnancy tests, faecal occult blood)
2. *Haematological tests* (routine, e.g. FBC, or special, e.g. tumour markers)
3. *Radiological tests* (e.g. CXR, ultrasound or CT)
4. *Special investigations* (e.g. gastroscopy, V/Q scans)

It is easy to shout out 'Full blood count', 'Chest X-ray' or 'Calcium' as an answer to the question 'How would you investigate such a patient?' However, if you think of and give the above answers every time you are asked such a question, going through the categories one by one, you will never leave out something by mistake. You may be asked to justify your choice of investigation. Often we send off investigations as a baseline since the patients are being admitted to hospital. This is justified in the elderly but is usually a waste of resources in young, fit patients. A full blood count is justified in young females, to check for anaemia. U & Es should be sent for patients on diuretics.

Management

'Discuss the treatment of benign prostatic hypertrophy' is a different question from 'Discuss the management of benign prostatic hypertrophy.' In the former the examiners want you to purely concentrate on treatment and not on diagnosis. In your answer you should define BPH (benign prostatic hypertrophy) and perhaps say one or two sentences on the condition and its investigation, but do not spend too long on this as you will get no extra marks. Management involves discussing all of the steps that deal with a clinical problem, including the history, examination, investigations, formation of a diagnosis and treatment.

When discussing treatment you can again break down your answer into subheadings. For example: treatment can be conservative, medical or surgical. For example, in this case:

Conservative. This usually means ruling out cancer. A prostate specific antigen (PSA) <4 and a normal examination would help the doctor reassure the patient and a policy of watchful waiting may be adopted until the symptoms get worse.

Medical. For example, drugs such as α1-adreno-receptor blockers or 5-α-reductase inhibitors.

Surgical. For example, trans-urethral resection of the prostate (TURP).

Answering an Essay

Essay questions nowadays are not common, but if they do feature tend to be quite generalized; for example, 'Minimal access surgery — discuss.' There will, however, always be the odd question based on a detailed knowledge of one condition.

The following is a guide for the headings you can use in writing such an essay; some surgeons refer to this as the pathological sieve.

- Definition
- Aetiology (incidence, age, sex, geography)/risk factors
- Histology (macro and micro)
- Clinical features (signs and symptoms)
- Diagnosis (and differential)
- Clinical staging (if appropriate)
- Investigations/treatment/management
- Complications
- Prognosis

Remember that management depends on diagnosis and that diagnosis depends on history, examination and special investigations. Therefore 'management' refers to all of the steps of clinical assessment and investigation as well as treatment.

Never forget the steps of management which occur early on as the patient is being admitted to hospital. For example, if asked how you would manage a case of acute cholecystitis, you need to say that you would give the patient adequate analgesia, arrange admission to a surgical bed, put up a drip, keep nil by mouth, etc., before talking about liver function tests or ultrasound scans (which would not normally be available immediately). It is often a good idea to try and imagine that you are actually the doctor in A & E who is trying to sort the patient out. What would you actually do? What observations would you ask the nurses to take? When would you review the patient? Would you inform someone more senior? Would you put in a urinary catheter, etc.? By mentioning such points you not only increase the content of your answer, you also demonstrate that you have become aware of the practical aspects of being a junior doctor as well as of the textbook theory.

As part of your management add the word 'POSSET' at the end of an essay if appropriate — *P*hysio, *O*ccupational therapy, *S*pecialists (e.g. stoma care, breast care, speech therapists), *S*ocial workers, *E*ducation and *T*erminal care. The last two are of the utmost importance. Education involves explaining things like when the stitches will come out, what you can and cannot do (such as when you can drive, have sex), etc. Terminal care means involving the Macmillan Nurses, arranging the syringe pump to deliver analgesia, speaking to the GP, etc. This last paragraph can be the difference between a good essay and an excellent one.

History of a Lump

Surgery is full of lumps. No matter where the lump is, there are only five questions you need to remember when taking the history of a lump:

- When and how did you first notice the lump?
- How has the lump changed since you first noticed it?
- What symptoms does it cause you?
- Have you got any more or have you had this before?
- What do you think it is?

You *must* learn this list. These are the vital questions and they apply to any lump, whether it be in the neck, in the breast or in the groin.

For example, was it *noticed* incidentally, whilst looking in the mirror, or did your partner point it out to you? Remember — this is when the lump was first noticed and not when it first appeared! *How has it changed?* Has it got bigger, smaller, stayed the same size, or has it come and gone? Has it changed its appearance and consistency, does it get bigger during a period? *What are the symptoms?* Is it painful? (Patients often wrongly equate this to cancer.) Symptoms usually are related to anatomical site. For example, in breast lumps, is there a nipple discharge? A lump in the neck could affect voice, respiration or eating. If you think this is a thyroid lump, ask relevant questions about hypo- or hyperthyroidism.

Have you got any more/had it before? If the patient has many lumps, are they the same? If he has had this before, what happened to it the last time, and what did the doctor say it was? Does it come periodically (for example, with every menstrual cycle)?

What do you think it is? This is an important question, since the answer may be 'Cancer, doctor.' You are then aware of the patient's anxieties. You may be able to reassure the patient even if you do not know the exact diagnosis. For example, you may be able to reassure a 20-year-old girl with a painful breast lump that breast cancer is rare at her age and usually is not painful, etc.

History of a Pain

Again, there are only a few questions you need to remember:

- Where is the pain?
- What is the nature of the pain?
- How did the pain start and what has happened to it since?
- What relieves and what exacerbates the pain?
- Are there any associated symptoms?
- Have you ever had this before? Previous history.
- What do you think it is?

As seen with the history of a lump, this set of questions can apply to any pain, whether cardiac in origin or due to appendicitis.

Site. Remember that visceral pain is referred along the somatic nerves; for example, diaphragmatic irritation is felt at the shoulder, and early appendicitis is felt around the umbilicus.

Nature. This includes character, severity and radiation. Colicky pains feel like the contents of a tube are being squashed or pushed forward. They originate from a hollow viscus, and usually come and go in a regular pattern. Severity is difficult to standardise, since everyone has a different threshold of pain, but saying something like 'The pain is worse than labour pains' or 'This is the worst pain they have ever had' is often helpful.

What has happened to the pain? This includes onset, progression and end. Was the onset sudden or gradual? Has the pain got better or worse since it started? Does it come and go? How is it now compared to when it started? It is sometimes helpful to get the patient to draw a graph of the pain against time.

Aggravating or relieving factors. Asking the patient for aggravating or relieving factors often leads to a blank and you may have to ask more direct questions in this context. For example, 'Does the pain want to make you writhe about or lie very still?' Classically, colicky pains make you move about trying to get comfortable, whereas if there is inflammation involving the peritoneum, then moving about makes the pain worse. This distinction is helpful in differentiating biliary colic, where the patient may be moving about during an episode, from cholecystitis, where the patient will tend to lie still.

Associated symptoms. Again, this will depend on the cause and site of the pain. For example, nausea, vomiting and signs of sympathetic stimulation all go with cardiac pain. Anorexia, weight loss, change in the bowel habit and, perhaps, rectal bleeding would be suggestive of a bowel cancer, etc.

Past history. If the patient has had this pain before he can usually tell you if this feels the same as the last episode — for example, an alcoholic with repeated episodes of acute pancreatitis or the angina sufferer, with an MI. Ask about the past medical history and what drugs the patient is taking.

Answering a Question

By the time finals come along, almost everyone knows how to answer a viva question with the boring words 'I would take a thorough history, examine the patient and investigate according to my findings ... .' The examiner hears this statement time after time, and when the candidate cannot back it up with something more substantial, the examiner rightly becomes annoyed. A better approach which will make you stand out from the rest of the candidates is to apply your answer directly to the question. So, if, for example, you are asked how you would manage someone with a breast lump, you could say, 'In my history I would find out about the history of the lump and ask in particular for risk factors for breast cancer or for factors suggestive of benign breast disease .... On examination I would inspect the breasts, followed by palpation, examining the normal side first, etc. ... My investigations would then be tailored to my findings from the history and examination, but should involve an imaging technique plus or minus a fine needle aspiration. The patient would then require counselling about the disease, and treatment could be divided into medical and surgical options (which can be subdivided into curative and palliative).'

This is not meant to give you the full answer — it only highlights the approach you would use (the correct answer is in the chapter on breast surgery). It is clear that this answer shows that you are thinking properly and not merely giving stereotypical responses. If the examiner wants to test you further he may then go on, 'Good, so tell me what questions you would like to ask in taking the history of this lump?' or 'What are the risk factors for breast cancer?' This way, you are forcing the examiner into asking you questions that you want to hear, and hence you are always one step ahead. Likewise, if the examiner asks you for the complications of thyroidectomy, do not spend too much time on the general complications; rather, use perhaps a simple sentence like 'Any operation has both general and specific complications and each can be divided into immediate, early and late. The specific complications of thyroidectomy are ... .' If he wishes to know the general complications he can then ask you — this way, it shows that you understand the question being asked.

It may be possible to give an adequate performance even when you are unsure of the exact diagnosis. A clear history or good clinical examination technique will go a long way towards persuading the examiners that you should pass. Often, if you have accurately reported the history and physical signs, the examiners will give you a hint towards the correct diagnosis if you do not get it immediately.

2

FLUID BALANCE AND PARENTERAL NUTRITION

Ian Nesbitt

During your first ever night on call as a doctor, it is almost a certainty that you will be asked to write up intravenous (IV) fluids. Fluid balance is one of the most important subjects in medicine. Sadly, however, it is a subject that is poorly covered in most textbooks and so in this chapter we start from first principles to help you understand and remember the topic.

BASIC FACTS

The human body is composed of approximately two-thirds water. The contribution of water to body weight depends on how much fat you carry, because fat contains very little water. People gain fat as they grow older. Women also tend to have a greater proportion of fat and so females and the elderly will have a smaller proportion of total body water.

If we assume body water is 60% of our weight, then a 70 kg man will carry 42 l water. Of this 42 l, two-thirds (28 l) will be intracellular fluid (ICF), and one-third (14 l) will be extracellular fluid (ECF). The ECF is subdivided into plasma (3 l), interstitial fluid (ISF — an aquatic habitat for the cells, about 10 l) and transcellular fluids (CSF, ocular, peritoneal and synovial fluids, about 1 l).

Osmotic pressure is the pressure needed to reverse osmosis (through a semipermeable membrane, i.e. a cell wall). Simply put, it is the ability of a solute to attract water. Oncotic pressure on the other hand is the pressure exerted by proteins to draw fluids back in.

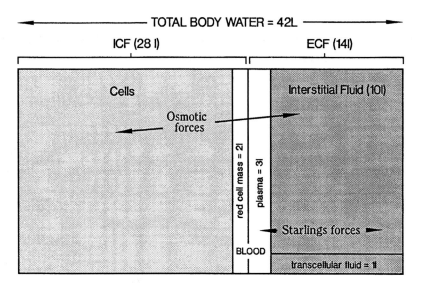

Figure 2.1. Distribution of fluids within the body spaces.

The osmolalities (reflecting the osmotic pressure) of the ICF and the ECF are similar, although the main cation in the ECF is sodium, whereas in the ICF it is potassium. Fluid distribution between the ECF and the ICF is governed only by changes in the osmotic pressure. This means that isotonic fluid (which has the same osmolality as plasma) administered into the plasma will not enter the ICF, since there is no difference in the osmolality.

Within the ECF, fluid distribution between the plasma and the ISF is only governed by Starlings forces, i.e. hydrostatic pressure (pushing fluid out of the blood vessels) versus oncotic pressures (sucking fluid back in). Therefore, fluid administered into the plasma would increase the hydrostatic pressure and dilute the oncotic pressure until the fluid was evenly distributed throughout the ECF (Figure 2.1).

TYPES OF FLUID

Crystalloids are essentially electrolytes in water. Because they have no large molecules (and thus have no oncotic pressure), they are easily distributed to the extracellular spaces and so can be used as maintenance fluids. Examples of crystalloids are normal saline (which is isotonic, i.e. 0.9% saline) and 5% dextrose, which is hypotonic. There is also a solution called Hartmans, which contains lactate, potassium and calcium in addition to sodium chloride, and is therefore described as 'physiological'. Colloids contain larger molecules which stay in the circulation for longer. They increase the oncotic pressure and thus can draw fluid back into the circulation. They are good for maintaining blood pressure, although they do not have oxygen-carrying capacity. Examples of colloids are Haemaccel, which contains gelatin, and Dextran, which is a solution of high molecular weight dextrose.

Why is this important? Well, if for example one gave 1 litre of isotonic saline intravenously, it would initally only be distributed into the ECF (which includes the plasma). As plasma is only 3 litre of the whole ECF, which is 14 litre, only 3/14 or 214 ml would remain in the plasma (the distribution takes minutes). In contrast, 1 litre of 5% dextrose (which is hypotonic and so initially dilutes the ECF relative to the ICF) administered intravenously would be equally distributed throughout the body, and so 3/42 litre or 70 ml would remain in the plasma. However, of 500 ml of a colloid given intravenously, all of it will stay in the plasma initially as there is no change in osmotic pressure and so no distribution into the cells (ICF).

It is clear that different situations require different types of fluid replacement, and you can see why crystalloid preparations are of little use in acute blood loss when colloids or blood may be more appropriate.

THE FLUID BALANCE EQUATION

The simplest way to think about fluid balance is that it is an equilibrium where input must equal output. In order to live we must excrete all of our waste products. The main route for this is via the kidneys. The minimal volume of urine we need to produce in order to be healthy is about 1 l a day (0.5–1 ml/kg/h). This is the minimal obligatory volume of urine (MOVU). If less urine than this is produced, the patient is oliguric, and if no urine is produced, anuric.

At rest, we also have other fluid losses that we are unaware of and these are called insensible water losses. Insensible losses occur from the lungs and in faeces, which amount to about 500 ml, and from the skin by sweating, which is also about 500 ml. If we add up MOVU to the insensible losses, then our minimal daily fluid replacement is therefore about 1.5–2 l.

This figure, however, relates to a healthy adult lying in bed; if we got up and moved around, then the requirements will go up. In view of this we usually estimate that the average adult will require about 3 l of fluids a day.

As well as water, we also lose about 60 mM potassium and 100 mM sodium per day; these salts will also need replacing. In a normal person, large amounts of fluid are recycled in the body and must be accounted for in the so-called equilibrium. These include gastric juice (3–4 l), bile (about 1 l) and intestinal secretions (succus entericus, about 3–4 l). This enteric recycling accounts for about 8 l/day and is mostly reabsorbed further down the GI tract.

It is common sense that any fluid and electrolyte losses must be replaced, if we are to remain in equilibrium. This is usually achieved by our daily dietary intake of food and drink, although a small proportion of water is derived as a by-product of metabolism (Figure 2.2).

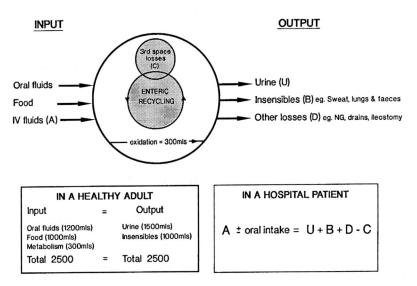

Figure 2.2. The balance between fluid input and fluid output.

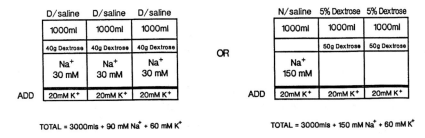

Figure 2.3. Typical daily requirement of intravenous fluids: two alternative regimens.

When patients come to hospital they may be unable to have sufficient oral fluid intake either because they are 'nil by mouth' (perioperatively or through illness) or because they are vomiting.

Such patients require intravenous fluids and these can be any of the available crystalloid preparations. As highlighted above, the average adult will need about 3 l a day. This amount of dextrose saline would do (each litre bag contains 30 mM of sodium). Another method would be to give 1 l normal saline (containing 150 mM sodium) and 2 l of 5% dextrose. The dextrose is quickly metabolised, leaving water. In either of these two methods you have replaced 3 l of water with either 90 or 150 mM of sodium. If you add 20 mM of potassium to each litre bag (some bags come with this already added), then you will have also replaced the necessary 60 mM of potassium. If you request each bag to run over 8 h, then the 3 l will last the full day (Figure 2.3).

In cases where patients are on fluids for several days, it is inadvisable to prescribe dextrose saline alone, because after a few days of replacing too little sodium, the patient could well become hyponatraemic. This is easily avoided by adding in normal saline in every third bag.

These are the standard regimens given to most normal adults; there are, however, many exceptions to the rule, including the following.

The Postoperative Period

The metabolic response to the stresses of surgery involves a rise in various hormones, including circulating catecholamines, ADH and, through stimulation of the hypothalamo-pituitary-adrenal axis, cortisol and aldosterone. The overall result of these is the renal conservation of salt and water, with somewhat increased losses of potassium and hydrogen ions. These effects usually last for about 24–48 h. Despite the high potassium losses in the urine, the serum potassium is usually maintained or may even transiently rise, through release of cellular contents by damaged tissues. Therefore, unless serum potassium levels are very low, it is probably best to avoid potassium supplements in the first day or two postoperatively.

In addition, since water is being retained it is usual to reduce the fluid replacements to about 2 l in the first postoperative day, especially in patients prone to heart failure. It is important to remember that a patient going to theatre is likely to have starved for several hours beforehand and may not have been given any fluids intraoperatively or whilst in recovery.

This patient will probably need extra fluids to maintain the fluid balance equilibrium. It is easy to see why one cannot rely on standard regimens when calculating how much fluid to give someone and so urine output is the best indicator, aiming for greater than 50 ml/h. The nursing staff should document urine output on the charts by the patient's bed. Young, fit adults can usually tolerate excess fluids and so as long as the urine output is satisfactory, you are probably doing okay. The minimum urine output is about 30 ml/h (remember MOVU). Obviously, the urea and electrolytes (U & Es) can be checked, to help assess renal function.

Third Space Losses

As mentioned before, about 8 l of secretions per day are reabsorbed in the bowel. A patient who has undergone abdominal surgery is likely to have a transient ileus postoperatively, where the bowel temporarily stops working. In such patients this is usually due to mechanical handling of the bowel, although any patient can suffer a transient ileus, due to an electrolyte disturbance or even the effects of anaesthesia. When an ileus is present, the fluid secreted into the bowel simply lies there, and is not reabsorbed completely. These 'third space' losses mean that the patient effectively has a reduced volume of the ECF, and hence is fluid depleted.

In such patients, extra fluid needs to be given to allow for the third space losses. Unfortunately, you will not know how much extra fluid is needed and so must rely on urine output as an indicator. You will usually notice a sudden diuresis on day 2 or 3 postoperatively, explained by recovery of the ileus and reabsorption of the fluids from the bowel.

Similarly, in pancreatitis, patients can lose several litres of fluids rich in electrolytes and plasma proteins into the peritoneal cavity. Really, the only way to effectively gauge these losses is by vigorous replacement to maintain their urine output and correcting any electrolyte disturbances according to daily U & Es. If after 2 days 10 l have been put in with only 3 l of urine produced, then assuming 1–2 l of insensible losses, this equates to about 5 or 6 l of fluid sequestered into the peritoneal cavity.

Other Losses

If a patient has a nasogastric tube or a wound drain or is draining via a fistula, these losses need to be calculated daily and replaced (usually as normal saline) in addition to the standard losses.

Ileostomy patients can have huge losses, especially several days postoperatively. It is advisable to assess the ileostomy output at least twice daily, replacing these fluids and electrolytes accordingly to prevent acute dehydration.

Patients with pyrexia require more fluids. One can lose 3 l, maybe more, in certain circumstances. A rough estimate is to increase the fluid replacement by 10% for each degree of fever. Similarly, losses through vomiting or diarrhoea need replacing; remember that large-intestinal juices contain high concentrations of potassium and gastric juice contains a lot of hydrogen ions.

Heart or Liver Failure

Because the renin–angiotensin system is already working overtime, conserving sodium, you should avoid giving fluids which contain sodium, hence you should mainly use 5% dextrose in these patients.

In heart failure, the patient is fluid overloaded, the usual cause in surgical patients being poor management of the fluid balance by the doctor. If you look at the fluid balance charts you will probably see a positive balance over the previous few days. Therefore, you will need to reduce their input, maybe even stop the fluids altogether and consider diuretics. Obviously, you should examine the patient regularly, measuring their JVP, listening to their chest and watching for oedema. Very sick patients on the ward usually will have a CVP line, and this makes the assessment of these patients a little easier. Ask the nursing staff to chart the patient's daily weight as this will help in monitoring progress.

Acute Renal Failure

This can be prerenal (e.g. hypovolaemia), renal (e.g. acute tubular necrosis) or postrenal (e.g. a blocked catheter). After surgery both pre- and postrenal causes are the commonest, and so should be looked for and treated first. If the patient is fluid depleted, you may respond simply by correcting the dehydration. Look over the fluid balance charts from the previous days to decide whether the patient is in negative fluid balance. If you think that a renal cause is likely, you should avoid potassium loads, stop any drugs that may affect renal function (such as NSAIDS, ACE inhibitors, etc.) and involve the renal team in the management early on. Usually, they advise replacing the previous days' output plus 500 ml to cover insensible losses. Alternatively, one could measure hourly urine output and replace 100% of this every hour.

In summary, input should equal output unless the above exceptions apply. Look over the fluid balance charts (remember to bear in mind that in practice these are often very inaccurate) and the daily weight charts. Assess the patient's state of hydration (dry lips, skin turgor, etc.) and check their blood results for renal function and haematocrit. Finally, do not forget the temperature, both the patient's and that of the room.

We have deliberately gone into a lot of details on this subject, perhaps more than you need to know to pass the finals. This is because it is not really a topic that one can waffle about in the exam — either you understand the principles or you do not.

NUTRITION

Patients who are malnourished are prone to many complications, such as delayed wound healing, muscle weakness and an increased tendency to infection. There is evidence that patients with poor nourishment prior to surgery will benefit from preoperative supplementation and do better after their operation. One caveat of this is that intervention must be for a reasonable period of time (more than 10 days) in order to be of significant benefit.

There are a lot of reasons why hospital patients become malnourished. They may have a decreased appetite due to the illness itself. They may have increased nutritional demands or their digestion may be impaired. Another reason could be due to the hospital stay itself, i.e. dislike of hospital food, being rushed off for an X-ray or ultrasound at noon, or being nil by mouth.

If oral intake is not anticipated within 7–10 days of surgery, then nutritional support is indicated (perhaps 5 days in a previously malnourished patient). The main indication for preoperative nutritional support is severe malnourishment (greater than 10% weight loss).

Nutritional support can vary from mere supplementation of vitamins, or protein in a high-protein diet, to a complete replacement of all essential foodstuffs. In this section, we only cover the latter.

Enteral versus Parenteral Nutrition

Enteral diets are those given via the gut, including oral intake. Obviously, the ideal situation is one where the patient takes in all the required nutrition orally; if this is not possible, then *enteral feeding* is the next option. This involves passing the food into the gut, allowing it to be absorbed normally, either through a nasogastric tube or, if required for longer periods, via a gastrostomy or jejenostomy. The commonest indication for enteral feeding is where there is a problem with swallowing, caused by a stroke or oesophageal obstruction.

Parenteral nutrition bypasses the gut and involves a specialised feed directly into the patient's bloodstream. Parenteral nutrition may be used as a supplement to enteral feeding when it is usually given through a cannula in a peripheral vein. Alternatively, total parenteral nutrition (TPN) can be used to deliver the complete nutritional requirements. As TPN has a high osmolality it is toxic to veins and is usually given via a central line. The buzz words would be to insert 'a small cannulae into a large vein with a high rate of blood flow'. Hence, a central venous pressure (CVP) line is usually used. For longer-term use, a Hickman line is preferred, which is a modified CVP line usually tunneled under the skin to make it more secure and has a Dacron cuff to prevent infection from entering. Unfortunately, parenteral feeding has some complications, including an increased risk of infection:

- It is not uncommon for a house officer to get called to see a patient with parenteral feeding who has recently spiked a temperature. Obviously, your management would be as for any pyrexia (see page 36); however, if you suspect that the feed is the likely source of the infection, the correct thing to do is to stop the feed. If indeed this is the cause, then the temperature usually settles quickly, despite the fact that the CVP line is still *in situ* and may be infected. It appears that the running feed may be responsible for introducing the bugs from the infected line into the bloodstream. The CVP line will, however, ultimately need to be removed and replaced.
- Another complication of parenteral feeding is villous atrophy in the gut. Since the gut luminal cells (enterocytes) derive their nutrition from the lumen, long periods of rest can lead to atrophy. This makes the gut wall more permeable to bacterial flora and there is evidence that this can increase the risk of 'translocation' of bacteria into the bloodstream.
- Electrolyte imbalances are likely and, therefore, the urea and electrolytes should be checked daily and adjusted accordingly.
- Hyperglycaemia is another problem and the patient may need to be given insulin temporarily whilst on TPN. Other disturbances of liver function are common (possibly because of fatty infiltration of the liver) and a cholestatic picture may be seen with raised alkaline phosphatase, and hence LFTs should be measured every few days.

- The take-home message must be that parenteral feeding should be reserved for patients in whom enteral feeding is impossible, such as patients with short gut syndrome, where large pieces of their gut have been surgically removed. Otherwise, enteral feeding should be your first choice.

Requirements

1. *Water.* See section on fluid balance; roughly 2–3 l per day.
2. *Energy.* About 1800 calories per day. This is given as a mixture of carbohydrate and fats: roughly, in a ratio of two-thirds to one-third, respectively (but can be up to 50–50).
3. *Nitrogen.* About 14 g/day in protein, but the requirement may change (8–20 g/day) according to the metabolic state.
4. *Vitamins.* The fat-soluble vitamins are stored and so the levels are carefully adjusted to avoid overdose. Water-soluble vitamins being excreted are therefore given more generously.
5. *Minerals.* Sodium, potassium, calcium, magnesium, phosphate, etc.
6. *Trace elements.* Zinc, copper, iron, selenium, iodide, etc.

The management of nutrition should be multidisciplinary, including the surgeon, the dietician, the pharmacist, who makes up the feed, and the nurses, who actually administer it. Nowadays, the feeds are usually made up into one complete sterile 3 l bag (even if it contains only 2 l) in the pharmacy department according to the specific requirements of the individual patient, hopefully with the dietician's advice. The most important step is the connection of the feed to the patient as this is when infection is likely to occur, and hence it should be a sterile procedure.

Monitoring assessment of nutritional status is best done on a clinical basis. The patient's appearance and weight are the best indicators. Other anthropometric measurements, such as skin fold thickness, are not ideal but may be of benefit in monitoring progress.

Daily measurement of albumin is pointless, since its half-life is long (about 21 days) and its level can be altered for many other reasons, although it is helpful in long-term monitoring.

Other biochemical tests are available, such as transferrin, which is better than albumin in the short term. But probably the best day-to-day biochemical measurement is prealbumin (a liver protein), which is a good marker of nutritional status. Obviously, electrolytes should be measured daily and LFTs should be checked every few days.

Finally, of much amusement on ward rounds are the other markers of nutrition, such as grip strength and stool length — but as to who does these, let alone how, I leave to your imagination.

3

PRE- AND POSTOPERATIVE MANAGEMENT

Ian Nesbitt

When you are a surgical house officer (or F1), part of your role preoperatively will be to clerk the patients and prepare them for the theatre or their investigations.

A clerking consists of the history of the presenting complaint, past medical history, drug history, family history and social history. You should then examine the patient fully, looking first at their general health and whether they are fit enough for the operation, and if not you should be thinking of ways to optimise their health, such as using preoperative nebulisers for an asthmatic. The clerking also allows other problems to be picked up.

If, when the patient arrives on the ward, you feel that the diagnosis made in the out-patient clinic has changed, you should inform a senior colleague before the operation is booked. For example, if a patient was admitted for an excisional biopsy of a lymph node that has completely disappeared when you examine them, you should inform your consultant, as the operation might need to be cancelled.

In the main, appropriate investigations should be performed before surgery and this is often a good question for a viva examination. For example, before a laparascopic cholecystectomy is performed the patient should have had an ultrasound to confirm the presence of gallstones, and a set of liver function tests.

The house officer should discuss the order of patients on the operating list with the operating surgeon. Usually, children are placed first on the list, as this is nicer for the child and the parents; also they find it hard to go without food for long periods. If special equipment is needed in the theatre, such as the image intensifier for X-rays or laparascopic equipment, then these should be discussed with the theatre staff (and radiographers) the day before.

Specialist nurses who have expertise in certain areas such as breast disease, wound management and stomas should be involved preoperatively in all appropriate cases. For example, a patient who is likely to need a colostomy or ileostomy should be seen by the stoma nurse specialist several days before the operation. This allows for patient education (i.e. answering of any questions and worries), and also the site where the stoma will be cited is marked (note that the patient should be standing, so as to position it in the most appropriate place).

Comorbidity

Many patients have problems other than the one that is being operated upon. These may be social and as such need a social work or occupational therapy referral. For example, if the patient has difficulty climbing stairs and there is no lift, then there may be a need to arrange for a stair lift or rehouse into ground floor accommodation.

The patients may have intercurrent medical problems such as diabetes, hypertension or chronic obstructive pulmonary disease (COPD). They may also be on drugs such as steroids or anticoagulants. When clerking the patient you should be looking out for these, and if you think they may affect the operation, then you should inform the anaesthetist or the consultant in charge of the patient.

As a house officer the tests you need to consider preoperatively include blood tests, such as a full blood count, a sickle screen if at risk (this includes anyone of Afro-Caribbean origin), and either a group and save or a cross-match. You should X-match any patient at risk of blood loss extensive enough to need replacing — for example, the anticipated blood loss from an anterior resection is about two units, but to be safe we usually X-match four units. The blood is kept in the refrigerator ready for use. If it is not used it goes back to the blood bank for storage.

A young healthy person, in general, requires no preoperative investigations, but if at all unsure then you should ask the anaesthetist what they would like performed (for example, some anaesthetists like to have a recent full blood count on all females of childbearing age). The National Institute for Clinical Excellence (NICE) have issued guidelines on preoperative investigation available on the Internet. If the patient is hypertensive or on diuretics then a U & E (urea, creatinine and electrolytes) to assess renal function must be performed. An ECG is necessary on anyone who is hypertensive or has a history of heart disease, and a chest X-ray on anyone with respiratory disease, including a personal or family history of TB. In most hospitals the requirement is to order an ECG and CXR as a baseline on the elderly (aged over 60), but check the policy in your hospital. The management of medical problems in surgical patients is essentially the same as that you read about in medical textbooks. We will, however, cover just a few topics.

DIABETES

Diabetics have an increased incidence of perioperative complications. The stress of surgery can lead to an increased production of catabolic hormones, such as glucagon and catecholamines, which antagonize the action of insulin, making control more difficult, especially as the patient will also be nil by mouth. These patients are at an increased risk of infection (wound, chest, IV access sites and urine), peripheral vascular disease, pressure sores and ischaemic heart disease. The aim is to maintain the patient's blood sugar level between 5 and 9 mmol/l. Preoperatively you should dipstick the urine to check for protein, send off a laboratory blood glucose, check the electrolytes and creatinine and order an ECG.

Management depends on the types of diabetes.

Insulin-dependent Diabetics

For anything other than minor surgery it is probably best to put these patients on an insulin sliding scale to establish good control. This means they are on a drip of dextrose or dextrose saline (as they are not eating), together with a continuous infusion of fast-acting insulin ('Actrpid'). The rate of infusion of insulin will depend on their blood sugar level, which can be monitored by hourly BM stix (a finger prick testing stick specific for glucose). If the BM is low the infusion is decreased or stopped, and if the BM is high the insulin rate can be increased to bring the sugar level down. It is important that you add potassium to each bag of fluids you give, since the insulin causes cellular uptake of potassium and can lead to hypokalaemia. The sliding scales regimen differs in different hospitals and you should try and get hold of a sliding scale protocol at your hospital. This is one example:

Sliding Scale for Insulin					
BM (mM/l)	0–4	4–8	8–12	12–16	>16
Rate of insulin (units/h)	0.5	1.0	2.0	4.0	6.0

Diabetics Controlled with Oral Hypoglycaemics

Long-acting oral hypoglycaemics such as metformin should be changed to a short-acting sulphonylurea (e.g. Gliclazide) a few days before the operation. Ask the diabetic team for advice. On the morning of the operation omit the dose of oral hypoglycaemic. This can be resumed once the patient starts eating postoperatively. The BMs should be measured, and if very high the blood sugar can be brought down by small doses of subcutaneous soluble insulin (e.g. 6 units of actrapid). If this fails to control the sugar level or in the case of major surgery, you cannot go wrong by simply converting the treatment to a sliding scale as above. Diabetics should really go first on the list, as the starting time is predictable and this allows better management of sugar levels.

Diabetics Controlled by Diet Alone

These patients rarely need any special measures. Remember that provided they have not been given any insulin or oral hypoglycaemics the patients cannot become hypoglycaemic (unless they have an insulinoma); if anything, their sugar level will be high. A BM stix will tell you where you stand if you are worried. If you find their control is poor, then you should refer the patients back to their diabetologist.

STEROIDS

Patients on steroids are liable to impaired healing and postoperative infections. Also, long-term corticosteroids can lead to adrenal insufficiency, where the adrenals are unable secrete the increased glucocorticoids necessary in response to the stresses of surgery. This can lead to an Addisonian crisis, where the patient becomes shocked. Patients who have been on long-term oral steroids should therefore be treated with perioperative steroids. This usually means intravenous hydrocortisone before and after the operation until the patient can resume their oral intake.

CHRONIC OBSTRUCTIVE PULMONARY DISEASE

Surgery and anaesthesia predispose patients to basal lung collapse (atelectasis), aspiration pneumonitis and chest infection. This is especially true of operations on the abdomen, since the patient may be in pain and therefore does not cough up the secretions. Any pre-existing respiratory disease, such as chronic obstructive pulmonary disease (COPD), increases the risk of chest complications, as do smoking, obesity and old age.

Preoperatively, therefore, you should arrange for a chest X-ray and lung function tests in any patient with pre-existing chronic airways disease. You should also do a baseline blood gas analysis if hypoxia or carbon dioxide retention is anticipated.

You can assess the degree of reversibility of the airway disease by measuring peak flows before and after bronchodilators are given by nebuliser. If there is a degree of reversibility, then prescription of nebulisers may help optimise lung function.

Physiotherapy is an important modality in these patients and preoperative breathing exercises can help prevent a chest infection.

Postoperatively physiotherapy should be initiated early to help remove airway secretions, especially in abdominal operations. Smokers should be encouraged to stop smoking at least 4 weeks prior to elective surgery.

DEEP VEIN THROMBOSIS

All surgical patients are at risk of deep vein thrombosis (DVT). In some hospitals prophylaxis with subcutaneous low molecular weight heparin injections and thromboembolic deterrent (TED) stockings is given to all surgical patients, whereas other hospitals only give this to patients at medium-to-high risk of DVT. Risk factors for DVT include previous thrombosis or pulmonary embolus, long periods of immobility, pelvic or hip operations, obesity, cancer and use of the oral contraceptive pill. Find out what the DVT prophylaxis protocol is in your hospital.

Intermittent limb compression is where an inflatable device is wrapped around the legs and periodically blown up, from the distal to the proximal end, encouraging venous return. Also available is low molecular weight (LMW) heparin, which is thought to work on the antiplatelet factor antithrombin III and therefore has little effect on the intrinsic clotting cascade. In normal prophylactic doses LMW heparin does not require monitoring; it is longer acting and thus only needs to be given once daily. LMW heparin is as effective as unfractionated heparins. Newer drugs such as direct thrombin inhibitors are also now available.

In most cases, early mobilisation in combination with one or more of the above options is acceptable.

ANTIBIOTICS

Antibiotic cover is necessary for surgery if there is an increased risk of infection. This could be due to patient-related factors or those related to the type of operation.

Contaminated operations, such as those where the bowel contents can leak out, carry a high risk of infection, as do operations where a prosthetic implant is used (e.g. joint replacement), and antibiotics should always be given in these cases. An example of a patient-related factor is mitral valve disease and the subsequent risk of developing endocarditis.

We usually give prophylactic antibiotics intravenously at induction of anaesthesia, so that blood levels are high during the operation, followed by two subsequent doses postoperatively (usually after about 8 and 16 h). If a tourniquet is being used, then the antibiotics must be given before the tourniquet is inflated.

You should have a rough idea of which organisms are likely to be responsible for the infection and which antibiotics should therefore be used. A common question concerns methicillin-resistant *Staphylococcus aureus* (MRSA), which is an increasing problem in many hospitals. It is especially worrying when it infects patients with prosthetic implants such as hip replacements or vascular bypasses.

Operations Involving the Bowel

Organisms

Mainly Gram-negative bacilli, i.e. *coliforms*, but also faecal *anaerobes* (bacteroides) and *S. aureus* from the skin. In the gut there is also *Enterococcus faecalis* (also known as *strep faecalis*), but this causes infection less commonly. In bile, the majority of infections are with gut bacteria, such as *Escherichia coli*, and, rarely, *pseudomonas*, which is more difficult to treat.

Prophylaxis

We tend to use a cephalosporin to cover the Gram-negative organisms together with metronidazole to cover anaerobes. If you are concerned about strep faecalis you should add amoxycillin, as the cephalosporins do not cover this well. For operations on the biliary tree, such as a laparascopic cholecystectomy, you could either use the same regimen as above or just use a cephalosporin alone, as most infections are with Gram-negative bacilli (mainly *E. coli*). One dose at induction is sufficient. For improved biliary penetration such as before and after an ERCP or for ascending cholangitis, a broad-spectrum β-lactam such as pipericillin is often used. This also covers for pseudomonas.

Operations Involving Prosthetic Implants

Organisms

Skin organisms are usually responsible. *S. aureus* is the commonest pathogen, but also *S. epidermidis* tends to colonise the newer plastic prostheses. Rarely, coliforms are responsible.

Prophylaxis

Either a broad-spectrum cephalosporin or flucloxacillin. Orthopaedic operations involving metalwork require a dose of intravenous antibiotics (usually a cephalosporin) at induction and for about 24 h postoperatively. Similarly, valve replacements are usually given amoxycillin (or a cephalosporin) and gentamycin. If MRSA is a particular worry, then vancomycin may be used. The British National Formulary contains up-to-date advice on this topic.

Remember that if ischaemic or necrotic tissue is involved, then spores of clostridium tetani may cause gas gangrene. Benzylpenicillin, to which the organism is highly susceptible, is the prophylaxis (and treatment) of choice against this (this includes penetrating wounds and compound fractures).

The mnemonic "ABCD LMNOPs" is helpful in remembering preoperative management:

A — Antibiotics/anaesthetist
B — Bloods (including X-match)/bowel preparation
C — Consent/CXR
D — Drug chart/DVT prophylaxis
E — ECG

F — Fluids (especially if NBM or if the patient is vomiting)
L — List (put in the theatre list)/lung function tests
M — Mark the area or limb (should be done by the operating surgeon)
N — Notes should be filed correctly
O — Operating theatre staff (e.g. book special equipment/radiology)
P — Physiotherapy
S — Specialist nurses (e.g. breast care or stoma care nurses)

POSTOPERATIVELY

The role of the junior doctor postoperatively is to check that the patient has recovered from the anaesthetic, look at their observation charts and check their fluid balance. The operation note should have a section on specific postoperative management written by the surgeon, and is a guide that should be followed. For example, following a vascular graft operation — say, to the leg — you should always check the pulses, capillary refill and toe movement in the involved leg to ensure that the graft has not blocked off.

A common question for exams concerns complications of surgery.

Complications

All operations carry a risk of complications. These can be divided into *general* and *specific*. General complications include those pertaining to the anaesthesia itself and those that can occur after any operation, such as a chest infection or DVT. Specific complications are those that occur because of the individual operation itself, such as cutting a nerve.

You can subdivide this classification by time, into complications that occur *immediately*, within the first 24 h; *early*, within the first week or so; *late postoperative*, occurring within the first month or so; and *long term*.

General immediate complications include those due to the anaesthetic, such as direct trauma to the mouth when intubating and reactions to the anaesthetic (inherited disorders or idiosyncratic reactions). Early complications include chest infections, urinary retention or infections, deep vein thrombosis and bed sores. *Specific* complications depend on the nature of the operation. In this category haemorrhage and wound infection are important.

Haemorrhage

This can be divided into primary, reactionary and secondary haemorrhage. Primary haemorrhage occurs during the operation, when a vessel is cut. Reactionary haemorrhage is when at the end of the operation the wound looks dry, but when the patient's blood pressure and cardiac output rise to normal levels, bleeding begins, presumably from vessels that were not properly ligated during the operation. Secondary haemorrhage, occurring several days after the operation, is usually attributed to infection that erodes through a vessel.

Wound Infections

These are most commonly caused by *S. aureus* (increasingly MRSA), although coliforms such as *E. coli* are also important. Wound infection is more likely if

- The operation is dirty (e.g. abdominal surgery)
- The duration of the operation is long (greater than 2 h)
- The patient is more susceptible (e.g. old age, immunosuppression, diabetes)

Minor wound infections, with a little redness and slight discharge, are relatively common and usually need just simple measures, such as regular wound dressing and perhaps antibiotics. More severe infections, common after abdominal operations, usually occur in the first week or so. The wound looks inflamed, and there may be cellulitis, discharge or localised abscess formation. The wound should be swabbed and maybe antibiotics started, but the only correct treatment for an abscess is drainage. This may mean simply removing a few of the surgical clips, and probing the wound, allowing the pus to discharge, or a further surgical procedure to open up the wound. The wound is then left to heal by secondary intention (i.e. to heal itself from within, with no further suturing).

Wound Dehiscence

This is an uncommon problem. It is usually due to an inadequate repair of the tissues (but infection, poor blood supply, malnutrition and steroids may all play a part in poor wound healing). Dehiscence usually occurs about a week after the operation. A warning sign is a sero-sanguinous discharge from the wound a few days before. The wound suddenly bursts open and in the case of a laparotomy the bowel protrudes outwards and is extremely alarming for the patient and the nursing staff. Sterile soaked swabs should be placed over the wound and the patient taken back to the theatre for repair.

An example of general and specific complications pertaining to a gastrectomy is outlined below.

	Specific	*General*
Immediate (within 24 h)	Haemorrhage Damage to adjacent structures	Broken tooth Reaction to anaesthesia Asphyxia

Early (first week or so)	Paralytic ileus
	Anastomotic leak
	Infection
	  wound
	  deep collection
		Chest infection
		UTI
		Pulmonary embolus
		DVT
		Bed sores

Late (first month)	Inability to eat normal-size meals Dumping syndrome Steatorrhoea/diarrhoea	Weight loss (combination of above)

Long term	Recurrence of ulcer
	Malignancy
		Osteoporosis
		Anaemia
		  Pernicious
		  Iron deficient

For further elaboration see the chapter on stomach operations. The general section will be the same for all operations. Try and draw up a list of the specific complications for other common procedures, such as operations on the colon, thyroid and breast.

The commonest reason that a junior doctor gets called to the ward is to write up fluids or to see a patient with postoperative pyrexia or poor urine output.

POSTOPERATIVE PYREXIA

A small rise in temperature is common postoperatively. If the temperature spikes above 38° or persists, then you should consider and look for the seven Cs as potential causes. This is a common viva question.

1. *Chest.*   Chest infection
2. *Catheter.*   UTI
3. *CVP line.*   Infected
4. *Cannula.*   Superficial thrombophlebitis (solved by removing the cannula)
5. *Cut.*   Wound infection
6. *Collection.*   Subphrenic or pelvic abscess (may indicate a failure of anastomosis)
7. *Calves.*   DVT (rumbling pyrexia in second postoperative week)

A *chest infection* is very common postoperatively, especially in patients who smoke or have pre-existing poor respiratory function. The mucus secretions are not cleared; these then clog up the smaller bronchi, which leads to collapse of the air spaces distal to the blockage (atelectasis). Inhaled organisms then infect the collapsed segments. In addition, thoracic and upper abdominal incisions cause pain and stop the patients from coughing up the secretions, and so they are much more likely to have basal atelectasis and develop chest infections. These patients should therefore be given adequate analgesia, have vigorous physiotherapy, and be encouraged to cough up the phlegm (ideally whilst holding their wounds — applicable for chest and abdominal wounds).

A deep collection, such as a *subphrenic or pelvic abscess*, can occur after the patient has had generalised peritonitis. The patient usually presents with general malaise, nausea, pain (a subphrenic abscess may also cause pain felt in the shoulder tip), a swinging pyrexia and localised peritonitis.

A pelvic abscess often occurs 4–10 days postop., whereas a subphrenic abscess usually occurs a bit later, 7–21 days postop. Clinically, the patient appears to be recovering well, but then develops a fever and starts to feel unwell. The white cell count may be raised and a collection is identified on ultrasound or CT. Treatment is by drainage, either percutaneously under ultrasound or CT guidance, or by an open procedure. A drain is usually left *in situ*.

A small anastomotic leak usually causes a localised abscess which becomes sealed off by the omentum and the bowel. Clinically, the patient is slow to recover, but usually improves with intravenous antibiotics and fluids and delayed return to food. A larger anastomotic breakdown causes the patient to be very unwell, with anything from local peritonitis through to a rigid abdomen and septicaemia. The abscess needs to be drained, the peritoneal cavity washed out, and the two ends of the failed anastomosis can be brought out as temporary stomas.

A diagnosis of DVT and pulmonary embolus (PE) in the first instance is essentially a clinical one, as treatment is usually instituted before definitive diagnosis is made. A PE usually presents with pleuritic chest pain (stabbing and worse on inspiration). The textbooks tend to describe the findings you would see in a massive PE, although more commonly in the smaller PEs the findings are less impressive. Usually, the patient is tachycardic, maybe with a low-grade fever and maybe tachypnoeic, but not much else and they may even be asymptomatic. The ECG usually shows sinus tachycardia (the classic S1Q3T3, which most students know about, occurs when there is a large amount of right heart strain, in a large PE, and is rarely seen). The CXR is usually unhelpful but may show a small area of linear atelectasis. Blood gas analysis is essential and you would expect to find a low PO_2 (due to ventilation/perfusion mismatches) and a low PCO_2 due to hyperventilation. Examination of the calves may or may not reveal evidence of a DVT. If a DVT or PE is suspected, a heparin infusion can be started before investigation but always check with a senior colleague before doing that, especially if the patient has had recent surgery.

To diagnose a DVT you can use duplex ultrasound (or a venogram). To diagnose a PE you can request a ventilation–perfusion scan, although the gold-standard is pulmonary angiography (note nowadays a spiral CT is used in some centres).

Other less common causes for a fever include infective diarrhoeas, drug reactions and blood transfusion reactions.

If faced with a patient with a pyrexia you would obviously find out a little history and examine the patient properly. In a viva situation you could answer along the lines of, 'I would listen to the chest, examine the abdomen, check the cannula sites, inspect the wound, etc. … My investigations would depend on my clinical findings but may involve sending a urine specimen, a full blood count and blood cultures, sending wound swabs or the tip of the central line for culture, etc.'

DRAINS

Collections within a wound (especially if they contain blood) are the perfect medium for colonisation of bacteria and hence infection.

A drain can be used to remove anticipated collections within a wound, but should never be used as a substitute for adequate haemostasis at the time of surgery.

Drains can be closed or open. Closed drainage includes suction drainage (e.g. Redivac) where the collection is attracted into a container either by gravity or suction. This can then potentially reduce the risk of infection when used for large spaces or cavities, such as after a mastectomy or joint replacement. Drains are usually removed as soon as possible (usually 24–48 h) or as soon as the losses begin to tail off. Drains can also introduce infections and so they should not be left in for any longer than needed.

Open drainage (e.g. a piece of corrugated tubing with one end in the wound and the other in the dressing), allows small losses to escape from the wound. This is often employed in established abscesses after incision and drainage to allow any remaining collection a passage out of the wound. Some surgeons like to withdraw this type of drain in stages to allow the track to collapse behind it.

Other drains commonly asked about in exams include chest drains, T-tubes and percutaneous nephrostomies (see relevant sections).

POSTOPERATIVE POOR URINE OUTPUT

This is a common exam question and can be classified as prerenal, renal or postrenal. The commonest causes of failure to pass urine postoperatively are postrenal.

Postrenal problems (commoner in males) include obstruction caused by a large prostate or a blocked catheter. Also, the patient may find initiation of micturition difficult for the following reasons:

1. Anticholinergic drugs or those with alpha adrenergic effects (e.g. the anaesthetic)
2. Pain (e.g. after a hernia repair)
3. Inhibition (e.g. because of strange surroundings or a nurse continually asking them if they have passed urine)
4. Opiates or epidural anaesthetics

Once the bladder reaches a certain volume of distension it fails to function properly and the patient goes into retention. Benign prostatic hypertrophy is an important predisposition and these patients are more likely to go into retention.

Prerenal causes are due to renal hypoperfusion because of either hypovolaemia or heart failure and will not be covered here.

Renal causes — Acute renal failure is usually due to acute tubular necrosis.

Junior doctors are commonly called to see patients who have failed to pass urine postoperatively. Often this will be a patient you are covering but have not met before. It is, therefore, worth spending a little time getting a history and reading the patient's notes. You should find out the type and date of operation and also search for clues pointing to whether the problem is prerenal or postrenal. Ask if there is any pain; an enlarged bladder causes suprapubic pain, although this is difficult to differentiate from pain in an abdominal wound (one exception is when there is an epidural *in situ* and there is no pain).

On examination you should look for signs of hypovolaemia (dry mucous membranes, decreased skin turgor, tachycardia, etc.), signs of heart failure (shortness of breath, tachycardia, raised CVP or JVP and bibasilar crepitations, peripheral oedema, etc.). A distended bladder palpable just above the pubis is dull to percussion and usually tender, making the patient want to pass urine, when compressed.

You can initially try conservative measures such as analgesia, privacy, sitting in a warm bath, etc., but if that fails then catheterisation is indicated.

If you suspect that the cause is postrenal (i.e., distended bladder and discomfort), then the diagnosis is proven by catheterisation. A large residual volume of urine should drain (usually about 500 ml or more).

If the patient already has a catheter *in situ*, then the catheter should be flushed to ensure it is not blocked. If the urine coming out of the catheter is small amounts of concentrated dark urine, then the cause is likely to be prerenal anyway. You could dipstick the urine, testing for a high specific gravity (>1020) to prove this.

You should check the fluid balance charts. Observe how much fluid has gone in before, during and since the operation and the measured urine output. Remember that a long laparotomy can lead to large losses of fluid by evaporation and this will not be measured on the charts. A urine output of less than about 30 ml/h is poor (oliguria). The patient should be catheterised anyway at this point to measure the hourly urine output. U & Es should be sent; if there is a prerenal cause, the urea will be raised. If from your clinical examination and your assessment of the fluid balance charts you think the patient has a prerenal cause, then you should try a fluid challenge — 250–500 ml of normal saline given as a stat dose (unless you suspect blood loss as the cause, in which case the patient may be shocked and should be given colloids and blood — see section on shock). Then, observe the urine output over the next hour. If the urine output picks up, you have shown the patient to be in need of more fluid and the next bag should be speeded up. If the patient has heart failure, the urine output will not pick up and the patient may become a little more breathless and the CVP might rise. If this occurs, a bolus dose of a loop diuretic, such as 40 mg of frusemide, will lead to a diuresis and a fall in the CVP. If the patient does not have a central line in at this point, you should ask a senior colleague for advice, as a central line is really necessary for knowing exactly what the state of vascular filling is and will help in the management.

Only after you have excluded a postrenal and a prerenal cause can you assume that there may be a renal problem and acute tubular necrosis has occurred. The creatinine will be raised and you should measure the urine and plasma osmolalities. The ratio of urine to plasma osmolality will be less than 1 (as opposed to prerenal oliguria, where the ratio will be >1). Advice from a renal physician should be sought early.

4

TRAUMA, SHOCK, HEAD INJURIES AND BURNS*

TRAUMA

Imagine yourself being faced with a multiply injured patient with trauma to the head, chest, abdomen and limbs. Where would you start? What if there were several injured patients, which would take priority?

The Advanced Trauma and Life Support (ATLS®) course was developed following a tragedy. In 1976 an orthopaedic surgeon who was piloting his own plane over rural Nebraska crashed in a cornfield. His wife died instantly and three of his four children sustained critical injuries. They were taken to the nearest medical facility, the surgeon was appalled at the poor quality of care that he and his family received and felt that a system was needed to improve the care of trauma patients.

Causes of Death in Trauma

There is a trimodal distribution of death following injury. The *first peak* occurs at the time of the injury, usually due to severe lacerations of the brain, heart or large blood vessels, and the patient is usually dead before arrival at casualty. Prevention by methods such as seat belts, crash helmets and speed limits is the only effective way of reducing these deaths.

---

*ATLS® Used/modified with permission by the American College of Surgeons Committee on Trauma, Advanced Trauma Life Support® Manual 1997. Third impression, Chicago.

43

The *second peak* occurs within minutes to hours of the injury. Injuries such as a tension pneumothorax, blood loss and intracranial bleeds account for this peak. These deaths are potentially reversible with immediate medical management.

The *third peak* of deaths occurs several days to weeks after the incident, due to sepsis and multiorgan failure. The care provided during the initial resuscitation and subsequent period directly affects the outcome of this group.

The concept behind ATLS® is to treat life-threatening injuries first and all other injuries in order of priority, and since a blocked airway kills within seconds this clearly should have first priority; likewise, a tension pneumothorax will kill before bleeding from a wound.

The ATLS® approach is divided into a *primary* and a *secondary survey*. In the *primary survey*, life-threatening injuries are identified. In this chapter we study *assessment* and *resuscitation* separately, although in reality they take place simultaneously (i.e. life-threatening injuries are treated as soon as they are identified). The *secondary survey* is a more thorough head-to-toe examination.

The patient is continuously *re-evaluated* until they are stable and a definitive care pathway can be instituted.

Primary Survey

As the patient arrives there is usually some history available — if not from the patient, then from witnesses or the ambulance crew. Their vital signs from when first seen by the paramedics until the time of arrival in the A & E department should be noted.

The primary survey is a rapid evaluation; the mnemonic ABCDE is used to allow one to think in an ordered and prioritised manner.

A — Airway with cervical spine control
B — Breathing and ventilation
C — Circulation with haemorrhage control
D — Disability
E — Exposure and environment

Airway with Cervical Spine Control

In anyone with an altered level of consciousness or injuries above the clavicles, suspect a cervical spine injury. The patient's head should be supported by a hand on either side to prevent any movement (in-line manual immobilisation), and when possible a semirigid collar should be applied with two sandbags on either side of the head with tape across them to hold them in place.

The airway should be checked to see if it is patent or if there are signs of airway obstruction. Listen for noisy breathing, look for obvious facial trauma, and inspect for foreign bodies.

Breathing

Assess the respiratory function. Inspect and palpate for tracheal deviation, expansion of the lungs and for any lacerations, rib fractures or flail segments. A flail chest, commonly asked about in exams, is a segment of the chest wall that, owing to multiple fractures, has no bony continuity with the rest of the thoracic cage. The flail segment moves paradoxically with the rest of the chest (i.e. it moves in on inspiration and out on expiration). The hypoxia that results is usually not due to the flail segment alone but more to the underlying contusion to the lung and hence mismatches between ventilation and perfusion.

Circulation with Haemorrhage Control

Assess the level of consciousness, pulse, blood pressure, respiratory rate, skin colour and capillary refill time (see page 55). Hypotension following injury must be assumed to be due to hypovolaemia until proved otherwise.

During the primary survey any external severe bleeding points should be controlled by applying a sterile pressure dressing or a pneumatic splint. Tourniquets are usually avoided, as they cause crush injuries and distal ischaemia.

Internal bleeding should be suspected and you should examine systematically for all of the common causes, such as an intrathoracic or intra-abdominal bleed or a fractured pelvis and/or femur. A bleed into the cranial cavity will by itself not cause hypovolaemia.

Disability

This is a rapid neurological evaluation assessing the patient's level of consciousness and the pupil size and response to light. The mnemonic AVPU is used as a quick assessment of the patient's level of consciousness. If, for example, the patient responds only to pain, then his AVPU score is P.

A — Alert
V — responds to Verbal stimuli
P — responds to Painful stimuli
U — Unresponsive

The Glasgow Coma Score (GCS) is a more detailed neurological evaluation that can be done during the primary survey although it takes a little longer, and because the life-threatening A, B and C take precedence in the primary survey the GCS may be performed in the secondary survey (see section on head injury for details).

A decreased level of consciousness may be due to many factors, including cerebral injury, hypoxia and shock. It may also be secondary to alcohol and drugs, although head injury, hypoxia and shock must be excluded first.

Exposure

Completely undress the patient (cut off the clothes as appropriate), inspect the entire skin surface for evidence of injury, such as bruising, abrasions or lacerations. A log roll should be performed with in-line cervical spine immobilisation (i.e. the head is supported and turned in line with the patient to prevent any displacement of the cervical spine). The entire vertebral column is palpated down to the coccyx for tenderness and a rectal examination is performed.

During the primary survey a series of X-rays are taken, called the 'Trauma Series', which include a lateral C-spine, chest and pelvic X-rays. An ECG is usually taken.

A nasogastric tube should be considered (note: contraindicated if a cribiform plate fracture is suspected as the tube could enter the cranial vault and an orogastric tube may be used instead) and urinary catheter should also be considered (note: during the rectal examination, a high-riding prostate or any sharp bony pelvic fragments might indicate a urethral transection which would mean trans-urethral catherisation is contraindicated). Other signs to suggest a urethral injury: blood at the urethral meatus or a scrotal haematoma. If a urethral transection is suspected then a retrograde urethrogram can be performed and a supra-pubic catheter might be needed.

RESUSCITATION

As mentioned above, this is carried out simultaneously during the primary survey.

Airway

Every injured patient should receive supplemental oxygen; however, the airway must be patent and protected in all patients. There are five things you can do to ensure a patent airway; always start with simple measures, such as the chin lift, and progress through the following list until oxygenation is adequate. Apply an oxygen mask with a reservoir (to allow about 85% oxygen).

1. *Chin lift or jaw thrust.* In the supine position the tongue naturally falls back, obstructing the hypopharynx. These procedures bring the tongue forward, opening up the airway. In the chin lift the chin is grasped between the first finger and the thumb. The chin is then lifted gently

and brought anteriorly (being careful not to hyperextend the neck). In the jaw thrust manoeuvre the angles of the mandible are grasped by hand on each side and the lower jaw is brought forward.

2. *Guedel airway.* If breathing is still noisy, you can maintain the airway by inserting an oropharyngeal airway, such as a Guedel airway (an S-shaped plastic tube). The size should correspond to the distance from the centre of the patient's mouth to the angle of the jaw. It is sometimes put in upside down and rotated when it is past the tongue.

3. *Nasopharyngeal tube.* If the patient is conscious and has a gag reflex, they will be unlikely to tolerate an oropharyngeal airway. In this case a nasopharyngeal airway can be tried, as it is better tolerated and less likely to induce vomiting, although many conscious patients will not tolerate either and may need to be anaesthetised and intubated.

4. *Intubation.* This is called a definitive airway, which means a tube is inserted into the trachea with a cuff inflated to prevent aspiration; the whole thing is secured with tape and oxygen is connected. A definitive airway can be an orotracheal tube, a nasotracheal tube or a surgical airway (see below). A definitive airway is needed if the patient is not breathing, or is unable to maintain an airway with the above measures, or if there is impending airway compromise (as in inhalation injuries) or in a head injury requiring hyperventilation. Since CO_2 is produced in the lungs you can confirm that the tube is in the trachea by measuring the end tidal CO_2 tension. If the tube was mistakenly placed into the oesophagus then the CO_2 gas pattern would be absent. Proper placement of the tube is also checked by listening for bilateral air entry (i.e. if the tube is in the right main bronchus, then no air entry will be heard on the left).

5. *Surgical airway.* If you are unable to intubate (for example, in severe facial trauma) then a surgical airway is indicated. A tracheostomy is difficult to perform and is time-consuming, and so a needle cricothyroidotomy can be performed [a large-caliber cannula is inserted through the cricothyroid membrane into the trachea (feel for Adam's apple, and move your finger downwards till you come to the first gap between the thyroid and cricoid cartilages)]. Oxygen is then connected to the airway.

A needle cricothyroidotomy will only buy a short amount of time and must be converted to a surgical cricothyroidotomy by widening the incision and placing a cuffed endotracheal tube into the space between the thyroid and cricoid cartilages (if you are ever asked about the difference between tracheostomy and a surgical airway, note that a tracheosttomy is placed into the trachea at about the level of the second or third tracheal ring and is a much longer procedure as the thyroid gland has to be divided and is therefore performed in theatre when the patient is stable).

Breathing

The mnemonic 'ATOMIC' has been used to list life-threatening chest injuries, which should be identified in the primary survey:

*A*irway obstruction
*T*ension pneumothorax
*O*pen pneumothorax
*M*assive haemothorax (greater than 1500 ml)
*I*ntercostal disruption (some people modify the mnemonic to ATOM FC, where *F* stands for 'Flail chest')
*C*ardiac tamponade

A *tension pneumothorax* occurs when air enters the pleural space either from outside or from inside the lung. A one-way valve is formed by the pleura, which allows air to enter the pleural space during inspiration, but does not allow it to escape during expiration. The lung collapses, and the mediastinum and the trachea are deviated away from the affected side. The patient becomes very short of breath and cyanotic. The venous return to the heart is impaired and the signs are similar to those of cardiac tamponade (i.e. raised JVP and falling BP, but they can be differentiated by listening for breath sounds). The diagnosis is made clinically — a distressed, tachycardic patient with a deviated trachea, hyper-resonance to percussion and absent breath sounds on the affected side. You should never see a chest X-ray on patients with a tension pneumothorax, as they should have been treated immediately before waiting for an X-ray to be taken. Treatment is by placing a cannula (venflon) into the second intercostal space, midclavicular line, and hearing a hiss as the air escapes. Once this is performed the tension pneumothorax will be converted to a simple pneumothorax and the immediate threat to life is over. A chest drain should be inserted as soon as possible.

Insertion of a Chest Drain

A chest drain is inserted under aseptic technique anterior to the midaxillary line, in the fifth intercostal space. If possible (provided no cervical spine injury is suspected) the patient is sat up at 45° and the hand is placed behind their neck on the affected side to expose the field and open up the intercostal space.

If sitting up is not possible, then the procedure should be performed with the patient supine and again the arm on the affected side is placed behind the patient's neck. The area is prepared with antiseptic (e.g. betadine) and draped. Local anaesthetic is infiltrated into the skin, subcutaneous tissues and down to the pleura. A 2 cm transverse incision is made in the fifth intercostal space (aiming above the rib as the intercostal bundle sits in the groove just below the rib). Blunt dissection is then performed down to the pleura with a pair of forceps which then are pushed through the pleura into the pleural space.

A finger is placed in the hole and swept around to free any adhesions and create the space for the tube. A chest drain is inserted using a pair of forceps, usually French gauge 24–28 (if a haemopneumothorax exists a larger tube size, Fr. 38, is usually used). The drain is fixed with a stitch and a purse-string or mattress suture is placed in the wound (to allow it to be closed when the drain is removed). The chest drain is connected to an underwater seal (this allows air to escape during expiration, but no air to enter on inspiration). Ensure that the underwater seal is below the level of the patient, otherwise the water will enter the chest. Re-X-ray the patient after the procedure to ensure correct positioning of the tube.

If you are ever asked how you can check if a chest drain is blocked, a top tip is to ask the patient to cough and you will see bubbles escaping if it is patent and no bubbles if it is blocked.

In an open pneumothorax, if the opening is approximately two-thirds of the diameter of the trachea, then air passes through the wound in preference to the airway during inspiration (taking the route of least resistance). This is also called a 'sucking chest wound'. The management is to close the wound with a sterile dressing taped on three sides to form a flap valve.

Circulation (see page 55)

Two large-bore cannulae should be inserted, one into each antecubital fossa of all patients exposed to major trauma. Blood should be taken for a cross-match, a full blood count and urea and electrolytes.

The ATLS® system recommends giving two litres of warmed physiological fluids (Hartmann's or Ringer's lactate) immediately, although some surgeons in the UK often start colloids (such as haemaccel) if there is definite blood loss. Obviously, it is important to get the blood as soon as possible. O negative blood is used if necessary (the universal donor), whilst awaiting the X-match.

Recognise the signs of shock, and look for a cause. The chest, abdomen and pelvis are the likely causes if there is no obvious haemorrhage from a wound. A bleed into the abdomen causes distention and signs on examination, such as tenderness, guarding and perhaps absent bowel sounds. If intraperitoneal bleeding is suspected (say, in a stab wound) and the patient is shocked despite immediate resuscitation, then no time should be wasted and the patient should be taken straight to theatre for a laparotomy to 'turn off the tap'. If the findings on examination are equivocal and the patient is not unstable, then a diagnostic peritoneal lavage (DPL), ultrasound or CT scan can be performed (in the USA an ultrasound is often available in the emergency room).

Diagnostic Peritoneal Lavage

For finals you probably just need to know that this involves an incision in the midline, below the umbilicus, and dissection down to the peritoneum, into which a catheter is placed.

A litre of normal saline is run into the peritoneal cavity. The bag is then placed on the floor and allowed to fill. If there is no obvious blood, then a sample of fluid is sent for microscopy to count the red blood cells.

A urinary catheter and nasogastric tube must be inserted prior to the DPL in order to avoid damage to the stomach and bladder during the procedure. The findings of this procedure, however, are often equivocal.

An unstable fractured pelvis can cause profuse blood loss and stage IV shock. The cause is usually venous bleeding. During the primary survey the chest and abdomen will have been examined to look for other causes of the shock. An orthopaedic surgeon can place an external fixator onto the pelvis, and this usually stops the rapid blood loss (by tamponade, and also stops any shearing forces on the vessels).

Disability

See section on head injury (page 59).

Exposure/Environment

The patient is completely exposed so that a full examination can be performed. In order to protect them from heat loss, both the patient and the resuscitation room should be heated. Methods for heating the patient include the use of warmed fluids and blood and the use of blankets. A *log roll* may be performed here or it may be performed in the secondary survey.

In this procedure one person holds and turns the head and neck and three people roll the body. This allows the patient to be turned with in-line cervical spine immobilisation to examine the back of the body for any signs of trauma (stab wounds, bruising, abrasions), palpating for any tenderness, and a rectal examination is performed.

Secondary Survey

A quick history should be ascertained, from witnesses, family or the ambulance men. The mnemonic AMPLE is used for the following vital questions:

*A*llergies
*M*edication

*P*ast medical history
*L*ast ate or drank
*E*vents prior to the accident

The secondary survey is the head-to-toe or full examination. Check the head (eyes, ears, scalp — run your fingers through the hair), cervical spine, chest, abdomen, limbs and perform a full neurological examination.

If the log roll has not been performed in the primary survey, it should be performed here. At the end of the secondary survey the patient should be re-evaluated by starting again at the ABCs. Once you are sure they are fully stabilised you can begin to make arrangements for definitive care (this usually means an admission).

Cervical Spine — X-Rays and Management

A cervical spine injury is almost always accompanied by pain in the neck; however, it is important to know that the absence of a neurological deficit does not rule out a fracture of the cervical spine. Under A for 'airway' with cervical spine control, the neck should be immobilised and a lateral 'shoot through' X-ray should be taken. If a motorcycle helmet needs to be removed or intubation is required, these should be performed with in-line manual immobilisation.

Assessment of the Cervical Spine X-Ray

Yet again, think of the mnemonic ABCs — *A*dequacy and Alignment, *B*ones, *C*artilages and *S*oft tissues.

> *Adequacy.* An adequate C-Spine X-ray is one in which you can see the junction between the body of C7 and T1. If given a cervical spine X-ray in an exam and all you can see is C1-6, tell the examiner that this is not acceptable and you would like a further view. If they tell you that this is the best they could get and asks you what other methods you could use to improve the view, then say that you would like to repeat

the X-ray with someone pulling down on the arms from the end of the bed or would like a swimmer's view (where the arm is abducted fully).

Alignment. Assess four lines — the line that runs down the anterior vertebral bodies, the anterior vertebral canal, the posterior vertebral canal and the tips of the spinous processes. These should be curved with a slight lordosis. A step along this line or a loss of the lordosis is abnormal (note: whether the X-ray was taken with a hard collar on, because that can often be a cause for loss of lordosis). If the anteroposterior spinal canal space is narrowed, there is possibly spinal cord compression.

Bones. Look at the shape of the individual vertebral bodies (which should be rectangular), the lateral mass (the pedicles, facets, laminae and transvere processes) and the spinous processes.

Cartilages. Assess the intervertebral discs (should be of equal height) and facet joints.

Soft tissues. Just anterior to the vertebral bodies are the soft tissues of the pharynx. If there is damage to the cervical spine, there is likely to be associated soft tissue swelling (haemorrhage). Look at the shadow of the prevertebral space for any swelling. In front of the upper cervical vertebrae its normal width is about half that of the vertebral body (or less than 5 mm). At about C4 the soft tissues take up more space with a width about equal to that of the vertebral body (as the larynx and oesophagus are here). If the space between the spinous processes is widened, this implies a torn interspinous ligament.

SHOCK

Shock is defined as an inadequate perfusion and tissue oxygenation of the vital organs (brain, heart, kidneys and skin). There are several causes of shock and they can be divided into haemorrhagic and nonhaemorrhagic.

The nonhaemorrhagic causes include cardiogenic, anaphylactic and septic shock (they should be known about but are not covered here).

Tension pneumothorax is another cause of shock due to mediastinal shift and impairment of the venous return.

Haemorrhagic Shock

Haemorrhage is the commonest cause of shock after injury. The most important step is to recognise and treat shock early even if the blood pressure is normal. As a rule, any patient who is cool and tachycardic should be assumed to be shocked until proven otherwise.

The normal adult blood volume is 7% of body weight (about 5 l for a 70 kg man), whereas in a child it is about 9% of body weight, or 80 ml/kg. The body has excellent compensatory mechanisms to deal with volume loss (although as age increases these mechanisms become less efficient) and there may be no changes in the blood pressure until the loss is considerable. On examination you should assess the appearance of the patient, the pulse, blood pressure, pulse pressure (the difference between the systolic and the diastolic blood pressure), respiratory rate, capillary refill time (normally less than 2 s), mental status and urine output.

There are four stages of shock based on the percentage of blood loss. If you play tennis you will have no problem in recalling the percentages, as they are the same as in the tennis scoring system.

Stage I Shock (0–15%)

This is up to 750 ml blood loss (based on a 70 kg man). This is the group that catches people out, as signs of shock are minimal. The patient is usually a little anxious; however, the pulse rate is usually less than 100 and the blood pressure and pulse pressure are normal.

Stage II Shock (15–30%)

This is 750–1500 ml volume loss. Again, the patient is anxious and the pulse is now above 100, with an increased respiratory rate. The systolic blood pressure is still usually maintained (by vasoconstriction and increased cardiac output); however, the pulse pressure is now decreased, mainly because of a rise in the diastolic pressure.

Stage III Shock (30–40%)

Up to 2000 ml. Now you see all the classic signs of inadequate perfusion, including a marked tachycardia and tachypnoea and a drop in the systolic blood pressure. There may be evidence of CNS impairment, such as confusion. It is therefore important to recognise shock in stages I and II in order to prevent the patient from going into stage III shock.

Stage IV Shock (Greater than 40%)

With a loss of greater than 2 l the condition is immediately life threatening. The pulse is weak and thready, there is a significant drop in the systolic blood pressure (the diastolic blood pressure may be unrecordable), and the patient is pale, cold and clammy, with a depressed consciousness level.

Stage	Stage I	Stage II	Stage III	Stage IV
Blood loss (%)	<15	15–30	30–40	>40
Blood loss (ml)	<750	750–1500	1500–2000	>2000
Consciousness	Slightly anxious	Agitated	Confused	Depressed
Pulse rate	<100	>100	>120	>140
Blood pressure	Normal	Normal	Decreased	Decreased
Pulse pressure	Normal	Decreased	Decreased	Decreased
Respiratory rate	14–20	20–30	30–40	>35
Urine output (ml/h)	>30	20–30	5–15	Negligible
Replacement	Crystalloid	Colloid	Colloid + blood	Colloid + blood

Management

Under C for 'circulation', insert two large-bore cannulae (brown or grey), preferably one into each antecubital fossa. According to Poiseuille's law, flow is proportional to the fourth power of the internal radius of the tube and inversely proportional to the length, and so a short fat tube is essential. Note that a central line, although important for monitoring, is usually long and very thin and hence not effective for fluid resuscitation. If IV access is difficult in the antecubital fossae, then a femoral approach or a cut-down on to the saphenous vein can be attempted (this is 2 cm above and anterior to the medial malleolus). In a child less than 6 years old, an interosseous needle can be used (this is a needle inserted directly into the tibia (just below the knee), allowing access to the vascular marrow, and can be used to replace blood and fluids in the same way as a venous cannula inserted into any other site).

Blood should be taken for laboratory analysis, including a cross-match, FBC, U & Es, glucose, toxicology studies and a pregnancy test in females of childbearing age. Blood gases are often useful at this stage. A central line (a catheter in a large central vein) may be inserted to help monitor fluid replacement or if cardiogenic shock is suspected.

Insertion of a Central Line

There are in use two approaches. The first is known as the infraclavicular approach into the subclavian vein and the second into the internal jugular vein. A guide wire based on the Seldinger technique is employed. In the infraclavicular approach the patient is supine with the head down (about 15° — this helps distend the neck veins and prevents an air embolism). The head should be supported by another helper if a cervical spine injury is suspected. An aseptic technique is used. Some local anaesthetic is infiltrated into the skin. A needle attached to a saline-filled syringe is introduced 1 cm below the junction of the middle and inner thirds of the clavicle. The needle is advanced medially and slightly upwards behind the clavicle (aiming for the sternal notch) as the plunger is slowly withdrawn. When venous blood enters the syringe, the syringe is removed leaving the needle in the vein. A guide wire is inserted through the needle into the vein. The needle is removed, leaving the guide wire in the vein. The central line is then inserted over the guide wire and into the vein. The central line is fixed to the skin with a suture and is dressed. If necessary, the central line is then connected to a manometer to measure the central venous pressure.

The internal jugular approach is similar but via a different vein. The carotid pulse is felt just anterior to the midpoint of the sternocleidomastoid muscle (the high approach) and a needle is inserted lateral to this, aiming posteroinferiorly and towards the nipple on that side (the internal jugular vein lies posterior to the carotid artery at the base of the skull; the vein then twists around the carotid and lies lateral to it half-way down the neck and in front of it just below the clavicle).

In the low approach the needle is inserted between the two heads of sternocleidomastoid just above the clavicle.

After the central line has been inserted it is important to get a check X-ray to confirm the position of the line and rule out a pneumothorax.

Complications of central line insertion include

- Pneumothorax and haemopneumothorax (especially in the subclavian approach)
- Arterial puncture (it is easier to apply pressure to the internal jugular if it is hit by mistake, than it is to the subclavian artery which is hidden deeply)
- Haematoma formation
- Infection

Recent evidence has suggested that real-time ultrasound guidance for central line insertion, with or without Doppler assistance, improves catheter insertion success rates, reduces the number of venepuncture attempts prior to successful placement, and reduces the number of complications.

The ATLS® system recommends starting two litres of crystalloid fluids as the initial resuscitation for every major trauma patient. The response to volume expansion is monitored by the same signs and symptoms that are used to diagnose it. The urine output is the best indicator of the adequacy of resuscitation.

There are three types of response to the initial fluid resuscitation:

1. *Rapid response.* Here, the patients respond rapidly to the fluids and remain haemodynamically stable once the fluids are stopped or slowed. These patients have usually lost minimal blood volume (<20%) and

can be observed but do not necessarily need any further intravenous fluids.

2. *Transient response.* There is an initial response with a rise in the blood pressure and a fall in the pulse rate; however, as the fluids are slowed down, the indices used to measure shock start to deteriorate again, indicating that the blood loss is ongoing or resuscitation has been inadequate. The response to the fluid will indicate those patients who are still slowly bleeding (as may other clinical findings).

3. *No response.* This could be exsanguinating haemorrhage and blood is needed rapidly. Type-specific blood (where the ABO and Rhesus groups are compatible, but there may be some minor antibodies that are incompatible) takes about 10 min to process and should be given initially in life-threatening bleeding whilst waiting for the full cross-match, which may take as long as 40 min. As a last resort, Group O negative blood can be given, which is the universal donor.

Failure to respond to the fluid resuscitation and the blood indicate the need for immediate surgical intervention to control the haemorrhage ('turn off the tap'). Less commonly, a failure of response may be due to the fact that there is a nonhaemorrhagic cause for the shock, such as myocardial contusion or tamponade, and a CVP measurement may help differentiate the causes. If blood is given (usually packed red cells without plasma) it should be warmed to prevent hypothermia and, after a large transfusion, platelets and fresh frozen plasma may be needed to correct the lack of clotting factors. The main aim of transfusion is to correct the oxygen-carrying capacity, since crystalloids and colloids can both correct the lack of intravascular volume but have no oxygen-carrying capacity.

HEAD INJURIES

Introduction

Head injuries are common and range from the minor bump on the head that usually warrants simple advice but no investigation or treatment, through to the multiply injured patient with an associated head injury and a depressed level of consciousness. The majority of head injuries fall somewhere between these two extremes, and the difficulty for the doctor is in deciding who needs to be admitted for observation and who can be sent home. Questions on head injuries are common in the finals.

Anatomy

The scalp has five layers, described by the mnemonic SCALP — Skin, Connective tissue, Aponeurosis, Loose connective tissue and Periosteum (pericranium). It is highly vascular and can lead to large blood losses. Beneath the scalp is the skull, which contains the meninges, and then the brain. In a head injury any of these structures can be damaged.

Intracranial Pressure

The pressure within the skull is known as the intracranial pressure (ICP) and is actually the pressure which the subarachnoid space is under. Normally, the ICP is less than 10 mmHg.

There is a simple, yet vitally important, concept relating to ICP dynamics, which is that the total volume of the intracranial contents must remain constant (known as the Monroe–Kellie Doctrine), which should be obvious since the skull in an adult is essentially a rigid structure that cannot expand.

The skull contains cerebrospinal fluid (CSF), blood and the brain. If the volume of one of these components increases, then the other two must decrease to compensate or the ICP will rise (Figure 4.1).

The ICP is usually maintained at a constant level by excellent autoregulatory mechanisms that can accommodate changes in the blood flow and so a normal ICP should not exclude a mass lesion.

We can accommodate a mass of about 50–100 ml without a significant rise of ICP. However, as the mass expands further, the autoregulatory mechanisms fail and the rise in ICP is rapid (as is the patient's deterioration) and can lead to brain herniation.

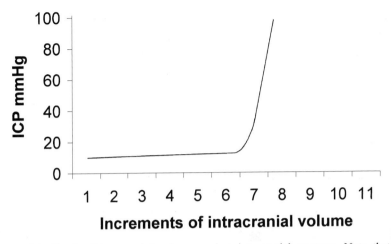

Increments of intracranial volume

Figure 4.1. Graph of intracranial volume against intracranial pressure. Note that an expanding mass can initially be compensated as blood and CSFs are squeezed out. However, the ICP rises rapidly after the period of compensation.

Cerebral Perfusion Pressure

The cerebral perfusion pressure (CPP) is just as important as ICP as it is a measure of the amount of oxygenated blood reaching the brain:

$$CPP = \text{mean arterial BP} - ICP.$$

Large increases in the ICP lead to a decrease in the CPP.

As the CPP falls there is initially electrical followed by structural brain damage and a prolonged CPP of less than 70 mmHg is usually associated with a poor outcome following head injury.

Cerebral blood flow is dependent on both the arterial PCO_2 and the systemic blood pressure. As the arterial PCO_2 rises, cerebrovasodilatation occurs, worsening the raised ICP. In reverse, reducing the arterial PCO_2 reduces the cerebral blood volume and hence the intracranial pressure. Therefore, in cases of raised ICP the patient should be hyperventilated to keep the PCO_2 low.

Maintenance of CPP is one of the priorities of management of a patient with a severe head injury.

Types of Injury

Scalp Laceration

Lacerations of the scalp can bleed profusely and lead to major blood loss, especially in children.

Skull Fracture

Skull fractures are common. It is possible to have one without severe brain injury, and likewise, you can have an intracranial injury without accompanying skull fracture, especially in children, whose bones and joints are more supple. The only significance of X-raying head injury patients and looking for a skull fracture is that such patients have a statistically higher probability of developing a bleed into the brain, and hence they get admitted for observation. The types of fracture are:

- *Linear (nondepressed) fracture.* This appears as a lucent line.
- *Depressed skull fracture.* Management will depend on the underlying brain injury. The fragment may need to be elevated if depressed more than the thickness of the skull or if there are focal signs.
- *Open skull fracture.* This usually requires operative intervention. A broad-spectrum antibiotic should be started, the patient taken to theatre for wound debridement and the fracture dealt with.
- *Basal skull fracture.* This fracture cannot usually be seen on a plain X-ray of the skull, although it should be suspected if there are fluid levels in the sphenoidal sinuses. The diagnosis is made on clinical findings of the CSF leaking from the nose (rhinorrhoea) or the ears (otorrhoea). The CSF is usually crystal clear, unless it is blood-stained. It can be tested for by allowing a drop to fall onto a piece of filter paper. The blood remains at the centre and the CSF soaks around it in concentric rings of clear fluid, called the 'halo sign'. Other clinical signs of a basal skull fracture include the *battle sign* (bruising around the mastoid region due to tracking of blood under the skin) and *haemotympanum* (blood behind the tympanic membrane), which together with

CSF otorrhoea are indicative of a middle fossa fracture through the petrous temporal bone. The *badger sign* (bruising around both orbits), together with rhinorrhoea, is associated with a fracture of the cribriform plate. The badger and battle signs may, however, take several hours to develop.

Brain Injury

Injuries to the brain can be primary, occurring at the time of impact, or secondary to hypovolaemia, hypoxia, hypo-glycaemia and raised intracranial pressure. Prevention of primary brain injury can only be brought about by measures to stop the accident happening in the first place, such as having road speed limits and the wearing of motorcycle helmets, etc. The main aim in the management of a head injury is, therefore, to prevent or limit the damage that occurs due to secondary injury.

Primary brain damage can be diffuse or focal.

Diffuse Injuries

- *Concussion.* This is a brain injury accompanied by a temporary loss of neurological function. The changes are reversible and are often resolved by the time the patient arrives in hospital. They may have just been confused or dazed at the scene or may have lost consciousness. Afterwards they may complain of a headache, feel dizzy, be amnesic or nauseous, and generally if the patient has been unconscious for more than 5 min it is probably best to admit them to hospital for observation.
- *Diffuse axonal injury.* This is a more severe injury, with microscopic structural damage throughout the brain tissue. It is often characterised by prolonged coma and can last from days to weeks. Such patients can develop autonomic dysfunction and hence have high fevers, hypertension and sweating. The mortality is high.

Focal Injuries

- *Contusions.* These are focal areas of brain injury. They can be *coup* injuries, where the brain is damaged directly by the skull at the point of impact, or *contre coup* injuries, where the brain is squashed by the skull at a remote point from the impact.

  The patient may have a focal neurological deficit, depending on the site of the contusion. Oedema may develop at the site of damage and cause a neurological deterioration. The patient is usually managed conservatively; however, due to the risk of delayed bleeding into the contusion, careful observation is needed to observe for deterioration (especially in alcoholics).

- *Intracranial haemorrhage.* This can be meningeal or into the brain tissue.
  - *Acute extradural/epidural haemorrhage.* This is due to a bleed from the arteries that supply the skull and dura — usually the middle meningeal artery, which sits just under the skull in a region called the pterion (or temple). This type of bleed is quite rare, accounting for less than 1% of coma-producing head injuries; however, it can be rapidly fatal. There is usually an associated skull fracture of the parietal or temporal bone, often caused by a direct blow — for example, being hit over the side of the head by a baseball bat.

    The typical picture is loss of consciousness (concussion), followed by a lucid interval. During this lucid interval the haematoma is expanding into the extradural space and compressing the brain inwards, stripping the dura off the skull as it expands (hence the convex appearance of the clot on the CT). As mentioned before, the ICP does not rise initially as the mass is accommodated; however, once the clot reaches a critical volume the ICP increases rapidly.

    The rapid rise in the ICP causes a secondary lapse in the consciousness level. As the ICP rises further, the uncus (the medial aspect of the temporal lobe) herniates through the tentorium (the layer that divides the cerebral hemispheres from the brain stem and cerebellum). The third nerve passes through this opening and can be compressed at this point. The patient initially develops a constriction of the pupil on the affected side, which then begins to dilate up (Hutchinson's pupil). The fixed dilated pupil on the affected side is usually accompanied by a hemiparesis on the opposite side (remember the corticospinal fibres cross over). As the pressure continues to increase, the opposite pupil dilates up and eventually the brain stem 'cones' through the foramen magnum.

This injury requires immediate surgical intervention. The patient should have a CT as early as possible if this type of injury is suspected. Neurosurgical advice should be sought and the patient transferred if necessary for surgical evacuation of the clot. If the injury is treated, early the prognosis is excellent.

○ *Acute subdural haemorrhage.* This is much more common than an extradural haemorrhage, and occurs in about 30% of severe head injuries. It is usually due to rupture of a bridging vein between the cerebral cortex and the dura (but it can also be due to laceration of the cerebral cortex), and is often caused by a rotational injury. The elderly are more susceptible, as their brains are often shrunken and hence the bridging veins are put under tension. The bleeding is typically less brisk than an extradural haemorrhage, but clinically it can present with symptoms of an expanding mass as above. The prognosis is much worse and the mortality high.

○ *Subarachnoid haemorrhage.* This can be associated with trauma, although it is usually due to hypertension and bleeding from berry aneurysms. The symptoms are those of meningeal irritation similar to meningitis.

○ *Brain haemorrhages and lacerations.* These are tears to the brain substance with bleeding into them. The deficit will depend on the site of the damage. These injuries are therefore similar to strokes, and surgery cannot help the patient. Rehabilitation can be very slow.

Assessment of Severe Head Injuries

As the patient is brought into casualty you should attempt to get some history, finding out as much as possible about the incident. If they are unconscious, the history is taken from witnesses or the ambulance crew, etc. Perform the primary survey according to ATLS® guidelines — ABCDE.

The *Glasgow Coma Score* (GCS) is a quantitative measure of the patient's level of consciousness. It is divided into three parts: assessing the best motor response, the best eye-opening response and the best verbal response. It was devised to allow comparisons to be made (if necessary by different observers) to see if the patient's consciousness has improved or deteriorated. The minimum score is 3 and the maximum 15.

A GCS of 8 or less implies coma and a severe head injury. If the score is greater than 8, then the patient is not in a coma. A GCS of 9–12 implies a moderate head injury and a GCS of 13–15 shows a minor head injury.

Glasgow Coma Score

	Score
Best Eye Opening	
Spontaneous	4
To voice	3
To pain	2
None	1
Best Verbal Response	
Orientated	5
Confused	4
Inappropriate speech	3
Incomprehensible speech	2
No speech	1
Best Motor Response	
Obeys commands	6
Localises to pain	5
Withdraws from pain	4
Flexes to pain	3
Extends to pain	2
None	1
Total	3–15

The vital signs and the GCS should be repeated at regular intervals, and deterioration by more than two points should be taken very seriously and a neurosurgical consultation sought. Remember that although bleeding from a scalp wound can cause shock, bleeding into the skull cannot, and therefore never assume that hypotension is due to an intracranial bleed or to brain injury (as this is a terminal event on failure of the medullary centres). Look for another cause.

The Cushing response is a combination of progressive hypertension, bradycardia and a decreased respiratory rate (the opposite of hypovolaemic shock). It is due to a lethal rise in the ICP, usually by an intracranial bleed needing urgent decompression. Hypertension alone or with hyperthermia suggests central autonomic dysfunction caused by diffuse brain injury.

Under D for 'disability', document the patient's level of consciousness using the AVPU score. If the airway, breathing and circulation are under control, then the minineurological examination can be performed in the primary survey; otherwise it is performed in the secondary survey.

The mini-neurological examination involves three components:

1. *Level of consciousness.* The GCS.
2. *Pupillary function.* Are the pupils equal and reactive to light?
3. *Lateralising neurology.* Swiftly assess the tone, power and reflexes of all four limbs.

The purpose of this is to detect those with a severe head injury who are likely to need surgery (i.e. those with abnormalities of all three components).

Remember that the initial neurological examination is only a baseline for comparing the results of repeated examinations, in order to determine deterioration or improvement of the patient's condition.

Management of Severe Head Injuries

This involves, first, dealing with the life-threatening injuries (ABC); then, assessing the severity of the head injury, whilst preventing secondary brain damage from occurring, by ensuring optimal cerebral metabolic supplies and preventing intracranial hypertension.

Cerebral Metabolism

The brain requires oxygen and glucose to function, and so adequate substrates must be present in the circulation to meet this requirement. The oxygen content depends on both the arterial haemoglobin and the PO_2.

The PO_2 can be measured by blood gases, and oxygen can be supplemented as necessary. If the haemoglobin is low, a transfusion may be required to improve the oxygen-carrying capacity.

Raised Intracranial Pressure

This may be due to a mass lesion or brain oedema and should be treated.

In cases of raised ICP the patient should be hyperventilated to keep the PCO_2 low (see section on ICP). To do this it is usually necessary to intubate and ventilate the patient and so early involvement of an anaesthetist is essential. Remember that a decrease in the PCO_2 leads to a decrease in the cerebral blood flow and so the PCO_2 must be kept at about 3.5 as a compromise.

Intravenous fluids may be needed in the management of other problems, such as shock, and the risk is that overhydration may make cerebral oedema worse. Therefore, isotonic fluids such as Hartmann's should be administered rather than hyposmolar fluids such as dextrose.

Diuretics such as mannitol are often used to reduce intracranial pressure and are given if a mass lesion is suspected whilst awaiting transfer to a neurosurgical unit, although a neurosurgical consultation should be obtained prior to giving any diuretics (if diuretics are used, a urinary catheter is required to aid fluid balance measurement). Steroids have no place in the acute management of head injury.

Management of Mild to Moderate Head Injuries

The problem for a casualty officer when he sees what appears to be a minor head injury is in deciding who needs admitting for observation. In general, the history is very important.

Falls from a height should be taken very seriously, as they have a much greater risk of an intracranial bleed than road traffic accidents. For a fall, inquire about the height of the fall and whether it was onto concrete or grass, etc. If the patient was driving a car, inquire about the speed of the car and whether a seat-belt was worn, whether any of the other passengers were injured or dead and whether alcohol or drugs were involved. Was consciousness lost and if so for how long? Has the patient regained consciousness since the accident or have they remained unconscious ever since? Has the patient fitted since or complained of visual disturbances, dizziness or a worsening headache?

Document the amnesia, for the events that led up to the incident (retrograde amnesia) or for the events that followed the incident (anterograde amnesia). The length of anterograde amnesia has been shown to be a good indicator of the severity of the head injury (less than 1 h — mild; 1–24 h — moderate; more than 24 h — severe), although this is not much help in the initial assessment, which takes place soon after the incident. With children it is also worth noting whether they cried immediately, as this is a good sign (i.e. normal behaviour), or whether they were limp and unresponsive.

Examination is essentially the same as above; however, in some cases it is difficult to decide what investigations are needed and whether or not you can safely send the patient home. For example, let us say the patient has walked into the department after a head injury sustained in an assault where he was hit over the head by a brick. His speech is slurred from drink and he has a bump on his forehead, but there is no focal neurology to find on examination (within the limits of the cooperation of this patient).

A large proportion of patients present like this. Should you X-ray these patients?

X-rays may help in deciding who will be admitted for observation, but not much else. Statistically, if there is a skull fracture, then the risk of an intracranial bleed is significantly higher.

Rough Risk of Intracranial Haematoma in Adults

	No Skull Fracture	*Skull Fracture*
Fully conscious	<1/1000	1/30
Depressed consciousness	1/100	1/4

Indications for performing a skull X-ray include (but do check the protocol at your hospital):

1. Loss of consciousness for more than a few minutes
2. Neurological symptoms or signs (unless a CT is indicated) such as visual disturbances, dizziness, weakness, persistent vomiting, etc.
3. Signs of a basal skull fracture
4. Suspected penetrating injuries (X-rays are essential in this case)
5. Common sense, i.e. history of significant injury or obvious significant scalp wound
6. Difficulty in assessing the patient (young/old, drunk, postepileptic)

The indications for admission are

1. Skull fracture
2. Depressed level of consciousness or confusion when examined
3. Neurological symptoms or signs
4. Difficulty in assessing the patient
5. Social circumstances (e.g. patient lives alone, with no responsible adult to observe)

If the patient is admitted, they are usually given nonopiate analgesia (or codeine phosphate, which is safe to use) and taken to the ward. Regular neurological observations are performed, initially on an hourly basis.

The observations include the vital signs, the GCS, pupils and motor function and are represented schematically on a graph to detect any deterioration.

If the patient is not admitted, they should be sent home with head injury instructions (go to your casualty department and get a copy) and accompanied by a responsible adult who will bring him back should his condition deteriorate.

BURNS

Different types of burns tend to affect different age groups. Toddlers tend to be scalded, for example, by pulling the kettle wire or the pan off the stove, kids tend to set their clothes on fire and the old tend to suffer domestic accidents at home. The majority of adult burns however, are associated with industrial accidents (or are drug- or alcohol-related).

Pathology

The damage is caused by coagulation of proteins with cell death. The burn can affect any depth of skin. The superficial burn causes vasodilatation with diffuse erythema, kinins are released and pain is felt. As the depth increases, the capillaries become damaged and therefore more permeable, leading to blistering and oedema formation. As the dermis becomes involved, the nerve endings which lie here are damaged and sensation is lost. Once the germinal layer is damaged, the skin will never regrow, and these burns heal with fibrosis and contractures. The damaged necrotic tissue lying in a protein-rich exudate is an ideal medium for infection. The increased capillary permeability can lead to the exudation of protein-rich fluid from the surface of the burn and oedema into the surrounding tissues. The patient can very quickly become hypovolaemic.

Types of Burns

1. Thermal — can be dry (fire) or wet (scald)
2. Chemical
3. Electrical
4. Friction

Chemical burns result from exposure to acids, alkalis or petroleum products. In general, alkali burns are more serious than acid burns as they penetrate more deeply. The chemical should be flushed away from the skin with copious amounts of irrigation with water (20–30 min). If dry powder is present, brush it away before irrigating. The neutralising agents are no better than water.

Electrical burns are more serious than they appear. The overlying skin may look normal, but deeper tissue may be damaged. Rhabdomyolysis leads to myoglobin release and the risk of acute renal failure. The patient can also develop cardiac disturbance due to acidosis and changes in potassium concentration. A cardiac monitor and a urinary catheter are therefore necessary. The patient will have dark urine due to the myoglobin and require large amounts of fluids to ensure a high urine output. If necessary, mannitol can be used to maintain a diuresis and flush out the myoglobin.

Management of the Burns Patient

The management of the burns patient, as with any trauma patient, is to exclude any life-threatening injuries first (i.e. ABCDE, according to ATLS® guidelines). The main priorities with burns patients, however, are

1. Securing the airway
2. Management of fluid loss
3. Prevention of infection

Immediate Resuscitation

Secure the airway, and stop the burning process by removing all clothing.

Airway

The supraglottic airway can rapidly become obstructed due to oedema and swelling following a burn injury. It is therefore important to suspect involvement of the airway, even if the patient is breathing normally when first examined. Apart from the obvious signs of airway injury, such as stridor or hoarseness, any of the following should alert the doctor to the likely presence of an acute inhalation injury:

1. Facial burns
2. Singeing of the eyebrows or nasal hairs
3. Carbonaceous sputum
4. Altered consciousness
5. History — such as long exposure to smoke or gases, or an explosion

An anaesthetist must be called immediately. Early endotracheal intubation is better than adopting a wait-and-see policy, as the airway can become obstructed rapidly.

Breathing

Apart from direct thermal injury, which causes upper airway oedema and obstruction, inhalation of toxic fumes and smoke can lead to chemical tracheobronchitis, oedema and pneumonia. You should always assume carbon monoxide (CO) exposure if the patient was confined to an enclosed area. CO has an affinity for haemoglobin that is about 240 times that of oxygen, and hence oxygen is displaced and the oxygen dissociation curve is shifted to the left. The CO dissociates very slowly when the patient is breathing room air (with a half-life of about 6 h). If 100% oxygen is breathed the half-life is shortened to about 40 min. Therefore, the patient should have arterial blood gases taken for assessment of the carboxyhaemoglobin concentration and 100% oxygen should be commenced. Symptoms may include a headache, nausea, vomiting, or confusion at high levels of exposure, but the classic cherry-red skin appearance is rare.

Circulation

It may be difficult to get a reliable blood pressure owing to the burns, and the urine output is probably the best indicator of circulating blood volume.

Establish intravenous access if necessary through the burnt skin, and start two litres of Hartmann's solution immediately. The fluid losses can be huge and a 50% burns patient can lose up to half their plasma volume in about 3–4 h.

A rough guide is to replace 2–4 ml of crystalloid fluid for each kilogram body weight per percent burn in the first 24 h. So a 70 kg man with a 50% burn will require 7–14 l in the first 24 h ($2 \times 70 \times 50 = 7000$ ml = 7 l). Half the fluid should be given in the first 8 h from the time of the burn (not from the time of arrival to casualty), so if the burn occurred 2 h before arrival, they will need at a very minimum 3.5 l of fluids in the next 6 h.

In some departments the policy is to replace colloids such as human albumin solution (HAS), and in this case the Muir and Barclay formula can be used. This determines how much plasma volume is needed in terms of colloid replacement.

Volume of colloid needed (per unit time) = weight (kg) × percent burn/2

So, for a 70 kg man, with a 50% burn this would be 1.75 l of colloid per unit time (70 × 50/2 = 1750 ml). The first amount is given in the first 4 h from the burn, then the same amount in the subsequent 4, 4, 6, 6 and 12 h. This would total about 8.75 l of colloid in the first day and in addition crystalloid maintenance (about 3 l) with, say, normal saline is required.

Remember that these figures are just guides and no matter whether crystalloids or colloids have been administered, the best indicator of sufficient replacement is an adequate urine output of greater than 30–50 ml/h. The haematocrit is also used to guide fluid balance.

Circumferential full thickness burns can impede the blood supply to the limbs owing to oedema in a confined space (a tourniquet effect), and are best treated by escharotomies (an incision through scar tissue). The incision is made along the line of the limb through the entire scar. As this is a full thickness burn, sensation is absent and in theory no anaesthetic is required. In practice, however, the escharotomy tends to be done with the patient anaesthetised (because there are some areas of partial thickness burns adjacent to the full thickness zones which will clearly cause pain). Cross-matched blood must be available, as this procedure can bleed profusely. Circumferential burns of the thorax may cause restriction of chest expansion, and bilateral escharotomies may be needed to improve breathing.

Assessing the Burn (History, Size and Depth of the Burn)

History

Note the cause and exact time of the burn (remember to ask about associated injuries — for example, did the patient jump out of a window to escape the fire?). Try to ascertain some past medical history, such as diabetes, hypertension, heart or lung disease, the medication the patient is on, allergies and tetanus status.

Depth of Burn

Superficial burns (also called first-degree burns) are not life-threatening and are simply painful red areas, such as sunburn. There is no blistering and long term they usually do not scar. In *partial thickness burns* (also called deep dermal or second-degree burns) there is associated swelling and blistering, and the skin is red and may be oozing fluid. These burns are very painful even to air current. Long term most deep dermal burns do not scar but it depends on the patient's skin type and whether or not they need a skin graft (for example, there have been cases of marked keloid scarring following a deep dermal burn in black patients even without surgery). In *full thickness burns* (also called third-degree burns) skin is dry, painless and insensate; it may appear pale, white or charred. Long term these will scar.

Body Surface Area

The 'rule of nines' is a useful way to determine the extent of the burn (Figure 4.2). The adult body is divided into regions that represent 9% of the body area. The genital region is considered to be 1% of the body surface area (BSA). The proportions are different in children whose head contributes more than the legs to the total area (as it does for heat loss). Another good guide is that the *patient's* palm (not your palm and not including the patient's fingers) represents about 1% of the body surface area. You can use these guides to estimate that, in an adult with a burn to one arm and one leg with a small area affected on the torso of about three palm sizes, the percent burn will be about 30 (9 + 18 + 3).

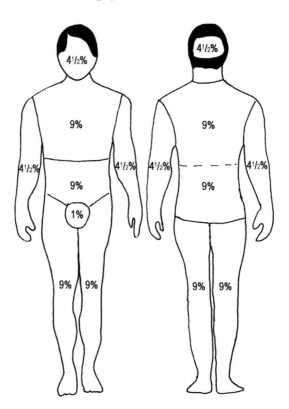

Figure 4.2. The 'rule of nines'.

Summary of Management of the Burns Patient

1. *Airway.* Look for signs of obstruction or signs indicating the risk of obstruction; inform the anaesthetist.
2. *Breathing.* Pulse oximetry; look for signs of CO poisoning, 100% oxygen, arterial blood gas analysis; request a chest X-ray.
3. *Circulation.* IV access × 2 — take blood for FBC, U & Es, glucose, X-match and carboxyhaemoglobin levels; start IV fluids, ECG; catheterise if necessary.
4. Assess the burn depth and BSA, adjust fluid requirements, consider escharotomies.

5. *Analgesia.* Usually opiates, titrated to the patient's pain.
6. Assess for associated injuries; a nasogastric tube may be needed.
7. Cover the burns — partial thickness burns are painful to air current; gently cover them with sterile towels. Do not apply any antiseptic and do not pierce the blisters.
8. Take extra special precautions to avoid infection, which after the initial resuscitation is the main cause of morbidity and mortality. The patient should be transferred to a regional burns unit if necessary, especially if there is
   - A partial thickness burn of greater than 20% BSA (in the very young or old a 10% burn should be referred).
   - A full thickness burn of greater than 5%.
   - Involvement of the face, hands, feet, genitalia or major joints.
   - Significant chemical or electrical burns.
   - An inhalation injury or other serious comorbidity.

The burns should be covered with clingfilm, then warm blankets should be applied before transfer as the use of agents such as sulphasalizine or paraffin gauze interfere with the assessment of the burn when the patient arrives at the burns unit.

5

LIVER, BILIARY TRACT AND PANCREAS

Richard M Charnley

Many of the pathological entities in this section appear in both medicine and surgery, and questions on them may therefore be found in either part of the examination. There is, however, often a different emphasis between the types of answer one should give in a medical examination and in a surgical examination, even when dealing with the same condition. Having said that, however, most surgeons now work closely with their physician colleagues and, despite differences of emphasis, will usually have similar views about management and the precise role of surgical intervention.

INVESTIGATIONS

The relevant investigations for most conditions of the liver, biliary tract and pancreas are blood tests (including liver function tests) and diagnostic imaging.

Liver Function Tests

These usually consist of:

Bilirubin	A rise of bilirubin is the definition of jaundice. It is bilirubin which makes the patient yellow.
Alkaline phosphastase	This enzyme tends to be raised more with obstruction of the bile ducts (i.e. obstructive jaundice).
Transaminases (e.g. ALT, AST)	These tend to be raised more with defective liver cell function (i.e. hepatocellular dysfunction).
Albumin	This is synthesised by the liver and is therefore low in patients with chronic liver disease and malnutrition.
Gamma GT	This enzyme is raised in both hepatocellular and obstructive disorders.

In addition, the prothrombin time or INR (INR = international ratio, i.e. the length of time the patient's blood takes to clot in comparison with that of a normal person) may be abnormal and should be checked in any jaundiced patient or when defective liver synthesis is suspected. If abnormal, it can be corrected by vitamin K (vitamin K is a fat-soluble vitamin and is not absorbed well in many forms of liver disease because of a lack of bile salts, which are required to emulsify fats in the intestinal lumen).

IMAGING TECHNIQUES

Ultrasound (Transabdominal)

This is noninvasive and is the first imaging investigation of choice in patients with hepato-biliary or pancreatic disease.

Computerised Tomography

Computerised tomography (CT) of the liver and pancreas, particularly if carried out on a helical or multislice scanner provides good views of the organs of the upper abdomen. It is very useful in diagnosing and staging suspected tumours and is also of importance in identifying the degree of severity in acute pancreatitis and complications in chronic pancreatitis.

Magnetic Resonance Imaging

Magnetic resonance imaging (MRI) is of value in imaging the bile duct and pancreatic duct (known as magnetic resonance cholangiopancreatography or MRCP). MRI of the liver is commonly used for the assessment of malignant tumours.

Endoscopic Ultrasound

With an ultrasound transducer on the end of an endoscope, endoscopic ultrasound provides good images of the gallbladder, bile duct and pancreas. It is useful for identifying bile duct stones and gallbladder microlithiasis as well as pancreatic tumours and chronic pancreatitis. Endoscopic ultrasound allows the early parenchymal and ductal changes of chronic pancreatitis to be identified. It is also safer than endoscopic retrograde cholangiopancreatography, particularly with regard to the risk of postprocedure pancreatitis.

Endoscopic Retrograde Cholangiopancreatography

A side-viewing endoscope is passed into the duodenum and the bile duct or pancreatic duct can be cannulated. In addition, endoscopic sphincterotomy and stone extraction can be carried out for biliary stones or a biliary or pancreatic stent can be inserted for relief of obstruction. The complications of endoscopic retrograde cholangiopancreatography (ERCP) include acute pancreatitis, bleeding, perforation and cholangitis. These complications can be reduced by investigating patients with endoscopic ultrasound or MRCP and by reserving ERCP for those patients who are likely to require a therapeutic procedure.

Percutaneous Transheptic Cholangiography

Percutaneous transheptic cholangiography (PTC) provides percutaneous access to the biliary tract and is mainly used in those patients with a hilar obstruction or in those where ERCP has failed to relieve the biliary obstruction.

Liver Biopsy and Pancreatic Biopsy

If a patient has a liver tumour or pancreatic tumour which is suspicious of malignancy, biopsy is usually not necessary and might risk causing peritoneal metastases. Liver biopsy is usually used for parenchymal disorders such as cirrhosis. Pancreatic biopsy is usually carried out at the time of endoscopic ultrasound in patients in whom the diagnosis is uncertain.

GALLSTONES

Gallstones are very common and are therefore frequently asked about in the finals. The majority are asymptomatic and require no treatment. They can, however, cause a wide range of clinical problems, depending on their position (see list). They are either made up of cholesterol and pigment (composed of bilirubin breakdown products) or a mixture of the two. Pure pigment stones are rare (<10%) and are found in conditions such as haemolytic anaemia. Most (75%) gallstones are predominantly cholesterol. Ninety per cent of gallstones are radiolucent, i.e. they do not show on a plain X-ray (unlike renal calculi, of which 90% are radio-opaque). Predisposing factors to gallstone formaton include female sex (three times more common), obesity, age (10% of >50-year-olds have gallstones, and 30% of >70-year-olds), haemolytic anemia, hyperlipidaemias and Crohn's disease. Some people also appear to have an innate tendency to form gallstones and are said to have 'lithogenic bile'. People often refer to the typical gallstone patient as fat, female, fertile and forty.

Complications of gallstones:

1. *In the gallbladder*
   - Chronic cholecystitis
   - Biliary colic
   - Acute cholecystitis
     - ○ Empyema
     - ○ Biliary peritonitis
     - ○ Abscess
   - Mucocele
   - Carcinoma of gallbladder
2. *In the common bile duct*
   - Obstructive jaundice
   - Cholangitis
   - Pancreatitis
3. *In the gut*
   - Gallstone ileus

CHRONIC CHOLECYSTITIS

Chronic cholecystitis is a term used to describe symptoms of upper abdominal pain, indigestion, bloating, burping, nausea and occasional vomiting. Sometimes this symptom complex is called flatulent dyspepsia. The patient may describe the symptoms as being precipitated by fatty food (fats stimulate the release of cholecystokinin, which causes gallbladder contractions). There is usually nothing to find on physical examination. The main differential diagnoses include peptic ulceration, hiatus hernia and irritable bowel syndrome. Because gallstones are common, it is important not to automatically ascribe such symptoms to them simply because gallstones are present on an ultrasound scan. A missed peptic ulcer or irritable bowel syndrome will obviously not be helped by unnecessary cholecystectomy and the patient will continue to get symptoms (sometimes called postcholecystectomy syndrome). If the symptoms are thought to be arising from the gallbladder and are significant, then the treatment is cholecystectomy, usually laparoscopic. Attempts to dissolve gallstones using bile salt therapy are possible only in patients with small, noncalcified stones and are reserved for those who refuse or are unfit for surgery. This treatment is not very successful.

BILIARY COLIC

Biliary colic is the pain caused by gallbladder muscle spasms against a stone stuck in the neck of the gallbladder (Hartmann's pouch) or the cystic duct. It may account for some of the symptoms of chronic cholecystitis. Unlike intestinal colic, the pain is continuous and not in waves. It is usually felt in the epigastrium or right upper quadrant and may radiate around both costal margins and into the back. The pain can be extremely severe and patients may be sweaty, pale and tachycardic because of it. They may also feel nauseated or vomit. They will usually be unable to get comfortable and will prefer to writhe around rather than stay still. Attacks usually last less than 6 h and examination is usually otherwise normal. Differential diagnoses include other causes of severe upper abdominal pain, such as perforated peptic ulcer, pancreatitis, ruptured aneurysm, etc. Management involves giving analgesia, investigation to confirm gallstones (ultrasound) and subsequent cholecystectomy in most cases.

ACUTE CHOLECYSTITIS

In its earliest stage this may appear to be biliary colic, and indeed many attacks of acute cholecystitis probably start with biliary colic. Most episodes of acute cholecystitis are caused by chemical inflammation within an obstructed gallbladder and the exact mechanisms are poorly understood. Bacterial infection probably is a secondary event in about one-third of cases and these may be the ones most likely to develop complications. Patients will typically have severe right upper quadrant or epigastric pain. Like biliary colic, this may radiate around the costal margins or into the back. Unlike biliary colic, patients will prefer to lie still and take shallow breaths (this is now a form of local peritonitis, not colic). They will usually have a temperature and tachycardia, and may also have nausea and vomiting. Murphy's sign may be positive and is often asked about in vivas. It is elicited by pressing in the right upper quadrant under the costal margin. The patient is then asked to breathe in, and winces or gasps with pain as the gallbladder moves down and hits the examiner's hand. The test should also be performed in the left upper quadrant to exclude nonspecific reactions due to other pathology.

A mass may be present in the right upper quadrant, but if so this is not usually the gallbladder itself but rather a 'phlegmon' (i.e. inflamed and adherent omentum and bowel around the gallbladder).

The treatment of acute cholecystitis is initial resuscitation with intravenous fluids and antibiotics. The patient will normally be kept nil by mouth or on sips of clear fluids, and initial investigations will be arranged, including basic blood tests such as an FBC (usually the white cell count is raised), U & Es, LFTs and amylase (as acute pancreatitis may be a differential diagnosis). The most important confirmatory test is usually an ultrasound scan. This can confirm gallstones, show thickening and oedema of the gallbladder wall and localise the tender spot to the gallbladder itself. It can also exclude dilatation of the common bile duct and other pathology, such as liver masses. Only very occasionally is a HIDA scan used to help confirm or exclude cholecystitis. The principle of this test is that HIDA (a radioisotope) is taken up by the liver and excreted into the bile. If the cystic duct is patent, it will fill the gallbladder effectively, excluding cholecystitis.

With conservative treatment approximately 80–90% of cases of acute cholecystitis will settle over the next 24–48 h (i.e. the pain settles, the temperature falls and the patient's abdomen becomes nontender). In about 10% of cases there will not be a prompt resolution of symptoms and signs, and in these cases surgery is usually advised. Particularly worrying signs are increasing temperature, tachycardia and the onset of increasing tenderness or the signs of peritonitis. These may indicate infarction of the gallbladder (gangrenous cholecystitis) or perforation, which may produce either a local collection or generalised peritonitis. A gallbladder full of pus (empyema of the gallbladder) usually leads to an unwell patient with the signs of sepsis (fever, tachycardia, hypotension, etc.) as well as pain, and tenderness in the right upper quadrant.

More controversial is the question of what to do with patients who do not absolutely require early surgery. Although conventional management is to allow the acute episode to settle down and to readmit the patient for elective cholecystectomy 6–8 weeks later, many surgeons now prefer cholecystectomy in the acute phase. This allows patients to recover quicker and to be spared further episodes of pain. Laparoscopic cholecystectomy can now be carried out in the acute phase by experienced surgeons.

CHOLECYSTECTOMY

Laparoscopic cholecystectomy has now replaced open cholecystectomy in the majority of cases. Open cholecystectomy may still be indicated in difficult cases or when laparoscopic cholecystectomy has been attempted and has failed. The open operation is usually performed through a right subcostal incision or occasionally through an upper midline. The gallbladder is dissected off the liver. The cystic artery and cystic duct are then identified, ligated and divided (note that there is no cystic vein). Great care should be taken not to damage the bile duct.

The first laparoscopic cholecystectomy was performed in 1987 by Phillipe Mouret (a gynaecologist!) in France and the procedure has since become accepted as the mainstay treatment of uncomplicated gallstone disease. The term 'laparoscopy' (peritoneoscopy) means insertion of a rigid endoscope into the peritoneal cavity, which is insufflated with carbon dioxide gas to provide a view of the abdominal contents. The advantages of minimal access surgery are attributable to the smaller wounds used for the laparoscopic ports. This results in less postoperative pain, less chance of wound infection, reduced postoperative chest complications and an earlier mobilisation and discharge from hospital as well as earlier return to work. The main disadvantage of laparoscopic surgery is the loss of tactile feedback and the potential for tumour implantation if an incidental carcinoma of the gallbladder is present. The only current contraindications to laparoscopic cholecystectomy are suspected cancer and patients with bleeding disorders or portal hypertension. Multiple adhesions may make laparoscopy difficult but not impossible.

The principles of laparoscopic cholecystectomy are as follows. Access to the peritoneal cavity is achieved at the umbilicus by direct exposure of the peritoneum and insertion of a blunt trochar. The pneumoperitoneum is created by insufflation of carbon dioxide. The intra-abdominal pressure is kept at about 15 mmHg, just enough to keep the anterior abdominal wall of the viscera. The camera is introduced through the umbilical port and three further ports are sited under direct vision, one in the epigastrium, one at the right costal margin and one in the right flank, to allow the instruments and graspers access.

The gallbladder is retracted upwards lifting the liver and allowing the whole gallbladder to be visualised. The position of the patient (head up tilt and rotation to the left by 15 to 20°) improves visualisation. The neck of the gallbladder is dissected off the liver by incising the peritoneum anteriorly and posteriorly. This allows a window to be created between the liver and the neck of the gallbladder. The cystic artery and cystic duct are then identified. It is mandatory to confirm that the right hepatic artery is not mistaken for the cystic artery. This artery must be shown to be passing only to the gallbladder. The cystic duct is then identified joining the gallbladder. Creation of the large window between the neck of the gallbladder and the liver is essential to avoid bile duct injury. If an operative cholangiogram is to be performed a cannula is inserted into the cystic duct and retained with a clip whilst the cholangiogram is carried out (dye is injected under an image intensifier). If the cholangiogram is satisfactory (normal anatomy, no bile duct stones and flow of contrast into the duodenum), the cannula is withdrawn and the cystic duct clipped and divided above two clips. The gallbladder is then dissected off the liver and removed through the largest port (usually at the umbilicus). The gallbladder bed is irrigated and haemostasis checked. The carbon dioxide is then removed from the abdomen, the fascia closed at the umbilicus and the skin closed with subcuticular Vicryl sutures.

The laparoscopic cholecystectomy is the best example of minimal access surgery (MAS) at the present time. MAS is essentially the same operation through a smaller wound. It encompasses laparoscopy, thoracoscopy, arthroscopy and endoluminal endoscopy. Although these techniques have been around for many years, it is only within the last two decades that laparoscopy has been used for surgical procedures such as laparoscopic cholecystectomy, colectomy, appendicectomy, hernia repair, etc.

Many would regard the other procedures as controversial and it would seem that with improved technology, expertise and training, many of these procedures will in the future become as widely accepted as laparoscopic cholecystectomy.

The proposed advantages of laparoscopic surgery are attributable to a smaller wound, and there will thus be less postoperative pain, the wound will heal quicker with less chance of infection, the patient will recover and mobilise quicker, return home sooner and hence return to work quicker.

The disadvantages of laparoscopy include the need for special equipment and extra training; the procedure itself is technically more challenging (hand–eye coordination), the complications are harder to deal with (e.g. haemostasis–the blood obscures the field of vision), and there is loss of tactile feedback. Recently, there have been reports of tumour implantation at port hole sites, leaving questions unanswered as to the role of laparoscopic techniques in the management of malignant disease. The question as to whether laparoscopic surgery is cheaper and quicker or slower and more expensive involves so many factors (the expertise of the surgeon, the length of the operations, the cost of the shorter hospital stay, etc.) that it is probably best just to say that this remains controversial.

There are relatively few contraindications to laparoscopy, although patients with cardiac or respiratory problems do not tolerate the pneumoperitoneum well owing to a decreasd venous return and increased strain on the heart. Laproscopy is best avoided for patients with bleeding disorders, as bleeding is more difficult to deal with, and also patients who are shocked must have an open operation. Relative contraindications include those patients with multiple previous abdominal scars who are likely to have multiple adhesions between the bowel and the anterior abdominal wall, making laparoscopy hazardous. Pregnancy, certainly in the later stages, is also a relative contraindication.

Complications of Laparoscopic Cholecystectomy

General

The increased intra-abdominal pressure when the pneumoperitoneum is created can lead to a decreased venous return and hence can cause strain to the heart and lungs. Rarely, a CO_2 embolism can occur, which causes the patient to become hypoxic and have a rapid reduction in cardiac output.

Specific Complications

- Bleeding from the cystic or hepatic artery can be much more difficult to deal with laparoscopically.
- The incidence of common bile duct injury in laparoscopic cholecystectomy is now similar to that in the open operation but may be more difficult to identify laparoscopically. This may, however, decrease in the future as surgeons become more experienced with the technique.
- Instrumental injury, for example thermocoagulation of tissues with diathermy is more common because of the use of diathermy dissection at laparoscopic surgery. Some laparoscopic operations are technically more difficult and this is most likely in those patients who have experienced recent acute attacks of cholecystitis.

Before performing a cholecystectomy the surgeon must establish whether there are any stones in the bile ducts as well as in the gallbladder. If the patient has been jaundiced, the liver function tests are abnormal or if ultrasound shows dilated ducts, there may be stones in the common bile duct. The options for identification and treatment of bile duct stones are as follows:

- Perform operative cholangiogram on all patients and explore the common duct laparoscopically if stones are found to be present. Laparoscopic bile duct exploration is an advanced laparoscopic technique.
- Perform ERCP on patients with confirmed bile duct stones after ultrasound or MRCP on those with suspected bile duct stones on ultrasound or as indicated by liver function tests, reserving ERCP for therapeutic removal of bile duct stones only. Diagnostic ERCP should be avoided if possible.

MUCOCOELE

A mucocoele of the gallbladder is a condition where the neck of the gallbladder is blocked by a stone, which has become impacted. There is no inflammation at this stage but mucus secreted by the gallbladder wall builds up and gradually distends the gallbladder, which may reach a large size. A mucocoele may be completely asymptomatic or may present as a mass in the right upper quadrant if it becomes infected and an abscess may form.

CHOLANGITIS

Cholangitis is a condition where there is infection within the biliary tract and it is rare unless there is associated obstruction. This is a demonstration of the surgical principle that obstructed tubes tend to get infected, i.e. appendicitis, pyelonephritis, etc. Cholangitis is clinically manifested by Charcot's triad of pain, jaundice and rigors (rigors means involuntary shaking in association with pyrexia). It requires prompt diagnosis and treatment, otherwise it can have a high mortality. Treatment consists of resuscitaton with fluids and the administration of intravenous antibiotics. If resolution is not rapid, then attempts to produce biliary drainage, endoscopically, radiologically or surgically, are required.

GALLSTONE ILEUS

Gallstone ileus is a misnomer; it is a small bowel obstruction and not an ileus (an ileus is a condition where there is absence of peristalsis in the intestine, such as usually occurs for a few days after a laparotomy). It is relatively rare but is frequently asked about in the finals.

In the normal anatomical position the gallbladder lies adjacent to the duodenum. A gallstone ileus is caused when a large gallstone (usually >2.5 cm) erodes directly through the wall of the gallbladder into the duodenum. Small gallstones will not cause obstruction, and they normally enter the duodenum by passing down the cystic duct and then the common bile duct. The erosion of a large gallstone directly into the duodenum is a process which probably occurs over a very long period of time. Surrounding inflammation seals the area such that no local abscess or peritonitis occurs in these cases. Once in the duodenum, the stone starts to be moved down the intestine by peristalsis. The narrowest part of the intestinal tract (after the gastro-oesophageal junction) is about 2 ft proximal to the ileocaecal valve and it is here that the gallstone may impact. The classical X-ray would show the signs of distal small bowel obstruction, air within the biliary tree (because of the fistula between the gallbladder and the duodenum) and the gallstone in the right lower quadrant of the abdomen. However, most cases are not diagnosed until surgery. Treatment is removal of the stone through an enterotomy (incision in the small bowel). The gallbladder is usually left alone, as removal can lead to a hole in the duodenum.

CARCINOMA OF THE GALLBLADDER

This is a relatively rare malignancy. Unfortunately most cases are advanced at the time of presentation. It is associated with long-standing gallstones, polyps of the gallbladder (if a gallbladder polyp is >1 cm in size, then a cholecystectomy should probably be performed) and calcification of the gallbladder (known as a 'porcelain' gallbladder), which is also an indication for cholecystectomy.

Incidental carcinoma of the gallbladder is found in 0.5 to 1% of laparoscopic cholecystectomies. If suspected preoperatively, the patient should be referred to a hepato-biliary surgeon and an open operation performed. If suspected following removal of the gallbladder at cholecystectomy, a retrieval bag should be used to avoid recurrence at port sites. In such patients a further radical operation including resection of the gallbladder bed of the liver, incision of the extra hepatic biliary tree and radical hilar lymphadenectomy should be performed as a second operation if there is no evidence of metastatic disease.

TUMOURS OF THE PANCREAS

Although ductal carcinoma of the pancreas is one of the most lethal of all gastrointestinal tumours, 10–15% of tumours of the pancreas (including those of the periampullary region) are not of the same histological type as ductal carcinoma and have a much better prognosis. This group of tumours includes ampullary carcinoma, islet cell tumours of the pancreas and cystic tumours of the pancreas. A tumour of the pancreas should, therefore, not be assumed to carry a poor prognosis.

Ductal adenocarcinoma of the pancreas is highly malignant and has usually metastasised by the time of diagnosis. Smoking is the only recognised aetiological factor and the disease is uncommon under the age of 40. The disease occurs in the head of the pancreas in 80% of cases. It presents with obstructive jaundice in 70% of cases but may also present with severe upper abdominal pain (which may radiate into the back), weight loss, anorexia, malaise, or rarely, thrombophlebitis migrans.

On examination, there may be cervical lymphadenopathy, an abdominal mass, hepatomegaly or ascites. The gallbladder may be palpable. Courvoisier's law states that if, in the presence of jaundice, the gallbladder is palpable, then the cause is unlikely to be gallstones.

Investigations include basic blood tests and specific diagnosis by ultrasound, CT or MRI. The ERCP may be helpful too, and may also allow therapeutic manoeuvres such as stent insertion (see section on obstructive jaundice).

Most tumours are treated palliatively by insertion of a biliary stent or bypass surgery. Resectional surgery is suitable for 15–20% of patients with a ductal carcinoma but 50–75% of patients with ampullary carcinoma, islet cell tumours or cystic tumours of the pancreas. Five-year survival following curative resection in ductal carcinoma is 10–15% although resection is also associated with good relief of symptoms. For those with ampullary tumours, islet cell tumours or cystic tumours, 5 year survival of 40% can be anticipated.

For tumours of the head of the pancreas or peri-ampullary region, pancreatico-duodenectomy (Whipple's operation) is the operation of choice (see Figure 5.1). The pylorus-preserving operation is the operation of choice. The mortality rate of pancreatico-duodenectomy is less than 5%.

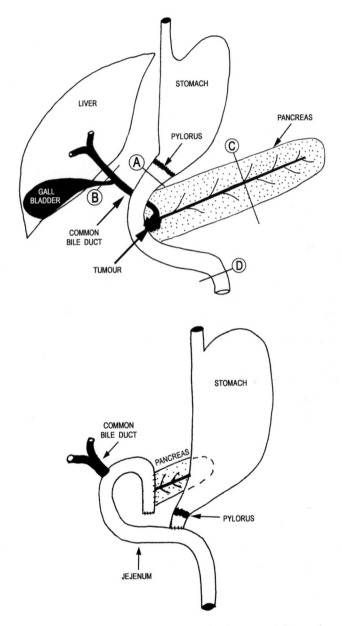

Figure 5.1. Whipple's procedure (partial pancreatoduodenectomy) for carcinoma of the head of pancreas (shaded).

ACUTE PANCREATITIS

In acute pancreatitis, pancreatic enzymes are released and activated leading to a vicious circle of events. The exact mechanism for this is unknown but the end result is that the activated enzymes autodigest the pancreas. There are four stages in the process and resolution can occur at any point in the sequence of events. Initially, there is oedema and fluid shifts which can lead to severe hypovolaemic shock (vomiting is usually present, which compounds fluid losses). Fluid and enzymes are released into the peritoneal cavity, which may lead to autodigestion of fats resulting in the development of fat necrosis within the peritoneal cavity. The second stage occurs when the autodigestion affects the blood vessels and can lead to haemorrhage into the retroperitoneal space. This may result in tracking of blood-stained fluids causing bruising in the flanks (Grey Turner's sign) and bruising at the umbilicus (Cullen's sign). Both these signs indicate a severe attack. In the third stage of the disease inflammation progresses to necrosis, which may affect part of the pancreas or, in severe cases, all of it. If the necrosis becomes infected this is associated with further deterioration and a high mortality rate.

Acute pancreatitis usually presents with acute onset upper abdominal pain associated with raised serum levels of amylase. There are many aetiological factors which cause acute pancreatitis. In the UK the most common cause is gallstones, accounting for 60% of cases. Alcohol is the next common cause (20% of cases). The mnemonic GET SMASH'N is often used by students — gallstones, ethanol, trauma, steroids (and other drugs including Asathioprine), mumps (and other viral infections including coxsackie B), autoimmune diseases (e.g. SLE), scorpion bites (rare and not seen in the UK), hyperlipidaemia (and hyperparathyroidism, hypothermia and hereditary causes) and neoplasia. All of these should be asked about in the history, especially alcohol intake and family history. A patient with acute pancreatitis will usually present with a sudden onset of severe upper abdominal or epigastric pain which may radiate directly through to the back. The patient may also have nausea or vomiting and the condition may rapidly progress to involve the whole abdomen and lead to shock. Usually, the abdomen is diffusely tender but soft with normal bowel sounds; however, with significant acute pancreatitis the abdomen can have an appearance similar to peritonitis with the patient preferring to lie still, with widespread guarding and rigidity and absent bowel sounds.There is no absolute test for a diagnosis of pancreatitis. The condition should be suspected in cases with the above presentation, but sometimes it can be impossible to exclude other causes of the acute abdomen, such as a perforated ulcer, without recourse to laparotomy.

The most useful test is the serum amylase level, but this can be normal in up to 30% of patients. If serum amylase is greater than three times the upper limit of normal, it is usually diagnostic of acute pancreatitis; however, the degree of elevation of the serum amylase does not bear any clear relationship to the severity of the pancreatitis. If a patient is strongly suspected of having acute pancreatitis but the serum amylase is normal, it may be because the earlier onset of the symptoms has resulted in the amylase returning to normal. In this case the measurement of serum lipase is useful because this stays elevated longer than the amylase. The measurement of urinary amylase is also useful since this remains elevated for 24–48 h longer than the serum amylase. In patients still suspected of having acute pancreatitis where diagnosis has not been confirmed a contrast enhanced CT scan should be carried out, which in severe cases is likely to show a tumour of the pancreas or pancreatic necrosis.

Early assessment of severity in acute pancreatitis is worthwhile because those patients with predicted severe acute pancreatitis should be monitored more closely, considered for prophylactic antibiotics and if the aetiology is gallstones, considered for an urgent ERCP and endoscopic sphincterotomy. Assessment of severity is carried out by a multifactorial scoring system such as the Ranson's scoring system (see list). Alternatively, measurement of the C reactive protein, particularly if carried out as repeated measurements, can also provide an accurate assessment of severity.

Ranson's Criteria for Acute Pancreatitis

One point for each variable; a score of 3 or more points indicates severe pancreatitis:

1. *At admission*
   - Age greater than 55 years
   - Blood glucose >11 mmol/l

- Serum LDH >500 IU/l
- AST >200 IU/l
- White blood count >16 × 10^9/l
2. *At 48 h after admission*
   - Haematocrit fall >10%
   - Blood urea >16 mmol/l
   - Serum calcium <2 mmol/l
   - Arterial pO_2 < 8 kPa
   - Base deficit <4 mmol/l

In the initial stages of treatment of acute pancreatitis the aims are resuscitation of the patient with intravenous fluids and oxygen and analgesia. The patient need not be kept nil by mouth and a nasogastric tube need not be inserted unless the patient is vomiting. Fluid balance charts must be kept and a urinary catheter is necessary to accurately monitor urine output hourly. It is usually necessary to give patients large volumes of fluid intravenously and it is essential that the urine output is maintained above 30 ml/h.

The development of renal failure is associated with a bad prognosis. Respiratory failure in the form of adult respiratory distress syndrome is also associated with a bad prognosis. There is still debate about the precise role of antibiotics in acute pancreatitis. For those patients with predicted severe pancreatitis most units give prophylactic antibiotics for 7 days. The agents in common usage include Meropenem, Imipenem, Ciprofloxacin or Cefuroxime. The use of antibiotics beyond 7 days is in response to positive cultures only. During treatment of acute pancreatitis, gastric acid secretion should be reduced by the administration of a proton pump inhibitor or H2 receptor antagonist. Early assessment of aetiology is also important. Ultrasound is carried out in the first 24 h to look for gallstones and if gallstones are present, the patient will require an elective laparoscopic cholecystectomy to prevent further attacks. If the patient has a biliary cause and also has severe pancreatitis, an urgent endoscopic sphincterotomy should be carried out as this has been shown to reduce mortality in severe acute pancreatitis.

The majority of patients with acute pancreatitis settle down after a few days and make a good recovery; however, in severe acute pancreatitis, patients may die early from multiorgan failure (often respiratory and renal failure). If they get over the acute phase, patients with severe acute pancreatitis may develop infected pancreatic necrosis. This is suspected if the patient has a positive blood culture, if there are changes of low density within the pancreas or if the patient's condition deteriorates with a high white cell count. The presence of infective necrosis can usually be confirmed by CT-guided aspiration. The conventional treatment of infected pancreatic necrosis is open surgery with necrosectomy and postoperative cavity irrigation. More recently, other techniques have been developed to treated infected necrosis, including retroperitoneal endoscopic necrosectomy, which is performed by a retroperitoneal approach using a modified nephroscope. An alternative technique, which is only suitable for walled-off collections behind the stomach is transgastric endoscopic necrosectomy, which is carried out using an endoscope. Infected necrosis is the most common cause of death in acute pancreatitis. If the necrosis does not become infected, other complications may occur such as pseudocyst formation. A pseudocyst is a collection of fluid in the lesser peritoneal sac. If a pseudocyst is persistent, drainage may be necessary and this can usually be carried out endoscopically or if not applied to the back of the stomach, laparoscopic or open cyst gastrostomy may be necessary.

Nutrition is a very important aspect of the management of acute pancreatitis. The majority of patients can be fed enterally from early on in the illness. This is usually achieved by placement of a naso-jejunal feeding tube.

OBSTRUCTIVE JAUNDICE

Jaundice can be classified in three ways. The most common is to divide it into prehepatic (caused by haemolytic anaemia), hepatic (caused by hepatitis) and posthepatic jaundice (which is also called obstructive jaundice or, sometimes, surgical jaundice). Prehepatic and hepatic causes of jaundice are usually dealt with as medical conditions not requiring surgery and will not be referred to further in this chapter. An additional type of obstructive jaundice should, however, be mentioned, namely drug-induced cholestatic jaundice, which is produced by drugs such as chlorpromazine. Clinically and biochemically, this can be impossible to differentiate from true obstructive jaundice without further tests, and it is important that all cases of jaundice have a careful drug history taken.

The classical symptoms of obstructive jaundice are, first of all, the yellow appearance of the skin and mucous membranes. Quite often, patients will have had this pointed out to them by a friend or relative rather than noticing it themselves. In addition, they may have noticed a change in their urine and stools, with the urine becoming darker and the stools becoming paler. The urine becomes darker because conjugated bilirubin appears in it and the stool becomes paler because no bilirubin is entering the bowel. In addition, the patient may complain of itching, which is caused by the deposition of bile salts in the skin (not bilirubin!). Pain is a variable feature in posthepatic obstructive jaundice. It is more common when jaundice is caused by gallstones. But it may still be a feature even with obstruction due to carcinoma at the head of the pancreas. These two entities, gallstones and carcinoma of the pancreas, are the main areas to be covered when answering questions about obstructive jaundice in surgical finals, as they each constitute about one-third of the causes of obstructive jaundice (the other two-thirds are due to cholangiocarcinoma, chronic pancreatitis and enlarged lymph nodes in the porta hepatis).

Clinical Assessment

Clinical assessment in obstructive jaundice consists, first of all, in taking a full history. The importance in noting any drug therapy has been mentioned above. The duration of symptoms, associated weight loss (which can be particularly marked in obstructive jaundice, due to difficulty in fat and vitamin absorption) as well as the specific features of obstructive jaundice (itching, pale stools, dark urine) should be noted. Physical examination will reveal jaundice itself. Jaundice is usually best seen by examining the sclerae of the eyes. Bilirubin levels above 50 μmol/l are usually clinically detectable (the normal range is up to 17 μmol/l). Other features to look for on physical examination include the stigmata of chronic liver disease (spider naevi, liver palms, Dupuytren's contracture, liver flap, gynaecomastia, testicular atrophy, etc.).

Examination of the abdomen should look for enlargement or tenderness of the liver and the presence of ascites. If the gallbladder is palpable, then Courvoisier's rule should be considered. This rule states that if in the presence of jaundice the gallbladder is palpable, then the cause of jaundice is unlikely to be stones. The reason for this rule is that when gallstones have been present for a significant period of time, chronic cholecystitis results in a thickening fibrosis of the gallbladder wall, making it unable to distend even when obstruction occurs. An exception is when there is dual pathology. A distended gallbladder will be felt underneath the right costal margin as a smooth convex, perhaps slightly tender, mass which moves down with the liver with inspiration. Basic investigations in patients with jaundice will include full blood count, U & Es, liver function tests, and a chest X-ray. The liver function tests will confirm the obstructive nature of the jaundice. Bilirubin will be raised, but the specific liver enzyme that will be raised predominantly will be the alkaline phosphatase rather than the transaminases. In addition, all jaundice patients should have their baseline clotting status checked. The next most important test is the ultrasound scan, which is a quick and cheap way of demonstrating whether there is extra hepatic biliary obstruction, whether gallstones are present and perhaps whether there is a tumour in the pancreas. Ultrasound is very good at determining dilatation of the biliary tree and common bile duct (the normal maximum upper limit for the width of the common bile duct is 7 mm). A diameter of up to 1.1 cm may be normal if there was previous obstruction which has now resolved. A width of the common bile duct greater than 1.1 cm is always abnormal. Ultrasound is also very good for looking at the gallbladder and for the presence of gallstones. Unfortunately, the lower end of the common bile duct and the head of the pancreas are often poorly seen on ultrasound, due to overlying bowel gas. This is a particular problem in an overweight patient. If further imaging is felt to be needed, then the type of imaging will depend on the findings at ultrasound. The options for further treatment are probably best illustrated by describing certain clinical examples.

Example 1: Obstructive jaundice with a stone in the bile duct on ultrasound

In this situation, ultrasound has clearly shown a stone in the bile duct and this is likely to be the cause of the obstruction. There are two ways of dealing with this scenario. One option is laparoscopic cholecystectomy and laparoscopic common bile duct exploration and this is a combination of procedures that is favoured by advanced laparoscopic surgeons. An alternative would be ERCP and stone extraction followed by laparoscopic cholecystectomy. ERCP should only be carried out if there is a strong suspicion that therapy will be possible. In the case of a stone, an endoscopic sphincterotomy is carried out and the stone removed using a basket or balloon. ERCP is associated with a 1% risk of serious complications, which could be acute pancreatitis, bleeding, perforation or cholangitis (infection). Open surgery for common bile duct stones is now performed rarely but may occasionally be necessary if the stones cannot be removed laparoscopically or endoscopically. In this case, the common bile duct is opened between stay sutures, the stones removed and either a T-tube placed in the common bile duct or the duct closed primarily. A T-tube is inserted, a T-tube cholangiogram is carried out 10 days after the operation and if the duct is clear, the T-tube can then be removed 14 days after surgery.

Example 2: Obstructive jaundice, ultrasound showing dilated common bile duct down to head of pancreas

In this situation, where obstructive jaundice is present but no gallstones have been seen, the patient is suspected of harbouring a tumour of the head of the pancreas or ampulla of Vater. The next test should be a contrast enhanced CT scan with fine cuts through the upper abdomen to look closely at the liver, biliary tract and pancreas. If a mass is present then features of unresectability (liver metastases, lymph node metastases or involvement of portal vein or superior mesenteric vein or artery) should be sought. If none of these features of unresectability are present, the patient should proceed to an endoscopic ultrasound to look more closely at the head of the pancreas and ampulla. Endoscopic ultrasound is a developing technique which is carried out by passing an endoscope down to the stomach and duodenum. On the tip of the endoscope is an ultrasound transducer which can take high-resolution pictures of the biliary tract and pancreas. Fine needle aspiration for cytology can also be carried out under endoscopic ultrasound guidance. If EUS suggests that the patient has an operable tumour, then the patient should ideally undergo surgery, if fit, before the bilirubin climbs above 300 mmol/l. Above this level complications are more likely and insertion of a biliary stent by ERCP prior to surgery is appropriate. Twenty per cent of patients with carcinoma of the head of the pancreas and 40% of patients with ampullary carcinoma are suitable for surgical excision. The operation which is carried out is a pancreatico-duodenectomy or Whipple's procedure. The pylorus-preserving modification of the original technique is now used although atnrectomy is still sometimes necessary. This is a major operation, which carries a mortality of 5% and is best carried out in major centres with high throughput to avoid the risk of complications. If staging suggests the patient has an operable tumour but at surgery the tumour is unresectable because of the presence of lymph node metastases or liver metastases or unsuspected vascular involvement, then a biliary and gastric bypass should be carried out. The biliary bypass should always be carried out onto the common hepatic duct after removal of the gallbladder (Figure 5.2).

Example 3: An unfit patient with obstructive jaundice and ultrasound showing a distal obstruction

In a patient unfit for major surgery and in whom a carcinoma of the head of the pancreas or ampulla is suspected, endoscopic insertion of a biliary stent by ERCP is appropriate. A plastic stent is likely to become blocked and, therefore, if the patient's life expectancy is greater than 3 months, then an expandible metal stent should be used.

Specific Complications of Surgery in Jaundiced Patients

Coagulopathy

Jaundiced patients often have impaired clotting. This is largely a failure to absorb vitamin K (one of the fat-soluble vitamins) from the gut. This is

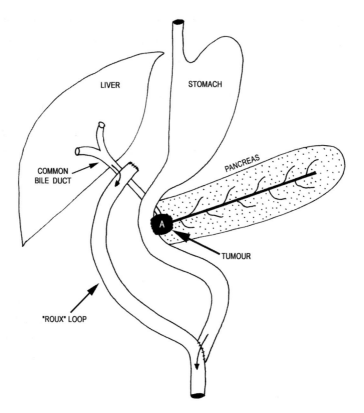

Figure 5.2. Biliary bypass with Roux loop (A = carcinoma in head of pancreas).

manifested as a prolonged INR. It can be reversed by the intramuscular administration of vitamin K preoperatively. Other clotting problems may also be present, and a careful coagulation profile should be done on a jaundiced patient who is undergoing surgery and clotting factors such as fresh frozen plasma should be arranged as necessary.

Renal failure (hepatorenal syndrome)

Patients with obstructive jaundice are much more prone to develop renal failure than patients undergoing similar degrees of surgery for other causes. The precise mechanisms underlying this are not well understood. The absorption of an endotoxin from the intestine (translocation), which is normally removed by the reticuloendothelium system of the liver, may be one factor. Additionally, there may be some as yet unidentified factor produced by the liver itself which helps modulate renal function. In order to overcome this risk, jaundiced patients undergoing surgery should be fully hydrated preoperatively. This will mean their having an intravenous infusion set up the day before. In addition, osmotic diuretics such as mannitol may be given during and after the procedure and dopamine infusion at 2.5 μg/kg/min may also be given via a central line in order to maximise renal function. The patient may have a central line inserted to monitor the central venous pressure and a catheter to monitor hourly urine output, which should be maintained at 40 ml/h or greater.

Nutrition

Patients with obstruction, especially due to carcinoma, are often very malnourished. There may be a history of marked weight loss. These patients may need nutritional support pre- or postoperatively. The most important factor, however, is to overcome the obstruction. There is no evidence that prolonged intravenous nutrition preoperatively is an advantage in these patients.

Infection

Patients with obstructive jaundice appear to have a greater incidence of infection problems including wound complications. This may be partly due to their poor protein status and there is a nonspecific effect of malignancy on the immune system. The patient should be appropriately covered with broad-spectrum antibiotics, preferably those which appear in the bile.

Cholangitis

Cholangitis is one of the most feared complications in obstructive jaundice. It is the cause of Charcot's triad, which consists of rigors or fever, abdominal pain and jaundice. It is caused by infection within an obstructed biliary tree. It should be regarded as an emergency: if left untreated it can result in severe shock, renal failure and death.

6

DISORDERS OF THE OESOPHAGUS, STOMACH AND DUODENUM

S Michael Griffin and Sarah Robinson

Disorders of the oesophagus, stomach and duodenum are dealt with by both medical and surgical gastroenterologists. It is the aspects of these disorders relating to surgery which are discussed in this chapter. Most upper gastrointestinal (GI) conditions give rise to symptoms rather than signs, and upper GI endoscopy is the mainstay of diagnosis.

DYSPHAGIA

Dysphagia is defined as difficulty in swallowing, whilst pain on swallowing is known as odynophagia. Most disorders of the oesophagus that are of relevance to surgical examination have dysphagia as a presenting symptom. The table below lists the most common causes and subdivides them into intraluminal, intra- and extramural and systemic causes.

Causes of Dysphagia

Intraluminal (inside the lumen)
Foreign body bolus obstruction (children and psychiatric patients)
Polypoid tumours
Oesophageal inflammation (oesophagitis)
Oesophageal infection (Candidiasis)

Extraluminal (outside the lumen)
Intramural (in the wall)
  Benign strictures (gastro-oesophageal reflux, ingestion of caustic substances)
  Malignant strictures
  Achalasia
  Oesophageal web (Plummer Vinson syndrome: middle-aged females with iron deficiency anaemia; the web consists of desquamated epithelium)
  Nutcracker oesophagus (characterised on manometry by high contraction pressures with normal peristalsis)
  Diffuse oesophageal spasm
  Scleroderma
  Presbyoesophagus (dysmotility associated with old age)
Extramural (outside the wall, pressing in)
  Pharyngeal pouch
  Rolling hiatus hernia
  Malignancy (bronchogenic)
  Retrosternal goitre
  Vascular structures: thoracic aortic aneurysms, congenitally abnormal vessels (dysphagia lusoria)
Systemic causes
  Myasthenia gravis
  Multiple sclerosis
  Parkinson's disease
  Pseudobulbar palsy
  Psychological

The mainstays of investigation of dysphagia include endoscopy, barium swallow and manometric assessment.

Endoscopy. Investigation of choice. Allows visual assessment, biopsy and histological review with the option of therapeutic intervention.

Barium swallow. Minimally invasive. Allows assessment of motility disorders in the absence of endoscopic findings.

Manometry. Adjunct to the above. Provides detailed assessment of the lower oesophageal sphincter and oesophageal peristalsis. This is of particular importance in achalasia.

OESOPHAGEAL CANCER

The incidence of oesophageal cancer is increasing faster than any other solid organ malignancy in the Western world. It is now the eighth commonest malignancy in the UK. The oesophagus is normally lined by squamous epithelium but gastric-type mucosa, termed Barrett's oesophagus, may develop at the lower end. In recent years, the relative incidence of squamous and adenocarcinoma has changed dramatically with adenocarcinomas now accounting for 65% of all oesophageal carcinomas in the UK. Most patients are middle aged and elderly, with a male to female ratio of 3:1.

Barrett's oesophagus is a condition in which the normal squamous epithelium in the distal oesophagus is replaced with glandular epithelium (columnar epithelium). It is secondary to gastro-oesophageal reflux of gastric contents, in particular, acid. It is associated with an increased risk of developing oesophageal adenocarcinoma. Consequently, many units adopt an endoscopic surveillance programme to detect malignant changes at an early stage. Other risk factors include obesity, high dietary fat intake, smoking, alcohol and male Caucasian origin. The principal risk factors for squamous carcinoma are alcohol intake and tobacco usage. The incidence is increased in northern China, Iran and South Africa in comparison to western countries. In addition, diets rich in nitrosamines and deficiencies in vitamins A and C and trace elements, achalasia, caustic strictures, hereditary tylosis and coexisting aerodigestive tract cancers are all implicated.

Most oesophageal cancers present with dysphagia, by which time spread has often occurred through the wall of the oesophagus and to lymph nodes. Without treatment the average survival from diagnosis is 9 months. Dysphagia is usually progressive: initially to solids (especially bread) and then liquids. Patients will often alter their dietary habits to increase their intake of liquids and soft foods in the earlier stages. This exacerbates the weight loss normally associated with malignancy. Significant weight loss is therefore common at presentation. Oesophageal obstruction may lead to overflow of oesophageal contents in turn predisposing to aspiration pneumonia. This risk is greatest at night when the patient is supine. Physical examination may reveal lymphadenopathy or hepatomegaly and ascites, but often there will be no abnormalities to detect other than obvious weight loss.

The mainstay of investigation is upper GI endoscopy. This allows biopsy or cytological examination of any lesions to confirm the diagnosis. In addition, dilatations, under X-ray control, can be performed to ease the symptoms of dysphagia. In the past, barium swallows were performed, with the typical appearance of a 'shouldered' stricture rather the smoother tapered narrowing seen with a benign stricture. This is now rarely used as a means of diagnosis. The patient will then undergo a more thorough staging process including CT scanning and endoscopic ultrasound (a special ultrasound probe attached to the endoscope) to assess invasion of adjacent structures and help predict resectability. Patient fitness is determined and further tests including bone scanning, MRI and PET scanning may rarely need to be performed. This will allow the stage of the tumour to be determined which will dictate the treatment options available. Staging uses the internationally recognised TNM method (i.e. tumour, node, metastases — see page 182).

The aim of treatment in carcinoma of the oesophagus is cure where possible and palliation where not. Surgery, where feasible, offers the greatest opportunity for cure. However, as a consequence of the advanced stage of the disease at presentation and the patient's coexisting disease (comorbidity), only one-third of patients have a technically resectable tumour at presentation. There is no role for palliative surgery in patients with proven distant metastases. There are several surgical approaches to resect the oesophagus (oesophagectomy). The principle is to resect all macroscopic tumour and mobilise the stomach so that it can be brought up into the chest or neck for anastomosis to the remaining oesophagus. To achieve this, abdominal, chest (thoracotomy) and neck incisions may be required. Trials are currently underway to evaluate the role of preoperative (neo-adjuvant) chemotherapy in oesophageal cancer. At least two-thirds of all staged patients will be inoperable, requiring palliative treatment. Repeated dilatations, oesophageal stenting, tumour ablation with laser or argon beam, chemotherapy and radiotherapy can be used to provide relief from dysphagia. Radiotherapy may be performed externally or within the lumen of the oesophagus (brachytherapy).

The prognosis for oesophageal cancer is poor. Surgically treated patients have stage-dependent survival. Palliatively treated patients have a median survival of 4 months. Overall, 5-year survival is 10–15%.

GASTRIC CANCER

Gastric cancer is one of the commonest cancers in the world. This is due to a high prevalence in Eastern Asia and Southern America. The incidence in western populations has actually decreased over recent decades. In the UK it is currently the sixth commonest cancer. In addition the commonest site of gastric cancer has altered from distal to proximal (cardia) over the previous three decades. The majority of gastric cancers are adenocarcinomas. Three per cent are lymphomas and, less commonly, GI stromal tumours and neuroendocrine tumours. Risk factors for developing gastric cancer include *Helicobacter pylori* colonisation, blood group A, smoking and diet. A high dietary intake of nitrate and salt containing foods, associated with pickling methods, is linked to gastric cancer, whereas increased vitamin C consumption is thought to be protective. There is an increased risk associated with pernicious anaemia and previous gastric surgery. A few cases of familial gastric cancer have been identified associated with abnormalities of E cadherin (a cellular adhesion molecule) expression.

Gastric cancer is classified in several ways. Early or late describes the depth of invasion of the tumour. Early gastric cancer (EGC) is confined to the mucosa or submucosa. In the late form the muscularis propria is breached. The incidence of EGC is 10% in the west and 40% in Japan. Histologically, gastric cancer is described as intestinal or diffuse, the latter having a worse prognosis. Linitis plastica (leather bottle stomach) is the description applied to diffuse gastric cancer affecting the entire stomach wall. Endoscopically this is recognisable as a non-distending stomach. Transcoelomic spread, throughout the peritoneal cavity, can occur with a predilection for the ovaries (Krukenburg tumour).

In the West, presentation is typically late and most often includes a history of weight loss and anorexia, epigastric pain, nausea and vomiting. Less commonly, patients may present with upper GI bleeding or gastric perforation. Abdominal examination may reveal an epigastric mass, a succussion splash (splashing of residual gastric fluid, caused by an obstructing antral cancer), ascites or hepatomegaly. A left supraclavicular lymph node may be palpable (Virchow's node); when present, this is known as Trosier's sign. Another association is with acanthosis nigricans (pigmented warty axillary skin). Pelvic deposits may be felt on rectal examination. These findings all indicate very advanced disease.

The diagnosis is usually made endoscopically at which time confirmatory biopsies may be taken. Further staging takes the form of thoracic and abdominal CT, endoscopic ultrasound and laparoscopy.

Treatment can be any of the following:

- *Surgical.* Surgery can be either curative or palliative. As with oesophageal cancer, surgery, where feasible, offers the greatest opportunity for cure. However, unlike oesophageal cancer, surgery can have a palliative role in the treatment of gastric cancer. Obstructing and bleeding tumours may be treated with by-pass procedures or palliative resections in an otherwise fit individual. With curative surgery, operation type is dictated by the position of the tumour. In most proximal tumours a total gastrectomy is undertaken but in more distal cases a subtotal gastrectomy is possible. A Roux en Y anastomosis is usually performed to prevent bile reflux. Early gastric cancers may be treated with endoscopic resection.
- *Chemotherapy.* The role of chemotherapy is predominantly palliative but research into neoadjuvant and intraperitoneal chemotherapy is ongoing.
- *Medical palliation.* That is, pyloric stenting (the passage of plastic tubes to allow stomach emptying), etc. may be used to relieve obstructive symptoms and proton pump inhibitors can reduce bleeding from ulcerating gastric tumours. Argon plasma coagulation (APC) is a new method of electrocoagulation. Using high-frequency electrical current it allows for the noncontact application of electrical energy to achieve

tissue destruction or hemostasis and may have a role in the palliative treatment of polypoid gastric tumours.
* *Radiotherapy.* This is of no value.

Overall, 5-year survival from gastric cancer in the UK is still in the region of 10%. Gastric cancer is often used as a classic model for the way in which tumours spread, namely:

* Spread within the wall of the organ leading to the so-called linitis plastica (also known as a leather bottle stomach)
* Local spread to adjacent structures, such as the pancreas
* Lymphatic spread such as occurs with spread to local lymph nodes and nodes further afield
* Transcoelomic spread, where the tumour seeds across the peritoneal cavity
* Blood-borne spread such as occurs with lung metastases

GASTROINTESTINAL STROMAL TUMOURS

Mesenchymal tumours of the GI tract originate within the bowel wall. They are divided into three groups with varying differentiation of neural and smooth muscle expression by immunohistochemistry:

* Leiomyomas and leiomyosarcomas express markers of smooth muscle differentiation.
* Neurofibromas are positive for S100 indicating a neural origin.
* Gastrointestinal stromal tumours (GISTs) are positive for CD34 and CD117, c-Kit protein, and originate from the interstitial cells of Cajal, the pacemaker cells of the GI tract. They comprise the largest group.

GISTs occur most commonly within the stomach (60–70%) and are rare within the oesophagus (2–3%) where leiomyomas predominate. They usually occur over the age of 40 with an equal male to female ratio. Three-quarters are benign with indicators of malignancy including tumour size

>10 cm, location (extragastric position), mitotic index >5/10, high-power fields and evidence of cystic degeneration on endoscopic ultrasound.

Many are found incidentally but may present as abdominal pain, as GI bleeding or with obstructive symptoms. Endoscopically they appear as well-demarcated spherical masses often with a central punctum. Superficial surface erosion may occur. Treatment is surgical resection based on clinical indications. These include size and physiological effects such as obstruction and clinically significant bleeding. Recently, imatinib, a Kit selective tyrosine kinase inhibitor, has demonstrated success in the treatment of metastatic c-Kit positive GISTs.

PHARYNGEAL POUCH

A pharyngeal pouch (also known as Zenker's diverticulum) is an out pouching of the pharynx, usually between the upper border of the cricopharyngeous muscle and the lower border of the inferior constrictor muscle of the pharynx. This corresponds with a weak area called Killian's dehiscence.

Pharyngeal pouches are thought to be 'pulsion' diverticulae, caused by peristaltic activity pumping against resistance resulting from uncoordinated muscle spasm. Although the deficit occurs posteriorly, any associated swelling usually bulges to the left side of the neck and may produce a palpable lump on examination. Food debris may collect within the diverticulum, which can in turn expand, pressing on the adjacent oesophagus causing dysphagia. Patients may also complain of regurgitation of food from the diverticulum, gurgling sounds, or bad breath (halitosis) due to the presence of decaying food in the diverticulum. Sometimes a patient will learn to empty the pouch by using external pressure on the neck. A further complication of oesophageal pouches is perforation at endoscopy should the scope enter the diverticulum rather than the oesophagus. Surgical treatment options include simple excision of the pouch by an open surgical approach. Endoscopic stapling of the bridge between the pouch and oesophagus opening up the pouch and allowing it to drain more freely is increasingly being considered the treatment of choice.

PERFORATION OF THE OESOPHAGUS

Oesophageal perforation may be caused by trauma at endoscopy or by ingestion of a sharp foreign body, such as a fish bone. Spontaneous rupture of the oesophagus (Boerhaave's syndrome) occurs with forceful or prolonged vomiting. Ingestion of corrosive agents (acid/alkali) and penetrating chest injuries are less common causes. Perforation will result in mediastinitis (infection and inflammation of the mediastinum as a result of food/fluid/micro-organisms entering the mediastinum). Prompt diagnosis is essential, taking the form of plain chest X-ray, contrast swallow, endoscopy and CT to evaluate the extent and position of the perforation. Iatrogenic perforations can usually be managed conservatively, due to minimal levels of contamination, with NG tube, proton pump inhibitors and antibiotics. Most other perforations require resuscitation of the patient, proton pumps inhibitors and antibiotics including anti-fungals. Surgery to debride the mediastinum and placement of a T-tube within the oesophagus, to provide drainage and the formation of a controlled oesophago-cutaneous fistula, is the mainstay of treatment. The oesophagus should rarely be repaired in the first instance in the presence of pleural soiling.

REFLUX DISEASE AND HIATUS HERNIA

The oesophagus passes into the abdomen from the thorax through the oesophageal hiatus of the diaphragm. Normally, about 2–4 cm of the oesophagus lies within the abdomen. Hiatus hernias may be sliding (85%), rolling (10%) or mixed (5%) (Figure 6.1). With a sliding hiatus hernia the oesophagogastric junction moves up into the thorax. The oesophago-gastric junction is in the normal position with a rolling hiatus hernia which is caused by the stomach rolling up beside the oesophagus.

Hiatus hernia commonly presents with retrosternal burning pains which may be worse on bending, stooping or at night on lying flat. Such symptoms are often called heartburn by patients and are due to the reflux of gastric contents (predominantly acid) into the oesophagus. This is termed gastro-oesophageal reflux disease (GORD). Regurgitation of acid fluid into the mouth may occur (water brash). Patients will normally

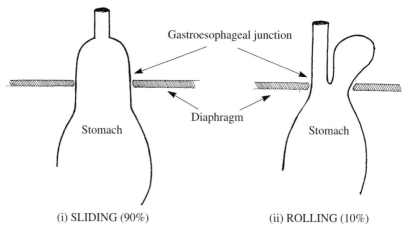

(i) SLIDING (90%)   (ii) ROLLING (10%)

Figure 6.1. The two main types of hiatus hernia.

report increased pain after meals (postprandially) and will usually have noticed some relief with proprietary 'over the counter' antacids. Severe reflux oesophagitis may lead to ulceration and bleeding or, if long-standing, benign stricture formation.

Treatment of hiatus hernia involves measures such as losing weight, stopping smoking, eating smaller meals earlier in the evening and raising the head of the bed. Antacids, H2 receptor antagonists, proton pump inhibitors and drugs which mechanically prevent reflux by forming a raft on top of the stomach, such as some of the alginate preparations, may be helpful. Where medical therapy has failed or where the patient is unhappy with the prospect of permanent medication, surgery may be indicated. Many operations have been described but the commonest is the floppy Nissen fundoplication. This involves mobilising the fundus of the stomach and wrapping it around the lower end of the oesophagus providing a high-pressure area designed to prevent reflux. This operation is increasingly performed laparoscopically. Prior to the surgical treatment of reflux it is important to perform pH and manometry studies. This will exclude a diagnosis of achalasia or dysmotility prior to performing a wrap. In addition, 24-hour ambulatory oesophageal pH assessment confirms the diagnosis of GORD.

ACHALASIA OF THE OESOPHAGUS

This is due to failure of relaxation of the smooth muscle at the lower end of the oesophagus secondary to an abnormality of its nerve supply. It usually presents in middle life and the precise cause is unknown. It has some similarities to the tropical disease trypanosomiasis (Chagas' disease), in which the nerve supply to the oesophageal muscle is also deficient. It usually presents with intermittent dysphagia with gradual progression. The patient may complain of fluid regurgitation, which tends to be worse at night and associated with pneumonia due to aspiration. Diagnosis is made on barium swallow with the typical features of a dilated oesophagus above a smooth tapering 'bird's beak' appearance. Oesophageal manometry provides manometric confirmation of a nonrelaxing sphincter. Achalasia is treated either by endoscopic dilatation of the lower oesophageal sphincter under X-ray control or by an operation termed a Heller's procedure in conjunction with an antireflux procedure. The former is a cardiomyotomy, i.e. an operation which involves dividing the muscle layer at the lower end of the oesophagus and entrance of the stomach down as far as the mucosa. The mucosa is left intact. It is similar in principle to the Ramstedt's operation for infantile hypertrophic pyloric stenosis. Squamous carcinoma of the oesophagus develops in 3–5% of patients with achalasia.

PEPTIC ULCERATION

Peptic ulceration is defined as ulcer formation associated with acid and can occur at several sites, namely the duodenum (commonest), stomach, oesophagus, jejunum (in Zollinger–Ellison syndrome), Meckel's diverticulum (if it contains ectopic gastric mucosa) and sometimes at the site of a previous gastroenterostomy. Obviously, duodenal and stomach ulcers form the vast majority of those cases seen clinically. However, in an essay answer it is important to be able to discuss these other areas if only in broad outline. Peptic ulcer disease, at any site, can present as:

- Pain (dyspepsia/indigestion)
- Bleeding (acute or chronic)

- Penetration into adjacent structures (into the pancreas for a posterior duodenal ulcer, gastro-colic fistula)
- Perforation (usually an anterior duodenal or gastric ulcer)
- Obstruction (i.e. severe scarring of the pylorus from chronic ulceration or acute obstruction of the pylorus from acute ulceration with oedema)

H. pylori gastric colonisation is the most important aetiological factor implicated in peptic ulcer disease. Ten per cent of patients infected with *H. pylori* will progress to ulcer development. The mechanism of injury is thought to be two-fold. A combination of the effects of toxins released by the bacteria and the body's inflammatory response to this leads to direct injury of the protective gastric mucosal barrier. Second, the associated gastritis and patterns of gastric re-colonisation by *H. pylori* is associated with increased gastrin-induced acid production. This effect is exacerbated by reduced production of the inhibiting peptide, somatostatin, due to a diminished D-cell mass associated with antral gastritis. More recently, different substrains of *H. pylori* have been identified. These are associated with differing effects on the gastric mucosa: gastritis, gastritis and ulceration or complicated ulcer disease. Host factors play a role. Lewis antibodies on the surface of gastric epithelial cells preferentially bind *H. pylori*. Lewis antibody involvement in the determination of the O blood group may explain a long recognised association between peptic ulcer disease and this blood type. Host inflammatory response will dictate the degree of mucosal damage elicited by *H. pylori*.

Nonsteroidal anti-inflammatory drug (NSAID) use is the second most common factor implicated in ulcer development. Smoking, increased acid secretion, coffee consumption and co-morbidity such as liver and renal failure and hyper-parathyroidism have all been implicated in the severity of the disease.

Duodenal ulceration occurs most frequently in men and has a peak in the age group between 45 and 55 years. Gastric ulceration tends to present later with a peak between 55 and 65 years of age. Ninety-five per cent of duodenal ulcers occur in the first part of the duodenum: within 2 cm of the pylorus. Patients often describe pain as being eased by food (unlike gastric ulcers, where it is often worsened by food). The pain is usually worse at night and may radiate through to the back. Patients with dyspepsia should undergo endoscopic assessment to confirm the presence of an ulcer and to test for the presence of *H. pylori*. Biopsy of all gastric ulcers is essential to avoid missing early gastric cancers. Repeat endoscopy following treatment is advisable to assess healing. Those colonised with *H. pylori* should undergo eradication therapy (proton pump inhibitor and antibiotic regime). NSAIDS and aspirin should be stopped and alternatives prescribed. Cessation of smoking should be encouraged. With this regime the majority of duodenal ulcers can be medically managed and relatively few progress to surgery.

GASTRIC AND DUODENAL ULCER SURGERY

Since the advent of medical management of peptic ulcer disease with H2 receptor antagonists and, more recently, proton pump inhibitors, with eradication of *H. pylori*, surgical treatment is predominantly of historical interest.

You may encounter patients who have undergone surgical treatment of peptic ulcer disease and are now experiencing the long-term complications.

In the surgical examination, in-depth knowledge of gastric physiology will not be required. However, the following principles are important. First, without acid there can be no ulcer formation and, in broad terms, whether or not an ulcer develops is the result of the balance between acid secretion and the mucosal protective factors which are reduced by drugs such as NSAIDs. Remember that the stomach starts at the oesophagogastric junction (cardia). There is a fundus, body and antrum which leads via the pylorus into the duodenum. The fundus and body contain cells that produce the acid, pepsinogen and intrinsic factor, whereas the major site of gastrin formation is in the antrum. Most peptic ulceration is found within the first part of the duodenum but may spread further down into the small bowel in Zollinger–Ellison syndrome (see page 121). Gastric acid secretion is stimulated by either gastrin or vagal nerve stimulation. There are two vagus nerves supplying the stomach, i.e. the right and the left vagus, which actually sit in a posterior and an anterior position close to the oesophagus as it enters the abdomen. Smaller divisions of the vagus nerves, called the nerves of Latarjet, supply the pyloric region and are responsible for relaxation of the pylorus to allow emptying of the stomach. Other branches of these nerves supply the acid-secreting areas of the stomach. This explains why a truncal vagotomy (division of the vagus nerves as they enter the abdomen) results in reduced acid secretion, but a stomach which fails to empty adequately. A truncal vagotomy operation, therefore, needs to be combined with a further procedure to enable emptying of the stomach, such as a gastroenterostomy or a pyloroplasty.

Previously performed operations include

- *Truncal or selective vagotomy.* Because the vagus nerve supplies the stomach and can stimulate the release of acid, division of these nerves can reduce the amount of acid produced. One downside is that a vagotomy will also cut the nerves that relax the pyloric muscle and produce a pyloric opening and so a truncal vagotomy also requires some form of drainage procedure [either a pyloroplasty (Figure 6.2) or a gastroenterostomy (Figure 6.3)].

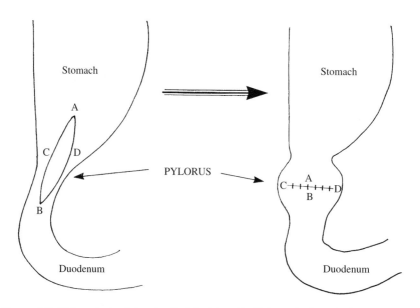

Figure 6.2. Pyloroplasty. A longitudinal incision (A–B) is made through the pylorus and then closed transversely (C–D) to widen it.

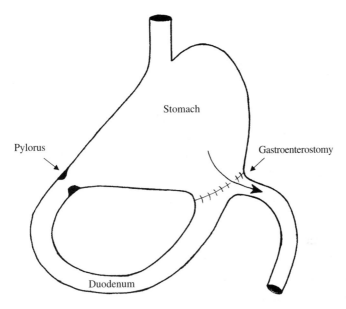

Figure 6.3. Gastroenterostomy.

- *Antrectomy with vagotomy.* In this procedure the distal half of the stomach is removed (i.e. partial gastrectomy) in combination with a vagotomy (see Figure 6.4). The stomach can then be reanastomosed either directly to the duodenum (Bilroth I procedure) or a duodenal stump can be closed over and a small bowel loop brought up for anastomosis on to the stomach (Bilroth II procedure, also known as a Polya gastrectomy).
- Subtotal gastrectomy with Roux en Y to restore intestinal continuity.

The latter operation is still occasionally performed for refractory ulcer disease or in the case of Zollinger–Ellison syndrome (see page 121).

COMPLICATIONS OF PEPTIC ULCER SURGERY

Although peptic ulcer surgery is nowadays rarely performed, the complications are specific and sometimes discussed in final exams. There are

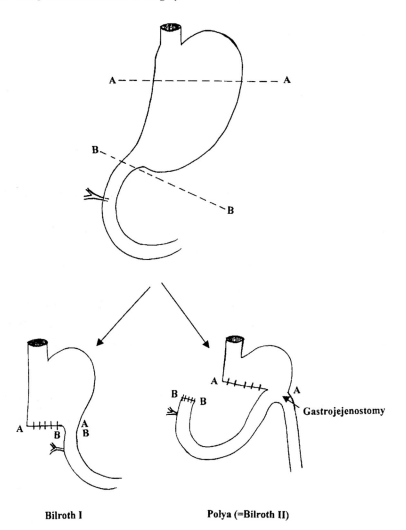

Bilroth I   **Polya (=Bilroth II)**

Figure 6.4. Gastrectomies. The distal part of the stomach (between A–A and B–B) is removed and the two main techniques for joining it up again are shown.

numerous ways of classifying these, an example of which is given below. Remember that complications can be general, to any operation, and specific to a particular operation. The following shows in detail only the specific complications related to the peptic ulcer operations (also see page 33).

Early Complications

- *Haemorrhage*
- *Duodenal stump leakage*
- Failure of the stomach to empty and *bilious vomiting* (occurs in 10% of patients)

Late Complications

- *Dumping syndrome.* Characterised by abdominal distension, flushing, sweating and nausea. This can be divided into early and late dumping. *Early dumping* occurs immediately after a meal and is due to food entering the small bowel too rapidly, drawing fluid into the bowel by osmosis, producing fluid shifts and hypotension. *Late dumping* occurs 1–2 h after a meal and is due to reactive hypoglycaemia caused by the wave of insulin produced in response to the rapid delivery of food into the small intestine. The treatment is predominately reassurance that most cases settle with time and dietary advice regarding small, more frequent low-carbohydrate meals.
- *Postvagotomy diarrhoea*
- *Blind loop syndrome.* Due to the long blind-ended bowel loop left in a Bilroth II gastrectomy. This allows proliferation of bacteria leading to anaemia and malnutrition and weight loss.
- *Biliary vomiting.* Occurs in 10% of patients.
- *Alkaline gastritis.*
- *Anaemia.* Can be due to a lack of the intrinsic factor, vitamin B_{12} and iron.
- *Osteomalacia due to lack of vitamin D and calcium.*
- *Recurrent ulceration and malignancy within the gastric remnant.*

ZOLLINGER–ELLISON SYNDROME

Zollinger–Ellison syndrome is the hyper-secretion of gastric acid due to a gastrin-producing tumour (gastrinoma). Most gastrinomas are within the pancreas but can occasionally be found in the duodenum, stomach or ovary. They are part of the Group of Neuro-Endocrine GastroenteropancreaticTumours

(NET) and MEN type 1 (see table below). Sixty per cent are malignant. They can be very small in size and hence difficult to find with investigations or at surgery. The classic feature of Zollinger–Ellison syndrome is refractory peptic ulceration, which may involve the whole duodenum and even the small bowel. The diagnosis is made by the demonstration of high gastrin levels in the presence of high acid secretion. Appropriate investigations include CT scanning, magnetic resonance imaging and angiography, which may be combined with venous blood sampling for gastrin levels. New investigations of interest include intraoperative ultrasound to look for small tumours in the pancreas. The treatment is essentially medical with drugs such as the proton pump inhibitors combined with surgery if the position of the tumour can be identified. Surgery has two roles: first, removal of the tumour and second, carrying out antiulcer operations such as subtotal gastrectomy.

Multiple Endocrine Neoplasia (MEN)

MEN Type I

- Hyperparathyroidism (parathyroid hyperplasia)
- Insulinoma of pancreas
- Pituitary tumours
- Zollinger–Ellison syndrome (gastrinoma), adrenocortical tumours and carcinoid tumours

MEN Type II

Medullary cell carcinoma of thyroid and phaeochromacytoma plus others, depending on the type, IIa or IIb.

MEN II	*IIa (Sipple's Syndrome)*	*IIb*
Medullary cell carcinoma of thyroid and phaeochromocytoma plus	Hyperparathyroidism	"Marfanoid" habitus
		Submucosal neurofibromata of the tongue, eyelids and lips

UPPER GASTROINTESTINAL BLEEDING

This is a commonly discussed topic in medical and surgical finals. Upper GI bleeding can present as haematemesis (vomiting of frank blood), coffee ground vomiting (blood altered by gastric acid) or melaena (black tarry stools with a distinctive aroma!). Occasionally, very brisk bleeding may present as haematochezia (fresh blood per rectum).

The following is a list of the most important causes of upper GI bleeding (note that peptic ulcer disease accounts for nearly 70%):

- Duodenal ulcer (30%)
- Gastric ulcer (20%)
- Acute erosions or gastritis (20%)
- Mallory–Weiss tear [at the lower end of the oesophagus due to vomiting (10%)]
- Oesophageal varices (5%)
- Oesophagitis (5%)
- Cancer of the stomach or oesophagus (< 3%)

The management of patients with upper GI bleeding includes a full history and examination to assess for signs of shock and stigmata of liver disease. Two large-bore intravenous cannulae should be sited (14 G) for fluid resuscitation. Blood should be sent for urgent cross-match of four units, full blood count, clotting and urea levels. Intestinal absorption of blood will lead to an elevated urea level. Haemoglobin levels may be misleadingly normal if the patient has not undergone fluid resuscitation prior to testing. A urinary catheter should be sited to monitor urine output (>30 ml/h). Correction of coagulopathies and prescription of intravenous proton pump inhibitors to decrease gastric pH should be undertaken. Depending on the severity of the bleeding further invasive monitoring (e.g. central venous catheterisation) may be necessary; such patient should be managed in a high dependency unit.

The group with the highest mortality risk from upper GI bleeding are those patients who rebleed as in-patients. Risk factors for this include patient age greater than 80 years, shock at presentation, haemoglobin less than 8 g/dl, endoscopic stigmata of recent bleeding and patient comorbidity. A scoring system has been devised to identify those most at risk (Rockall score).

Endoscopy is now the mainstay of treatment. This is performed to establish a diagnosis and to allow endoscopic intervention to stop the bleeding. This may take the form of injection therapy (adrenaline 1:10,000), which is the most established and frequently used method. Recent developments have included the use of thermal coagulation, laser ablation, fibrin glue application or the use of endoclips.

The indications for urgent surgical intervention include failure to stop the bleeding endoscopically and rebleeding during the current hospital admission. Surgery usually consists of opening the stomach or duodenum and under-running the bleeding vessel. Postoperatively patients should undergo *H. pylori* eradication therapy and be commenced on long-term acid suppression medication. All NSAID medication should be stopped.

The initial treatment of bleeding oesophageal varices, following resuscitation and correction of coagulopathies, is endoscopic band ligation or injection sclerotherapy. If this fails to control the bleeding, a Sengstaken tube should be inserted. This comprises two balloons: the gastric to anchor the tube and the oesophageal to tamponade the bleeding sites. The patient will require transfer to a specialist centre for further treatment.

PERFORATED PEPTIC ULCER

The commonest site of peptic ulcer perforation is the duodenum. The usual site for perforation is anteriorly within the first part of the duodenum (posterior perforation is more likely to either penetrate into the pancreas or erode the gastroduodenal artery causing haemorrhage). Surprisingly, many patients presenting with a perforated peptic ulcer have had little in the way of pre-existing symptoms of indigestion. Presentation is usually sudden at onset with severe epigastric pain and some vomiting. On examination the patient tends to lie very still avoiding abdominal movement. Tenderness is initially in the epigastrium but will spread thorough the abdomen if the leak is not contained. The abdomen may be rigid with rebound and percussion tenderness and absent bowel sounds.

The key investigation is an erect chest X-ray (not an abdominal X-ray). In 70% of cases this will demonstrate gas under the diaphragm. Treatment involves adequate resuscitation of the patient prior to proceeding to theatre for laparotomy. With a simple duodenal perforation peritoneal washout and simple closure of the deficit, with a re-enforcing omental patch, is the treatment of choice. In the case of gastric ulcer perforation it is advisable to excise the ulcer with a small ellipse of stomach and then repair of the defect. The specimen should then be sent for histological assessment to exclude malignancy: up to one-third of perforated gastric ulcers are malignant. Ninety per cent of peptic perforations are associated with *H. pylori* and as such eradication therapy with long-term acid suppression treatment is recommended.

HYPERTROPHIC PYLORIC STENOSIS

This condition affects 1–3 in 1000 live births. The male to female ratio is 4:1 with an increased preponderance in the first-born male. There is an increased prevalence in Caucasian populations and it is three times more likely if the child has a positive maternal history. The most common presentation is of vomiting between 3 and 10 weeks postdelivery, which may become projectile in nature. This will be associated with hypokalaemic, hypochloraemic metabolic acidosis. It is an acquired disorder of unknown aetiology.

Seventy to ninety per cent of cases can be confirmed by palpating the abdomen for a small epigastric or right upper quadrant mobile ovoid mass (the 'olive'). Visible gastric peristaltic waves may be seen going from left to right across the upper abdomen. Ultrasound or water-soluble contrast meal, demonstrating the 'string sign', will confirm the diagnosis.

Following appropriate resuscitation, a Ramstedt pyloromyotomy is performed, which involves dividing the muscle fibres of the pylorus down to the mucosa, which is left intact. This is increasingly performed using a laparoscopic technique.

7

SMALL INTESTINE AND COLON

Alan F Horgan

MECKEL'S DIVERTICULUM

Meckel's diverticulum is a remnant of the vitello intestinal duct, which normally disappears during embryological development. It is found in approximately 2% of the population and occurs approximately 2 ft proximal to the iliocaecal valve on the antimesenteric border (the border not attached to the mesentery) of the ileum. Some books suggest that it is usually 2 in. in length (hence 2, 2, 2), but in fact its length is very variable. Sometimes it extends as far as the back of the umbilicus on the anterior abdominal wall, and occasionally it may even present as mucosa protruding at the umbilicus when there is a so-called vitello intestinal fistula. This protruding mucosa is sometimes referred to as a raspberry tumour.

Meckel's diverticulum is usually completely asymptomatic. It can, however, present with

- A picture similar to appendicitis
- Bleeding
- Volvulus or intussusception

If the Meckel's becomes inflamed, it can produce a clinical presentation very similar to acute appendicitis. If a patient is taken to theatre for an appendicectomy and the appendix is found to be normal, a Meckel's should always be looked for. Occasionally, a Meckel's will contain ectopic gastric mucosa, which can cause bleeding and is in fact the commonest cause of major gastrointestinal bleeding in teenagers. A further complication that a Meckel's can cause is a volvulus of the intestine if it is tethered to the abdominal wall. Occasionally, it may also form the apex of an intussusception. Very often the diagnosis of a Meckel's is made at laparotomy, but occasionally it may be possible to use a technetium scan in cases of intestinal bleeding, which can reveal a Meckel's by targeting the gastric mucosa within it. Once Meckel's diverticulum is identified, the treatment is simple — surgical excision.

TUMOURS OF THE SMALL INTESTINE

Tumours of the small intestine are relatively rare, comprising less than 5% of all gastrointestinal tumours. Often an examiner tries to throw a student by asking about them. This is not because you are expected to know much about them but because it is a good question to ask to see if you can think and answer a question logically; for example, 'Tell me about small bowel tumours.' Approach this sort of question as discussed in the chapter 'Surgical Talk' as follows — small bowel tumours can be primary or secondary, benign or malignant.

Benign Tumours

These can arise from any of the elements of the bowel wall, such as

- Lipomas (arise from fat)
- Leiomyomas (arise from smooth muscle)
- Neurofibromas (arise from nerves)
- Adenomas (arise from glandular mucosa)
- Adenomatous polyps of the small bowel may be premalignant (as in the colon). As with colonic adenomas, they may also be associated with polyposis syndromes and Peutz–Jegher's syndrome (pigmentation around the mouth and small bowel polyps).

Benign tumours may be either found incidentally or present with bleeding or intussusception.

MALIGNANCY OF THE SMALL INTESTINE

Adenocarcinoma of the small intestine is occasionally seen and is believed in the majority of cases to arise from pre-existing adenomatous polyps (as in the colon). *Lymphomas* may also occur in the small bowel. *Carcinoid tumours* are of low-grade malignancy and are believed to arise from neuroectodermal cells embryologically. The commonest site for these is the appendix, but they can occur anywhere throughout the gastrointestinal tract and are also found in the lung (bronchial carcinoids). These tumours release serotonin (5-HT) and kinins, which can cause symptoms if they get into the circulation. Normally these hormones are broken down by the liver in the first-pass metabolism from the gut and so no symptoms occur. However, in the presence of metastases there is no first-pass metabolism and the patient may suffer from carcinoid syndrome which consists of flushing, bronchospasm and diarrhoea.

INTUSSUSCEPTION

An intussusception can be defined as a condition where a portion of intestine gets invaginated (by peristalsis) into its own lumen. The invaginated portion (the intussusceptum) can then be further propelled down the lumen for a variable distance (Figure 7.1).

Intussuscipiens

Intussusceptum

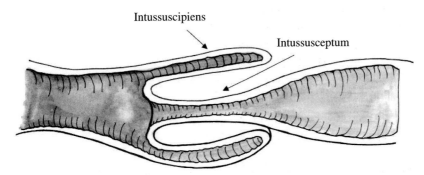

Figure 7.1. Intussusception.

A section through a piece of bowel containing an intussusception would contain two full layers of intestinal wall: the intussusceptum inside and the intussuscipiens outside.

Most intussusceptions are seen in children, usually infants under 1 year of age. They may present as colicky abdominal pain leading to obstruction. So-called redcurrant jelly stools may be passed (which consist of mucus and blood). The danger is that the intussusceptum may strangulate and infarct. Abdominal examination may reveal a mass and occasionally the apex of the intussusception may protrude from the anus or be felt on rectal examination.

In children most intussusceptions are thought to be caused by peristalsis acting on a hypertophied Peyer's patch. Meckel's diverticulum is another possible cause. Sometimes the intussusception can be reduced by a barium enema (so-called hydrostatic reducton), and if this is unsuccessful, surgical correction is required. If possible the intussusception is simply reduced and recurrence is then uncommon. If it cannot be reduced or if it is nonviable, then the affected segment needs to be resected.

If intussusception occurs in an adult (which is rare), then a tumour (benign or malignant) acting as the apex of the intussusception should be considered.

ACUTE APPENDICITIS

Acute appendicitis is the commonest emergency surgical presentation requiring operation. Most cases are thought to be caused by obstruction of the appendix with subsequent infection behind the obstruction. This concept of an obstructed system getting infected is also relevant to conditions such as cholangitis (infection of an obstructed biliary tree) and pylonephrosis (infection of an obstructed renal tract). In appendicitis the most common cause of obstruction of the appendix is either a faecolith (a piece of faeces within the appendix) or hypertrophy of lymphoid tissue within the wall of the appendix, presumably in response to an otherwise minor viral infection. Rare causes of obstruction of the appendix and, therefore, appendicitis include carcinoma of the caecum and carcinoid tumour.

To understand the way in which appendicitis presents clinically, one should realise that in its early stages the inflammation of the appendix is confined to the wall of the appendix itself and is therefore felt as a poorly localised visceral pain in the central abdominal (originates in embryological midgut). Because the essential feature is of an obstructed appendix, the pain will usually be colicky due to peristalsis in the appendicular muscle. As the inflammatory process progresses, the surrounding tissues and parietal peritoneum become inflamed and the pain is then felt locally in the right iliac fossa and is constant and typical of a localised peritonitis, worse on movement, etc. The typical patient will therefore present with an initial central colicky abdominal pain, which after a few hours progresses into a constant right iliac fossa pain (the pain moves; it does not radiate). By this time the patient will usually have a mild fever, be anorexic and may have nausea and vomiting. On examination there will be localised right iliac fossa tenderness and guarding with rebound tenderness or percussion tenderness. The diagnosis is essentially a clinical one and in straightforward cases no investigations at all are required.

The treatment of acute appendicitis is appendicectomy. It would be very reasonable of an examiner to ask simple questions about the operation, as it is the most common one performed as an emergency. For that reason the basic steps of an appendicectomy will be outlined.

First of all, an incision is made in the right iliac fossa. Conventionally, this would be centred over McBurney's point, which is two-thirds the way along a line drawn from the umbilicus to the anterior superior iliac spine. In practice, many surgeons make a slightly lower incision, which is cosmetically more acceptable. However, McBurney's point is often asked about in examinations because it marks the usual site of the base of the appendix. An incision is then made down through skin and subcutaneous tissues until the muscle layers are reached. The external oblique, internal oblique and transverse abdominus muscles are then opened. This is done by a muscle-splitting incision along the lines of the fibres with no fibres actually being cut. The final layer is the peritoneum, which is opened so that the abdominal cavity can be entered. The appendix and caecum are then identified and pulled up through the incision. There seems to be a misconception among many medical students that the retrocaecal appendix is unusual. In fact this is the commonest site of the appendix. After delivery of the appendix the blood vessels and mesentery of the appendix are divided and the appendix is ligated and removed at its base. Many surgeons then bury the stump of the appendix with a purse-string suture around the caecum. The caecum is then returned to the abdomen. Any fluid or pus is carefully sucked and swabbed out. If there is severe contamination a drain may be left. The layers of the abdominal muscles are then closed using an absorbable suture. The operation should be covered with prophylactic antibiotics, usually Metronidazole, given intravenously at induction of the anaesthetic.

Another misconception that many students (and indeed doctors) have relates to the presence of tenderness on rectal examination. Only 7% of appendixes lie in a pelvic position and most of these do not reach far enough into the pelvis to be in any way near an examining finger. Therefore, when patients have rectal tenderness in association with acute appendicitis, it is not because of the adjacent position of the inflamed appendix; it is in fact because inflammatory fluids and perhaps pus have tracted down from the area of the appendix in the right iliac fossa to the most dependent portion of the abdominal cavity, the pouch of Douglas.

Occasionally, acute appendicitis may present after it has been fully walled off by the omentum and small bowel. At this stage (usually greater than 72 h after the onset of symptoms) a mass is usually present on palpation. This may either resolve with antibiotics or develop into an abscess which may be amenable to radiologically guided percutaneous drainage. Most surgeons would advocate an 'interval' appendicectomy at about 3 months (Ochsner–Sherren regimen) on the premise that 20% of patients will develop recurrent appendicitis otherwise.

Causes of a Right Iliac Fossa Mass

1. Appendix mass
2. Gynaecological mass (e.g. ovarian cyst)
3. Caecal cancer
4. Soft tissue tumour, e.g. sarcoma
5. Lymph node mass

6. TB
7. Actinomycosis
8. Transplant kidney
9. Iliac aneurysm

MESENTERIC ADENITIS

Mesenteric adenitis is the main differential diagnosis for acute appendicitis. It is a condition where enlargement of the mesenteric lymph nodes occurs, causing pain and a temperature, as well as local tenderness. It is mostly seen in children and adolescents and is often associated with a viral or upper respiratory tract infection. Headache and photophobia are more common than in acute appendicitis. The temperature is often higher than in acute appendicitis and the tenderness and pain may not be as focal. Investigation shows a lymphocytosis rather than a raised neutrophil count. No specific treatment other than paracetamol is usually required. If operative exploration is undertaken to rule out appendicitis then the appendix should be removed whether or not it is normal in order to avoid confusion over any subsequent attacks of abdominal pain.

SMALL BOWEL OBSTRUCTION

The commonest cause of small bowel obstruction in the Western world is adhesions, secondary to previous surgery, and the second commonest cause is hernias. Other causes can be classified as in the following table:

Causes of Intestinal Obstruction

In the Lumen
Impacted faeces or food bolus obstruction
Swallowed foreign body
Large polyps
Intussusception

In the Wall
Tumours
Infarction

Crohn's disease

Benign stricture

Outside the Wall

Adhesions

Strangulated hernia

Volvulus

Extrinsic compression

The precise symptoms and presentation depend on the site of the obstruction, but the four cardinal features are

1. Pain
2. Abdominal distension
3. Vomiting
4. Absolute constipation

The pain is usually colicky in nature, i.e. intermittent spasms of pain due to peristalsis which wear off after a few seconds, only to return a few minutes later. The pain is often severe and makes the patient double up whilst it is present. Pain due to small bowel obstruction is usually found in the central abdomen (embryological midgut). Distension is variable and depends on the level of the obstruction, with more distal obstruction causing greater degrees of distension, as one might expect. Likewise, vomiting occurs early with high intestinal obstruction and late with low intestinal obstruction. Absolute constipation means that the patient is passing neither flatus nor faeces. In a high obstruction absolute constipation may not be present.

Abdominal examination may reveal distension and runs of hyperactive bowel sounds. Focal tenderness implies that strangulation might be occurring. 'Strangulation' refers to compromise of part of the intestinal blood supply due to twisting or kinking of its mesentery. It may also be suggested by findings of a temperature or raised white count and obviously in later stages will progress to gangrene and perforation of the bowel with signs of generalised peritonitis. A plain abdominal X-ray may be helpful in confirming the diagnosis of small bowel obstruction. The typical appearance would be of distended small bowel loops (remember that the small bowel usually has a diameter of less than 4 cm on a plain X-ray and is characterised by its central position within the abdomen and valvulae conniventes which go all the way across the bowel lumen).

Treatment of Small Bowel Obstruction

The patient should be carefully assessed and on abdominal examination particular attention should be paid to the presence of previous abdominal scars or the presence of hernias. The groin should be very carefully examined, as a small femoral hernia can be easily missed unless specifically looked for. If a hernia is found in a patient who is obstructed, then immediate surgery is required to repair the hernia and release the obstruction, as it is likely that the bowel is strangulated within the hernia. At operation the bowel should be carefully inspected, and if it is thought to be nonviable, a resection of that section of the bowel may be required. If the obstruction is thought to be due to adhesions and if there are no suggestions that strangulation has already occurred, then a period of conservative management may be appropriate. This usually consists of placing the patient 'nil by mouth', passing a nasogastric tube which should be left on free drainage with two-hourly aspiration in an attempt to decompress the bowel and giving intravenous fluids to avoid dehydration ('drip and suck'). The patient should then be carefully monitored and the resolution of the obstruction would be marked by a lessening of pain, a decrease in the NGT aspirate volumes, the passage of flatus and the resolution of signs on a repeat X-ray. Should the patient not settle within 24 h or should signs of strangulation develop, then surgery would be indicated. Surgery for adhesions normally consists of a laparotomy at which the adhesions are divided.

The term 'subacute bowel obstruction' is sometimes used to describe the condition where only one or two of the four cardinal signs are present. However, this term is really meaningless and obstruction should be classified as complete or partial. There is one other term used, which is 'pseudo-obstruction'. This means the patient is obstructed but no mechanical cause can be found and it may be due to many factors, such as electrolyte abnormalities, trauma or medications.

LARGE BOWEL OBSTRUCTION

The commonest causes of acute large bowel obstruction are carcinoma of the colon, diverticulitis and volvulus of the sigmoid or caecum. Unlike small bowel obstruction, adhesions and hernias are rarer causes. Like small bowel obstruction, large bowel obstruction gives rise to distension, colicky abdominal pain, vomiting and constipation, although vomiting may take longer to onset. In 20% of people the ileocaecal valve is competent and decompression of the large bowel back into the small bowel cannot occur. This is a dangerous situation, as pressure can rapidly build up in the colon, leading to a perforation, which is the major complication in large bowel obstruction. Perforation usually occurs in the caecum, as this is the thinnest-walled and most distensible part of the colon. Investigations would be blood tests (FBC, U & E, amylase and group and save) and X-rays. Sigmoidoscopy may show the site of the lesion and an emergency contrast enema may be helpful in differentiating true from pseudo-obstruction. Management is intravenous resuscitation and passage of a nasogastric tube. Immediate laparotomy is indicated if signs of peritonitis are present (indicating perforation has occurred) or if the caecum is greater than 10 cm in diameter or very tender, indicating imminent perforation. Recently, self-expanding metallic stents have proved useful in the treatment of large bowel obstruction. These stents can be inserted through the stricture under endoscopic or radiological guidance and are thus useful in the palliation of patients who are unfit for major surgery. They can also be useful to decompress acutely obstructing cancers and thus obviate the need for emergency surgery in an acutely unwell patient.

INFLAMMATORY BOWEL DISEASE

Inflammatory bowel disease is a term which includes both ulcerative colitis and Crohn's disease.

Crohn's Disease

Crohn's disease is a chronic relapsing, transmural granulomatous disorder (i.e. on histology the whole thickness of the bowel is affected and granulomas are seen) of unknown aetiology. It can occur anywhere in the gastrointestinal tract, from mouth to anus, but is commonest in the terminal ileum (hence its old name, 'terminal ileitis'). It can affect the colon, where occasionally it may be difficult to differentiate from ulcerative colitis. It will often affect separate areas of bowel with normal bowel in between (so-called 'skip' lesions). It tends to produce healing by fibrosis resulting in strictures and has a tendency to form fistulae to other structures, such as adjacent loops of bowel, the bladder, the vagina and the skin surface.

The way in which Crohn's disease first presents varies with its site and extent. The commonest presentation will be with a change in the bowel habit, usually diarrhoea, central abdominal colicky pains or pains in the right iliac fossa, fever, anorexia, weight loss and general malaise. On examination there may be tenderness or a mass in the abdomen, most often in the right iliac fossa. Often, however, there are no abnormal physical signs. Investigation consists of the exclusion of other possible diagnoses, including carcinoma. Blood tests may be helpful and show elevated acute phase proteins, especially C reactive protein. The mainstay of diagnosis, however, involves contrast studies (barium follow-through examination of the small bowel or barium enema for the colon) and endoscopic studies with biopsy (e.g. colonoscopy).

Most cases of Crohn's disease are initially managed medically by gastroenterologists, although about 65% will at some time require surgery. Drugs such as Mesalazine and steroids may be used. Severe cases where there is stricture formation, fistualisation or an inflammatory mass that is not resolving, may need surgical intervention.

The surgery for Crohn's disease depends on which part of the bowel is affected and the treatment can be divided into surgery for small and large bowel disease.

If the small bowel is predominantly involved, the main aims of surgery will be to perform stricturoplasties or resect the very diseased bowel locally but to minimise resection as much as possible. The reason for this is that occasional patients may require repeated surgery and end up with short gut syndrome if too much bowel is resected (the patients' main concern is liquid stools, although they also have all the vitamin and nutritional deficiencies). In large bowel disease the operation usually performed is panproctocolectomy with ileostomy (removal of the whole large bowel and anus) or subtotal colectomy with ileorectal anastomosis (if the rectum is spared of disease). Smaller, more limited resections of the large bowel in Crohn's are associated with high relapse rates requiring further surgery.

Detailed questions about Crohn's disease are most likely to come from gastroenterologists in medical exams. However, you should obviously know about the associated complications outside the abdomen, including the high incidence of perianal disease such as abscesses and perianal fistulae, the skin changes of erythema nodosum and pyoderma gangraenosum, the associated arthritis and ocular problems, etc.

Ulcerative Colitis

Unlike Crohn's disease, ulcerative colitis (UC) affects only the colon, and whilst Crohn's disease affects the full thickness of the bowel wall, UC affects only the mucosa. Another difference from Crohn's disease is that UC usually affects the rectum and as the disease gets more extensive it spreads proximally in a continual pattern (i.e. skip lesions should make one consider Crohn's disease). Like Crohn's disease, UC is a chronic and relapsing condition. The normal mode of presentation will be of blood-stained diarrhoea and abdominal pain, which is often eased by defaecation (NB: UC tends to be bloody diarrhoea whereas Crohn's tends to be painful diarrhoea). In most cases there are no abnormal physical signs. In more severe cases nausea, vomiting and distension may occur in association with pyrexia, and this should make one suspect the development of toxic megacolon.

In nonacute cases investigation consists of the elimination of other pathologies, and confirmation is usually made by biopsy on sigmoidoscopy or colonoscopy. It can sometimes be difficult for the histologist to differentiate Crohn's from UC, and he then terms the condition as 'indeterminate' or nonspecific inflammatory bowel disease. The other major difference between Crohn's disease and UC is that while the former appears to have only a small premalignant potential, the latter is most definitely premalignant. The figure usually quoted is that for ulcerative colitis involving most of the colon there is a 10% risk of developing a carcinoma for every 10 years that the disease exists. Because of this people with UC are advised to have regular routine screening colonoscopies with biopsies every 2–3 years. The particular feature looked for on the biopsy is the development of dysplasia, and if it is severe, consideration should be given to the possibility of an elective total colectomy to reduce the risk of cancer formation. The operation will normally be a proctocolectomy, which means that the whole of the colon and rectum will be removed so that no colonic mucosa will be left. After this the patient either is left with a terminal ileostomy or can have a new pelvic reservoir constructed ('a pouch'), which is made by joining several loops of small bowel together and sewing that directly down to the anal sphincters. A pouch operation would nowadays normally be offered to any person requiring a total colectomy for UC. Such an operation cannot be offered to patients with Crohn's colitis, because Crohn's disease often recurs in the small bowel used to construct the reservoir and the results of the operation are therefore poor.

The majority of UC patients (>85%) can be managed medically (antidiarrhoeals, steroids, Mesalazine, etc.), unlike Crohn's disease, in which about 65% will require surgery at some point. The principal acute complication of UC which you need to know about and which might require surgical intervention is toxic megacolon. This is diagnosed on a plain X-ray and is defined as dilatation of the transverse colon above 6 cm. The patient will normally be quite unwell with UC and will present with severe blood-stained diarrhoea and systemic signs such as fever, dehydration and tachycardia. There is usually abdominal tenderness and the white cell count may be raised. Initial attempts will usually be made to treat the patient conservatively with intravenous fluids, correction of electrolyte abnormalities and high-dose intravenous steroids. Repeated abdominal X-rays should be taken to watch the size of the colon (usually the transverse colon), and if it appears to be getting bigger despite appropriate medical treatment an operation is indicated before it perforates. Also, if a perforation is suspected or if the patient fails to settle within 24–48 h of medical treatment, then surgery will be indicated.

In this situation the usual surgical procedure is a total colectomy, an ileostomy and the rectal stump is usually oversewn or brought out to the skin so that it can be inspected (this is called a mucous fistula). Subsequently, when the acute problem has settled, the patient could be offered an ileal reservoir or completion proctectomy (i.e. removal of the rest of the rectum and anus, leaving them with a permanant ileostomy) according to discussions between the surgeon and patient.

It is not uncommon to get shown a barium enema during your viva, and the commonest diagnoses are ulcerative colitis or an apple core stricture indicating malignancy. You may also get shown a barium meal with follow-through which looks at the small bowel (you see some contrast in the stomach and hence you can tell it is a follow-through), and this may show the strictures of Crohn's disease.

COLON CANCER

Colon cancer is the commonest gastrointestinal cancer and questions are therefore common in surgical finals. Patients who have had previous operations for colon cancer are often brought up as long cases. The way in which colon cancer presents depends partly on its position within the colon. Tumours on the right side of the colon are more likely to present later with a mass or anaemia, since the faeces are still liquid in this region and thus are less likely to produce an obstruction to the flow. In contradistinction, tumours on the left side of the colon are more likely to present early with obstruction and a change in the bowel habit. Tumours in the rectum may give rise to tenesmus, which is a symptom where the patient feels as though there are some faeces which they need to pass even after they have just emptied their bowels. This symptom is actually a reflection of the mass present within the rectum. Examination may be entirely normal. Rectal examination is mandatory, as you may be able to feel a low rectal tumour. Sigmoidoscopy should also be performed, which will allow visualisation (and biopsy) of tumours in the last 15 cm or so of the intestinal tract (which may be missed on barium enema). Investigations — simple blood tests (FBC, U & E, LFTs) and CEA [carcinoembryonic antigen (CEA) — a marker for bowel cancer] — should be measured. Further investigation is usually with barium enema (apple core lesion) or colonoscopy, where a stricture or mass will be found. Colonoscopy allows biopsies to be taken. Ultrasound or CT may be indicated to stage and screen for liver metastases.

A common question relates to the staging of colon cancer. The classical way of staging such tumours is the Dukes staging. Initially, Sir Cuthbert Dukes (a pathologist at St Mark's Hospital, London) described three stages: Type A, where the tumour is confined to the mucosa and submucosa of the bowel wall (this has a 90% 5-year survival rate); Type B, where the tumour has invaded into or through the bowel wall into surrounding tissue but the lymph nodes are clear (this has a 60% 5-year survival rate); Type C, where the lymph nodes are involved, and this stage is usually divided into C1 and C2. C2 is where the highest lymph node in the surgical specimen is involved (implying further spread). Overall, stage C has a 5-year survival of about 30%. Although not originally described by Dukes, the further stage D is now usually mentioned where there is distant spread, and this has a 5–10% 5-year survival rate. Dukes' staging system has been largely superceded by the TNM classification system where T refers to depth of tumour invasion, N refers to lymph node involvement and M refers to the presence of metastatic disease. The treatment of colon cancer is surgery and resection of the tumour. Preoperatively, patients should have bowel preparation (except for right sided tumours). Tumours of the right colon usually undergo right hemicolectomy, the transverse colon undergo an extended right hemicolectomy, and the descending colon tumours undergo left hemicolectomy. When resecting bowel cancers attention is paid to the blood supply to the segment involved. There must be a good blood supply to the two cut ends and, therefore, the surgeon removes the entire part of the bowel supplied by the same blood vessels as those supplying the tumour (and hence are ligated when the tumour is resected). Thus a tumour of the caecum (supplied by the right colic artery) means a right hemicolectomy.

Tumours of the rectum are treated by anterior resection (this is where the rectal tumour is removed and the colon above the tumour is anastomosed to the remaining rectal stump). Usually, a primary anastomosis is performed using either sutures or a staple gun. If the immediate strength of the anastomosis is in doubt, then a proximal temporary stoma (usually an ileostomy or a transverse colostomy) may be constructed and closed a few weeks later. This is in order to divert the faeces away from the healing anastomosis. If the tumour is very low down and excision cannot be performed without damaging the anal sphincters, then an abdominoperineal (AP) resection (i.e. excision of the rectum and anus leaving the patient with a permanent colostomy) is required. This is a much more extensive operation and leaves the patient with two wounds (the perineal and the laparotomy) and a colostomy.

In terms of the latest developments in the understanding of rectal cancer, it is now thought that the presence of radial spread (in an outward direction from the bowel into the surrounding mesentery) is an important prognostic indicator and therefore many surgeons nowadays perform a careful total mesorectal excision (removing the mesentery of the rectum) during an anterior resection in order to reduce the incidence of local recurrence. Laparoscopic surgery for the removal of colorectal cancer is currently under scrutiny with several large multicentric randomised trials in order to determine the long-term oncological consequences.

The role of adjuvant therapy in colorectal cancer is still unclear. Many studies have been published and many more are still underway. At present it appears that systemic chemotherapy with 5-fluorouracil and levamisole leads to increased survival and decreased recurrence in patients with Dukes C cancers. The role of chemotherapy in Dukes B cancers is less clear.

Radiotherapy is of no value in colon cancer (as the tumour is too mobile and not particularly radiosensitive) but has been shown to be associated with improved outcome in some patients with rectal cancer if given preoperatively over a short (5 days) or long (5 weeks) course.

Stomas and Types of Colonic Resectons

Questions on these are common. The following is a simple guide. A stoma in the right lower quadrant is usually an ileostomy. Because small bowel content is irritant to the skin, ileostomies are usually constructed with a spout and they stand clear of the skin by a few centimetres. They may be either an end ileostomy in someone who has had a total colectomy or a loop ileostomy where the bowel has been temporarily 'defunctioned'. This latter type is usually performed after a difficult colonic resection to give the anastomosis time to heal before restoring intestinal continuity. Obviously, the end ileostomy will have only one opening whilst the loop ileostomy will have two. However, students will not usually be expected to remove ileostomy bags to confirm this in exams. There can be large fluid losses from an ileostomy and it is important to regularly measure these losses and replace them accordingly via the drip to prevent dehydration.

A stoma in the right upper quadrant is usually a defunctioning transverse colostomy. Like the defunctioning ileostomy, it will have two lumens, but will not usually have a spout and is therefore flush with the skin surface. Again, it will usually be a temporary stoma to cover an anastomosis.

Stomas are not usually constructed in the left upper quadrant; however, if there is one it is probably one of the types found in the left lower quadrant, which for technical reasons has been sited higher than usual.

Left lower quadrant stomas may be end colostomies, loop colostomies or double-barrelled colostomies. An end colostomy is produced after resection of the rectum or sigmoid colon (Figure 7.2). There is an operation called Hartmann's procedure, in which the sigmoid colon is resected and the rectal stump is left inside the pelvis and closed with sutures, while a temporary end colostomy is brought out in the left lower quadrant. This is most often performed for perforated diverticulitis, where the affected portion of bowel is resected but the contamination makes it unsafe to join the ends back together immediately. A permanent end colostomy is produced after complete excision of the anus and rectum (an abdominoperineal excision) for a very low rectal cancer. If after a resection it is thought unsafe to join the bowel ends together, but the distal end is long enough, then both ends may be brought out together to the surface. This is called a double-barrelled colostomy (Figure 7.3). If the bowel is long enough, it is preferred to a Hartmann's, because reversal does not require a full relaparotomy. Loop colostomy is when the apex of the sigmoid is brought out as a stoma without a resection having been performed. This is occasionally done for an inoperable carcinoma of the rectum that is likely to obstruct.

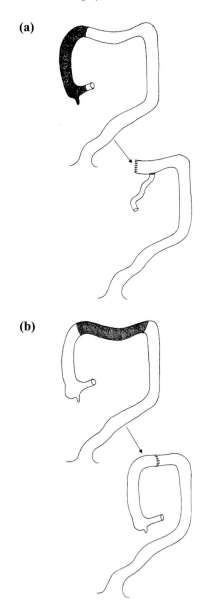

Figure 7.2. Colonic resections. **(a)** Right hemicolectomy. **(b)** Transverse colectomy.

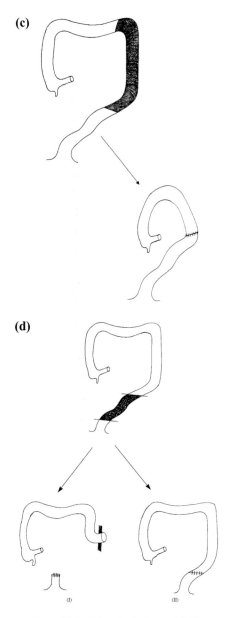

Figure 7.2. Colonic resections. **(c)** Left hemicolectomy. **(d)** Surgery for disease of the sigmoid colon or rectum — (I) Hartmann's and (II) sigmoid colectomy. The decision about which operation is performed depends on several factors, including the disease process, the skill of the surgeon and the general health of the patient.

(e)

(f)

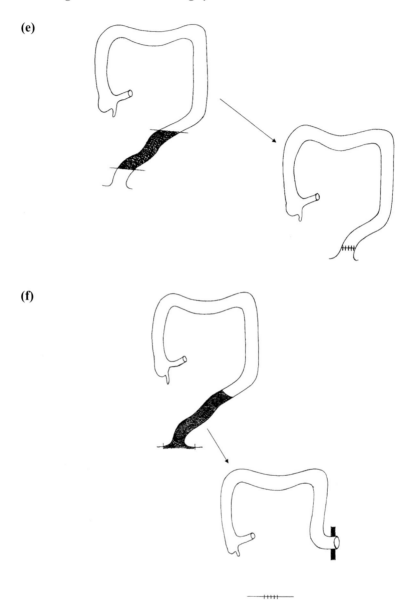

Figure 7.2. Colonic resections. **(e)** Anterior resection. **(f)** Abdominoperineal resection (note that there are two wounds — the laparotomy and the perineal wound — and a stoma).

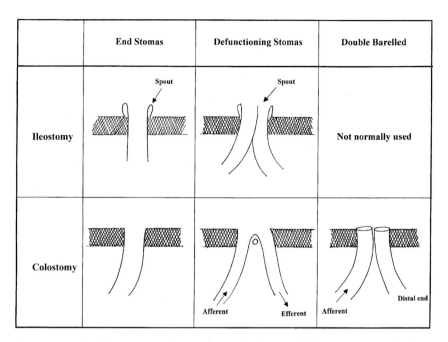

Figure 7.3. The different types of stomas. In the double-barrelled colostomy the distal end is sometimes known as a mucous fistula. This allows it to be inspected and reversal, if necessary, is easier.

Screening for Colorectal Cancer

Colonoscopy is the ideal test but is expensive. The haemoccult test, which looks for faecal occult blood, is one of the better and cheaper tests. However, it has a relatively low sensitivity and gives a high false positive rate; even so studies that are under way, looking at the haemoccult test, show early indications of a decreased mortality in the screened groups.

There are no clear guides as to who should be screened for polyps or colorectal cancer. However, the following should be screened:

1. Those with familial adenomatous polyposis (who usually have a colectomy early).
2. Those with strong family history (more than two close relatives).
3. Anyone with a personal history of polyps or colorectal cancer.

4. Patients with ulcerative colitis for more than 10 years, Peutz–Jeghers, juvenile polyposis, etc.

CEA is a serological marker for colorectal cancer. However, it is not usually elevated in early disease (less than 5% of Dukes A cancers have a raised CEA) and it also has low specificity, being raised in many other conditions (such as other inflammatory conditions of the GI tract, smoking or renal impairment). Therefore, it has little value in any screening programme. It is, however, used in the follow-up of patients with colorectal cancer. The level of CEA should fall to normal limits within weeks of the operation to remove the cancer. At the follow-up clinics a rise in CEA can be used to diagnose recurrence of the tumour, often before it is clinically apparent.

Colonic Polyps

A polyp is defined as 'a lesion which projects into the lumen of the bowel'. The relevance in the colon is mainly because of the tendency of some types of polyps to become malignant. The general term 'polyp', however, is purely a morphological term and in no way defines the actual diagnosis for which histology would usually be required (most often obtained by biopsy at sigmoidoscopy or colonoscopy). It is helpful to consider polyps under their different pathological headings:

Adenomatous Polyps

Adenomatous polyps are important because of their tendency to lead to colorectal cancer. Most authorities believe that the majority of adenocarcinomas of the colon develop from pre-existing adenomatous polyps. Evidence for this belief includes the fact that early stages of malignancy (severe dysplasia and carcinoma *in situ*) may sometimes be found in polyps and that patients with familial adenomatous polyposis die of cancer at a young age unless they have a prophylactic colectomy. In addition, carcinogens which produce adenomas experimentally also lead to cancer formation, and studies in which patients were followed up after previous colorectal cancer in which polyps were prophylactically removed at colonoscopy appeared to indicate a reduced incidence of subsequent new cancer development. The likelihood of an adenomatous polyp becoming malignant seemed to relate to its size. It appears to be rare for adenomas under 1 cm in size but occurs with increasing likelihood as the polyp gets bigger. Adenomatous polyps of the colon are usually subclassified into the better-differentiated tubular adenomas (75%), which are often on a stalk, and the less-differentiated villous adenomas (10%), which are often sessile (i.e. flat). Sometimes a polyp is described as tubulovillous (15%) when it has an appearance somewhere between these two extremes.

Adenomas can be sporadic or familial. The familial adenomas occur in conditions such as familial multiple polyposis coli and Gardener's syndrome, and they have a high if not inevitable chance of developing into cancer.

Familial multiple polyposis coli is an autosomal dominant condition with multiple neoplastic colonic polyps beginning in the second to third decade, and patients usually have a prophylactic colectomy in their early twenties.

Gardeners' syndrome is an autosomal dominant condition with multiple colonic adenomas in association with bony osteomas and epidermoid cysts.

Other than being premalignant, adenomatous polyps may present with the following:

- Bleeding which may be either frank blood or microscopic bleeding (present with anaemia).
- Polyps rarely present with change in the bowel habit, but a large benign polyp in the rectum can produce the symptoms of tenesmus (i.e. a sensation of incomplete evacuation due to the presence of a mass within the rectum).
- Some polyps may also secrete a large amount of mucus and the patient may complain of passing slime or jelly.
- Rarely, a polyp will prolapse through the anus or act as the apex for an intussusception.

Polyps may be diagnosed on imaging the colon with a barium enema, but if suspected the best investigation is usually a colonoscopy which gives the additional advantage of providing the opportunity for biopsy or complete removal of the polyp. Key points on histology, other than the diagnosis of an adenomatous polyp, will be whether or not there is any evidence of dysplasia of the cells on the surface of the polyp. Most histologists would classify this as mild, moderate or severe, with severe dysplasia being strongly suggestive that the lesion was premalignant.

Hamartomatous Polyps

A hamartoma (a lesion where there is an overgrowth of one or more of the cell types which are normal constituents of the organ from which they arise) is an unusual lesion defined as an abnormality of development. With regard to colonic polyps, there are two conditions in which hamartomatous polyps are normally described:

• *Juvenile polyps.* These have a low malignant potential. They may present with bleeding or intussusception and sometimes slough off spontaneously and actually present with material passed in the motion and noticed by the patient or parents. Usually, it is possible to deal with them colonoscopically.
• *Peutz–Jeghers syndrome.* This is a rare autosomal dominant condition where multiple hamartomatous polyps appear throughout the entire gastrointestinal tract and the affected individuals also have pigmentation of the skin around the lips and gums. Again the malignant potential of these polyps is small, although overall the patient is at a greater risk of developing carcinoma (both GI and non-GI tract).

Polyps Due to Protrusions of Mesenchymal Tissue

Conditions such as lipomas (benign tumours of fat), leiomyomas (benign tumours of smooth muscle), neurofibromas (benign tumours arising from nerve tissue) and haemangiomas (benign tumours of blood vessel origin) can all occur in the wall of the colon, and if they then form a lump which protrudes into the lumen, they are by definition polyps. These are all rather rare in clinical practice and their main importance is that they may mimic the presentation of a carcinoma.

Metaplastic Polyps

These are sometimes also called hyperplastic polyps. They are usually small, often multiple and slightly raised above the surrounding normal mucosa. They have a distinctive histological appearance and have no malignant potential whatsoever. Because of their small size they cause no symptoms and their only relevance is in distinguishing them from adenomatous polyps. They are often seen in inflammatory bowel disease or lymphoid hyperplasia (such as at the appendix). If they are found incidentally at appendicectomy, then usually no other treatment is required.

Inflammatory Polyps

Examples are those found in inflammatory conditions of the bowel, such as pseudopolyps in ulcerative colitis.

Diverticular Disease

Diverticula are defined as out-pouchings from a tubular structure (the opposite of polyps). Colonic diverticula occur where the colonic mucosa bulges out at the weakest point where blood vessels enter the colonic muscle. They tend to appear in middle and old age and are much more common in Western countries, where it is thought that they may be caused by lack of fibre in the diet leading to muscle spasm and hence increased intraluminal pressure and bulging out of the mucosa. They are usually found on the left side of the colon, although they can occasionally involve all of the colon around as far as the caecum. They are extremely common, being found in the majority of elderly patients, especially if there is a history of constipation. Many are asymptomatic, but diverticular disease can be responsible for a number of clinical problems:

1. Chronic symptoms of *gripey abdominal pains*, diarrhoea and passage of pellety stools are often ascribed to diverticular disease. Normal treatment is usually with antispasmodics and a high-fibre diet.
2. *Acute diverticulitis.* This is a condition where a diverticulum becomes inflamed, usually because of the presence of inspissated faeces within

it. In many ways it is similar to the process involved in acute appendicitis, and indeed diverticulitis is sometimes called 'left-sided appendicitis'. The typical presentation would be an elderly patient, perhaps with a previous history of problems with constipation, etc., who presents with pain and tenderness in the left iliac fossa, a fever, local signs of peritonitis and a raised white cell count. The majority of cases of acute diverticulitis can be treated successfully with conservative management consisting of resting the bowel, intravenous fluids and antibiotics. If they do not settle or their symptoms worsen, then they may require surgical intervention.

3. *Perforated diverticulitis.* Some patients may present with a more sudden onset of pain, perhaps preceded by signs and symptoms suggestive of acute diverticulitis, and have more generalised signs of peritonitis on examination. In addition, they may be shocked or have free gas on an erect chest X-ray, indicating a perforation. These patients will usually require laparotomy for confirmation of the diagnosis, washing out of contamination from the abdominal cavity and usually resection of the sigmoid colon, often as a Hartmann's procedure where the affected sigmoid colon is resected, the lower end (the rectal stump) is oversewn and left within the pelvis and the proximal end is brought out usually as a temporary left iliac fossa colostomy (which can be reversed after a few months) (see Figure 7.4).

4. *Diverticular abscess.* Sometimes a perforated diverticulum, rather than leading to free peritonitis, is walled off by surrounding anatomical structures such as bowel loops and leads to a local abscess formation. If a mass is felt on examination and this diagnosis is suspected, then the investigation of choice is probably a CT. Treatment is as for acute diverticulitis initially (the outline of the mass can be marked on the skin for regular reassessment), and if the patient fails to respond then drainage, either surgical or radiological, is needed. Sometimes the patient requires a resection and Hartmann's procedure as above.

5. *Haemorrhage.* This is usually sudden and painless, and there can be bright or dark red blood. It usually stops spontaneously, although if it persists, angiography and surgery may be required to remove the affected part of the bowel.

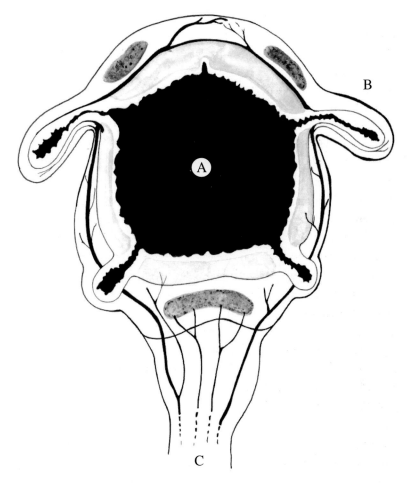

Figure 7.4. Diverticula. (A) Lumen, (B) diverticula and (C) mesentery.

6. *Stricture of the colon.* After the resolution of acute diverticulitis the colon may sometimes heal with a fibrous stricture formation. If severe this may require resection. Usually, when a resection is performed in the absence of acute inflammation or an abscess, it is possible to join the ends of the bowel together again immediately, with either sutures or staples, i.e. performing a 'primary anastomosis'. Other causes of a colonic stricture include a carcinoma, ulcerative colitis or Crohn's

disease, ischaemic colitis, post-radiotherapy changes or surgery — at the site of an anastomosis.

Lower Gastrointestinal Bleeding

This is caused by a number of possible conditions. It is, like upper gastrointestinal bleeding, a common question in the finals. The mainstay of investigation is colonoscopy and patients only occasionally require emergency surgery. Remember, if answering a question, to deal initially with rapid assessment and treatment of the shocked patient.

The causes of a lower GI bleed are

- Haemorrhoids
- Carcinoma
- Diverticular disease
- Angiodysplasia
- Infective colitis
- Polyps
- Anal fissure
- Ulcerative colitis

The age of the patient is important — for example, haemorrhoids, cancer, diverticular diease and angiodysplasia are the most common in elderly patients, whereas infective colitis and ulcerative colitis are more common in young people.

In the history note the frequency and amount of bleeding, the colour (bright red blood is suggestive of lower GI bleeding, whereas dark red blood could be both upper or lower GI bleeding), whether the bleeding was associated with the passage of faeces and if so whether it was mixed in, whether there was any mucus or slime and whether there was any abdominal pain (suggestive of inflammatory disease). Examination should always include a proctoscopy (and if possible a rigid sigmoidoscopy) to look for a local cause of bleeding (e.g. haemorrhoids). Resuscitation is the same as that for an upper GI bleed, although many cases stop bleeding spontaneously. If this is the case and there was a significant bleed, then the patient is admitted for urgent investigation. If the bleed was small and stops spontaneously, then the patient may be able to be investigated colonoscopically as an out-patient. Very occasionally, the bleeding continues and is rapid, requiring an urgent angiogram to find the source of the bleeding. If a region of the bowel is shown to have abnormal blood vessels (i.e. angiodysplasia), then surgery to remove the affected area may be required (occasionally, the bleeding vessel can be stopped by embolizing the vessel radiologically). The operation required will depend on where the cause of the bleeding is.

In some cases it is impossible to tell from the history whether the bleed was from the upper or the lower GI tract, and in these cases the patient needs a gastroscopy initially to rule out an upper GI lesion.

8

RECTUM AND ANUS

Alan F Horgan

HAEMORRHOIDS

There is much debate in surgical circles about the true nature of haemorrhoids. Unfortunately, this sometimes manifests itself in the finals by
questions such as 'What exactly are haemorrhoids?'. They are probably a
vascular cushion, covered in a layer of mucosa and containing a branch of
the superior rectal artery and a tributary of the superior rectal vein. The
key point that the examiners will want you to make is that haemorrhoids
are not simply dilated veins (when they bleed the blood is bright red).
Haemorrhoids occur at the point where the superior rectal branches enter
the muscle. Conventionally, their position is described in relation to the
anus imagined as a clock face visualised with the patient in the lithotomy
position (i.e. on his back with his legs up in stirrups). In this position the
penis or vagina is anterior at 12 o'clock. There are usually three haemorrhoids, at 3, 7 and 11 o'clock.

Haemorrhoids are classified as follows:

First degree. They do not prolapse from the anus

Second degree. They prolapse on defaecation or straining but return
spontaneously

Third degree. They prolapse and remain prolapsed unless manually
repositioned

Haemorrhoids may be asymptomatic, although if they do cause
symptoms this is usually bleeding or minor pain and itching. They are

usually not severely painful unless they are prolapsed and thrombosed. Bleeding from haemorrhoids is usually bright red and either on the outside of the motion or on the toilet paper. There is usually no change in the fundamental bowel habit and no other gastrointestinal symptoms or signs. Haemorrhoids can be treated by injection (with 5% phenol in almond oil); this works by shrinking the haemorrhoid through causing scar formation, by rubber band ligation or by coagulation with infrared devices. These procedures are usually performed in the out-patient department. If these methods fail, then it may be necessary to formally excise the haemorrhoids ('haemorrhoidectomy'), as a day case or an in-patient procedure.

Fissure *in Ano*

A fissure *in ano* usually starts with a tear in the anal canal caused by trauma or the passage of a constipated stool. In some cases this fails to heal and the inflammation it produces causes spasm in the sphincter muscle so that further trauma occurs when motions are passed and it eventually becomes a chronic fissure. Examination is often painful and it may be possible to see an external hypertrophic skin tag 'sentinel pile', which is indurated at the base where the fissure lies.

The initial treatment for a fissure is conservative, with advice to avoid straining on the toilet (and the use of bulk laxatives) and the topical application of local anaesthetic gels. A variety of agents have recently been developed in order to promote relaxation of the internal anal sphincter. These include the use of topical nitrates (0.2% GTN paste), calcium channel blockers (2% diltiazem cream), or the injection of Botulinum toxin into the internal anal sphincter. In the event of failure of the above conservative methods, then surgery may be needed. In the past the surgical treatment was manual dilatation of the anus under a general anaesthetic, but this was associated with high rates of long-term incontinence. Nowadays, chronic fissure is usually treated by the operation of lateral subcutaneous sphincterotomy, in which the external sphincter is partially divided through a small laterally placed stab incision.

Fistula *in Ano*

A fistula is an abnormal connection between two epithelial surfaces [NB: A sinus is a blind-ending tract joining an epithelial surface to a cavity lined by granulation tissue (e.g. an abscess)].

A fistula *in ano* has an opening internally to the anal canal and another opening externally onto the skin. Most probably start as a perianal abscess, but occasionally they are due to Crohn's disease, carcinoma, radiotherapy or tuberculosis. They can be classified as 'low' when they do not cross the sphincter muscles above the dentate line and 'high' when they cross the sphincters above this level (Figure 8.1). Low fistulae are usually treated by being laid open. This is achieved by inserting a metal probe into the fistula and incising through the tissue down onto the probe. The wound is allowed to heal from its depths upwards. This cannot be done with high fistulae, because the sphincters would be damaged, and so these fistulae may be treated with a seton. This is a thread which is passed

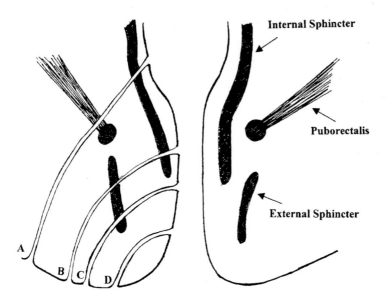

Figure 8.1. Perianal fistulae. Cross-section through the anal canal and lower rectum showing the normal anatomy on the right and the different types of fistulae on the left. (A) Pelvianal fistula, (B) high anal fistula, (C) low anal fistula, and (D) subcutaneous anal fistula.

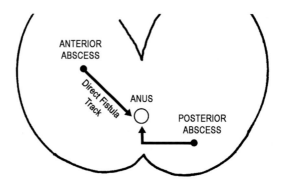

Figure 8.2. Goodsall's rule.

through the fistula track and is tied on the outside. It can then be gradually tightened so that over a period of weeks it cuts through to the surface, with the fistula healing by scar tissue behind it.

Goodsall's rule states that fistulae anterior to the anus usually open to the anus in a straight line, whilst posterior ones usually have a curving track and open in the midline posteriorly (Figure 8.2).

Rectal Prolapse

Rectal prolapse may be partial or complete. Partial prolapse is defined as involving the mucosa alone and obviously this rarely prolapses for more than a few centimetres. Complete prolapse involves prolapse of the full thickness of the rectum and can be much more sizable. It is most common in elderly females and presents with a mass that appears on or during defaecation. It may reduce spontaneously or require manual reduction and sometimes will present as a semi-emergency as a prolapse which has become oedematous and ulcerated, producing pain and bleeding.

Rectal prolapse is usually associated with poor anal sphincter function. Initial treatment is to reduce the prolapse manually, but this will often be only a temporary solution. Partial thickness (mucosal) prolapse may be treated by phenol injection (to induce scarring), rubber band ligation or by simple excision of the mucosa with plication of the underlying tissues

(Delorme's procedure); Full thickness prolapse usually needs surgical intervention such as an abdominal rectopexy (where the abdomen is entered and the rectum is stitched up, usually on to the sacrum, in order to prevent further prolapse). This can easily be performed laparoscopically with or without the use of mesh to fix the rectum to the presacral fascia. For those patients who may not be fit enough for abdominal surgery, a perineal approach (Delorme's procedure or perineal rectosigmoidectomy) has less morbidity but higher rates of recurrence.

Perianal Haematoma

A perianal haematoma is sometimes also called a thrombosed external haemorrhoid (which is a misnomer, as it is not actually a haemorrhoid). It is usually due to subcutaneous bleeding around the anal margin caused by the passage of constipated stool. It produces acute perianal pain which may be worsened by defaecation or movement. Examination will reveal a tense tender blue lump at the anal margin which can be simply treated by incision under local anaesthetic should the symptoms be too severe to be controlled by simple analgesia.

Anorectal Abscess

Anorectal or perianal abscesses are a common problem and are frequently seen as emergencies. They may either be perianal (Figure 8.3), ischiorectal or intermuscular (where they extend between the internal and external sphincters). Occasionally, they represent spread from a pelvic abscess down to the perianal region. It is thought that there are two main reasons for the development of these abscesses. Firstly, they may develop from infection in an anal gland, which then turns into an abscess. These will usually have intestinal-type organisms within them (e.g. *Escherichia coli*). Others may develop from simple skin infections, such as an infected sebaceous gland or hair follicle, and are therefore more likely to contain staphylococci.

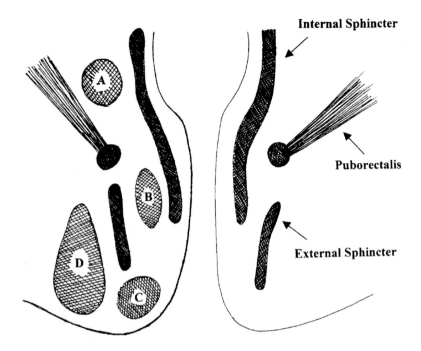

Figure 8.3. Perianal abscesses. (A) Pelvirectal abscess, (B) intersphinteric abscess, (C) perianal abscess, and (D) ischiorectal abscess.

The patient will usually complain of a severe throbbing pain, which gets worse on sitting, and may have signs of a fever, tachycardia, etc. The treatment is surgical drainage, packing and healing by secondary intention. The patient should be seen subsequently in the out-patient clinic to see if there is any evidence of an underlying fistula *in ano*, which occurs in up to 30% of patients.

Pilonidal Abscess/Sinus

The word 'pilonidal' comes from a Latin word meaning 'nest of hair'. A pilonidal abscess or sinus is usually found in the natal cleft. The exact aetiology is still not completely understood but they are thought to be an acquired rather than a congenital (as was once thought) condition. The hairs within the pilonidal cavity are thought to be hairs which have worked their way under the skin and not hairs growing within the sinus or abscess cavity. The condition is more common in people in their teenage and young adult years. It is more common in men than in women and, as one might expect, in those who are particularly hairy. It also seems to be more common in those whose occupation involves prolonged sitting, such as those who drive for a living.

The patient is usually unaware of the sinus until it becomes secondarily infected and presents as an abscess. Treatment of a pilonidal abscess is incision and drainage, followed by packing and healing by secondary intention. Later on a second procedure is needed to excise the sinus tract (which may extend for some distance away from the opening and which can be outlined by injection of methylene blue into the orifices of the sinuses at the time of surgery). If the excised area is small enough, it may be possible to close the area primarily. Alternatively, it may be necessary to leave the area open to heal by secondary intention. Pilonidal disease has a significant tendency to recur even after apparently successful surgery. Patients should be encouraged to be scrupulous with their personal hygiene and to keep the area clean and dry and free from any loose hairs.

9

THE ACUTE ABDOMEN

It is unlikely that any cases of acute abdominal pain will be seen as clinical cases in the finals. This is simply because of the difficulty of arranging such cases in advance. However, cases who have had previous acute abdominal problems may be included as long cases and questions on acute abdominal conditions will be commonly found in written papers and vivas. Indeed, the examiners will often place great importance on candidates having a good knowledge of diagnosis and management in the acute abdomen, as they know that the subject will be of immediate relevance when the candidate takes up his general surgical house job. The acute abdomen is usually defined as a case of abdominal pain with a short history (usually less than 1 week), presenting as an emergency with no history of trauma.

It is worth remembering, in answering questions, that such patients will usually be assessed in casualty departments and, as well as history and examination, simpler investigations such as blood tests and plain X-rays are likely to be all that is initially available. To a large extent the management of the acute abdomen is not, therefore, based on complex investigations but on clinical acumen.

ABDOMINAL PAIN

As with all pains, a certain number of features should be elicited, namely:

- Site (at onset and currently) (see Figure 9.1).
- What is the nature of the pain (character, frequency, radiation)?
- How did the pain start and what has happened to it since?
- What relieves and what exacerbates the pain?

- Are there any associated symptoms?
- Have you ever had this before?/Previous history.
- What do you think it is?

It is helpful to consider the underlying aetiology of the pain so as to try and classify types of acute abdominal pain further. In broad terms, pain in the acute abdomen is caused by one of the following:

1. Pain due to inflammation (i.e. peritonitis).
2. Pain due to obstruction of a hollow viscus (i.e. colic).
3. Referred pain (e.g. pain referred from nerve root compression).
4. Pain in a specific organ or mass (e.g. hepatitis).

Colic is defined as pain caused by obstruction of a hollow viscus and, in the context of the acute abdomen, may arise from obstruction of the small intestine, ureter, biliary system, colon, uterus or fallopian tubes and the appendix. When a hollow viscus with smooth muscle in its walls is obstructed, the smooth muscle contracts in peristaltic waves in an attempt to overcome the obstruction. These spasmodic contractions give rise to intermittent spasms of pain. The classical example is small bowel colic, where pain will come and grip the patient for a short period of time, be so severe as to double him up or make him cry out with pain and will then wear off before another attack occurs, usually a few minutes later. Pain from viscera is usually not well localised and probably travels along the autonomic nerves, which have no dermatomal distribution.

The gut developed embryologically from midline structures and hence pain is generally referred to the midline. Fore-gut structures (oesophagus to second part of duodenum) usually give rise to pain in the upper abdomen, mid-gut structures (second part of duodenum to transverse colon) give rise to pain in the middle of the abdomen, and hind-gut structures give rise to pain in the lower abdomen. Thus, small bowel colic is usually felt centrally, etc.

Peritonitis means inflammation of the peritoneum. In contrast to visceral pain, the parietal peritoneum is innervated by somatic nerves and hence pain is accurately localised to the site of inflammation. This type of pain is typically worse with movement, coughing or inspiration and therefore the patient lies still with shallow breaths (unlike colicky pain, where he moves about to try to get comfortable). Peritonitis is associated with guarding or rigidity of the abdominal muscles. There appears to be some difference in opinion as to the true definition of guarding and rigidity; however, most surgeons would agree that guarding is an involuntary (reflex) contraction of the abdominal muscles when the examining hand presses down over the inflamed area. It is sometimes difficult to differentiate true guarding from voluntary guarding, where the patient contracts his own abdominal muscles in anticipation of pain (especially seen in children). However, if you palpate the two sides of the abdomen at the same time while distracting the patient, you may find that the muscles appear tense on one side compared to the other. It is not really possible to do this voluntarily (where the two sides contract symmetrically) and hence this must be true guarding. If at rest the patient's abdominal musculature has an increased tone, then this is termed rigidity and is again due to underlying inflammation of the peritoneum. If peritonitis involves the whole abdomen, then the patient would typically present with a boardlike, rigid, tender abdomen with absent bowel sounds.

EXAMINATION OF THE ABDOMEN

Obviously, it is always important to do a general examination of the patient. In particular, attention should be paid to signs of shock or dehydration as manifested by peripheral shut-down, clamminess, pallor, tachycardia and hypotension. One can often tell, just by looking at the patient, whether he is unwell. The typical patient with peritonitis looks pale and sweaty, with sunken eyes and a weak thready pulse, shallow breaths and little movement — as first described by Hippocrates thousands of years ago.

Introduce yourself to the patient, ask if he minds your examining him and if he has any pain. Lay him flat (one pillow) and adequately undress him (ideally from nipples to knees, but in the exam you should try to preserve the patient's dignity). On inspection of the abdomen (from the foot of the bed) observe for any obvious scars or masses, distension and the movement with respiration. You may find it easier in an exam situation to comment on your observations as you go along (unless you are confident you can present it all at the end). It is sometimes difficult to differentiate fat from distension (which can be due to flatus or fluid or foetus or faeces).

Next, hold the hand and look for any nail changes (e.g. clubbing), liver palms, etc., feel the pulse, look into the mouth for furring of the tongue and for dry mucous membranes, look into the eyes for jaundice or anaemia (pale conjunctiva) and swiftly feel the neck for any lymph nodes.

On palpation of the abdomen (make sure the hands are warm) kneel down to the patient's right, so that you are roughly level with him. The abdomen can be divided into theoretical regions as in Figure 9.1. Starting at the furthest point from where he tells you the pain is, gently feel in each of these regions. This gives you a quick idea of any obvious masses or tender areas and whether the abdomen is soft. You should begin to think of what anatomical structures are under this area. Always look up at the patient's face (for grimacing). Next you can palpate a little deeper to build up on the findings of gentle palpation. Note if there is any guarding, rigidity or rebound. Rebound tenderness (most painful when the examining hand is removed) is not a good test, as it often causes the patient unnecessary pain and can give equivocal results. Tenderness on percussion is a more accurate and kinder way of assessing the same thing.

Examine the liver and spleen (starting in the right iliac fossa for both, with the patient inspiring each time you press in). In right upper quadrant abdominal pain, Murphy's test for cholecystitis is relevant, and if any masses or enlarged organs are palpated then the precise features need to be delineated. After palpation, percussion should be used before auscultation. Bowel sounds should be classified as being present (i.e. normal), absent (must listen for 3 min) or obstructive (high-pitched and tinkling).

Always finish your examination by palpating for an abdominal aortic aneurysm and check the hernial orifices and scrotum. A rectal examination is mandatory (although in an exam you usually just state that you would like to do it). The breast is really part of the abdominal examination, since if you were shown a case of ascites in the exam and you did not comment on the mastectomy scar, you would not receive any bonus points!

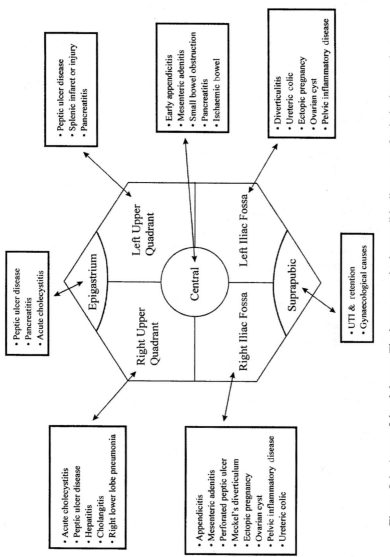

Figure 9.1. Areas of the abdomen. The boxes contain the possible diagnoses of pain in these regions.

ACUTE ABDOMEN: CAUSES

1. *Intestinal*
   - Acute appendicitis
   - Mesenteric adenitis
   - Meckel's diverticulitis
   - Perforated peptic ulcer
   - Gastroenteritis
   - Diverticulitis
   - Perforated
   - Nonperforated
   - *Intestinal obstruction*
   - Strangulated hernia
   - Adhesions
2. *Hepatobiliary*
   - Pancreatitis
   - Gallstones
   - Biliary colic
   - Cholecystitis
   - Cholangitis
   - Hepatitis
3. *Vascular*
   - Ruptured aortic aneurysm
   - Mesenteric embolus/thrombosis
   - Ischaemic colitis
4. *Urological*
   - Renal colic
   - Urinary infection
   - Torsion of testicle
   - Acute retention of urine
5. *Gynaecological*
   - Ectopic pregnancy
   - Ovarian cyst
   - Torsion
   - Ruptured

- Salpingitis
- Endometriosis
- Mittelschmerz
6. *Medical*
   - Pneumonia/pleurisy
   - Cardiac pain/pericarditis
   - Herpes zoster
   - Diabetes — ketoacidosis
   - Neurological pain
   - Hypercalcaemia
   - Sickle cell crisis
   - Syphilis/porphyria

TREATMENT OF THE ACUTE ABDOMEN

Most students learn each topic as it is laid out in the textbooks. However, in real life a patient does not present saying 'I have acute appendicitis', and neither does he always present with the classical textbook description. Instead, most patients tend to present with a variety of vague symptoms and signs that do not point to any specific diagnosis. The acute abdomen is the best topic for highlighting this fact, because a patient who presents with epigastric pain and vomiting could be having pancreatitis, cholecystitis, a perforated peptic ulcer or just gastritis, and it may not be possible to differentiate on the history alone. The examination and simple investigations add further clues to help make a diagnosis, but still it may not be possible to make an absolute diagnosis initially and management may consist of simple treatment such as resuscitation, analgesia and a period of observation whilst further investigations are performed. In other cases, although a specific diagnosis is not made, exploratory laparotomy may be needed (i.e. in cases of generalised peritonitis).

As a student, making the wrong diagnosis is not that important, because there will always be a doctor available to correct you. As a doctor, however, you need to ask yourself 'What if I am wrong?' with each decision made. Performing an appendicectomy on a patient with mesenteric adenitis is unlikely to be life-threatening; on the other hand, if you make a diagnosis of acute appendicitis in a female with right-sided pain without first performing a pregnancy test, then the surgeon may be left with an appendicectomy incision to deal with an ectopic pregnancy. For example, let us say a 14-year-old girl presents with right iliac fossa pain and nausea. The possible causes of this are appendicitis, mesenteric adenitis, a UTI, an ectopic pregnancy or any other gynaecological problem, or even just wind. You should, therefore, ask not only the pertinent questions that point to a specific diagnosis but also the questions that will rule out the other diagnoses. Thus, note the menstrual history and the history of the pain; for example, the pain of appendicitis usually starts centrally and moves to the right side after a few hours, whereas a torsion of an ovarian cyst gives a sudden onset of right iliac fossa pain. A UTI usually has associated urinary symptoms (frequency, dysuria and urgency).

Next, you derive further clues from the examination, looking for localised right iliac fossa tenderness or peritonism. Further clues are again derived from the simple investigations. A pregnancy test and urine dipstix and urgent microscopy must be performed to rule out an infection. A simple blood test such as a white cell count may help (although it is not that specific), and plain X-rays may give further clues (although not that helpful in this case, they would be if renal stones or bowel obstruction were on the differential).

At this point you may have narrowed the differential down to appendicitis, mesenteric adenitis or a gynaecological problem, but you still may not be exactly sure which it is. It is safe then to admit the patient, start IV fiuids and carefully observe her with repeated examinations. If the pain and tenderness appear to settle, no further treatment may be necessary. However, if they persist, then it may be necessary to investigate the patient further. An ultrasound can be helpful, as it can visualise the ovaries and look for any free fluid. It may even show up an enlarged appendix. In this situation an ultrasound is very sensitive although not that specific, and even if it shows no abormality it does not rule out appendicitis. Another option is to perform a diagnostic laparoscopy where the organs are visualised directly via a laparascope. If the appendix is inflamed it could be removed laparascopically (if the surgeon has

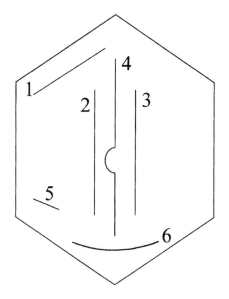

Figure 9.2. Abdominal incisions: (1) right subcostal or Kocher's incision, (2) right para-median, (3) left paramedian, (4) mid-line, (5) gridiron (Lanz), and (6) Pfannenstiel.

enough experience) or conversion to an open procedure can take place. In a male with the same history, symptoms and signs there is not much else it can be apart from appendicitis and mesenteric adenitis, and if the pain did not settle after a period of observation many surgeons would agree that an appendicectomy was indicated without any further investigation. Figure 9.2 illustrates the abdominal incisions possible.

If you are asked to write an essay on the acute abdomen, remember that whilst there are many causes of acute abdominal pain, most are relatively rare. Try to weight your answers to give the most prominence to the more common diagnoses. Obviously, treatment depends on the specific diagnosis made, but it usually consists of resuscitation (oxygen, IV fluids, analgesia, etc.), admission for observation (nasogastric tubes, catheters, fluid balance, repeated examinations, etc.) or even an exploratory laparotomy or diagnostic laparoscopy.

10

BREAST SURGERY

Alan Wilson

EXAMINATION

Examination of the breast should be practised many times before the finals. Breast cancer is very topical and frequently comes up in essays, vivas and long cases. Examination is difficult because it takes a lot of effort to make the patient, who will undoubtedly be anxious, feel at ease. You may be even more nervous or embarrassed than the patient, so always have a female colleague to chaperone you.

Inspection

Ask the patient to sit on the side of the bed exposing the upper half of her body. If the patient has found a lump ask her to point to it. With her arms relaxed at her side, observe for any obvious asymmetry or masses, skin dimpling, previous scars and inversion or eczema of the nipple. Then, ask her to raise her arms straight above her head; this strains the ligaments of Astley Cooper and may result in a skin dimple or inversion of the nipple if there is a breast cancer present. Now ask her to put her hands on her hips and press inwards. Check that pectoralis major is contracted and ask her to relax and contract whilst observing the breast for dimples and inversion of the nipple.

Palpation

Now ask the patient to lie down with arms by her side. Start with the normal breast first. Now ask her to put her hand behind her head. This spreads the breast tissue over the chest wall and makes it easier to examine the breast, particularly if it is large.

The breast is divided into five areas: the four quadrants and a central nipple area. Remember that the upper outer quadrant which includes the axillary tail is the commonest site for malignancies and that the breast extends from the second rib to the inframammary fold. Examine the four quadrants and then the central area.

Palpate each area using the flat surface of your fingers. Normal breast tissue varies between women and according to the stage of the menstrual cycle so by examining the normal breast you will have a good idea of the 'normal' breast tissue. Now examine the symptomatic breast.

If you find a lump, note its site, size (by measuring it with your ruler), shape, colour, contour, consistency, temperature, tenderness, tethering, transilluminance, etc. To assess if the lump is tethered more deeply, ask the patient to place her hands on her hips and push inwards. If the patient complains of a discharge from the nipple ask her to demonstrate it. Note the colour and viscosity of the fluid and whether it comes from one or more ducts.

Now ask the patient to sit up on the side of the bed and examine the axilla. Pectoralis major and latissimus dorsi need to be relaxed to allow proper examination of the axilla, so take her wrist, insert your fingers into the axilla (be gentle) and force her arm to her side. Now palpate the axillary fat pad against the chest wall and note any palpable lymph nodes. Do not push your fingers into the apex of the axilla — it is extremely painful. Now finish by examining the infra- and supraclavicular fossae.

Now turn to the examiner and describe your findings; for example, 'This lady has a 3 cm hard lump in the upper outer quadrant of the right breast. It has a smooth surface and a well-defined edge. It is mobile and not attached to the skin or underlying muscle and it is not tender. There are two nodes palpable in the right axilla. They are soft and mobile. There are no nodes palpable in the supraclavicular fossa. This is a cyst, fibroadenoma or possibly a breast cancer'. The order in which you give this differential diagnosis depends on the age of the patient and your findings.

BREAST CANCER

Breast cancer affects 1 in 10 women in the UK. The risk of developing breast cancer by the age of 50 is 1 in 50, by age 65, 1 in 17 and by age 85, 1 in 9.

The incidence of breast cancer increases with increasing age and has increased with the introduction of mammographic screening. It is the commonest cause of cancer-related deaths in females aged 15–54 (Figure 10.1).

Risk Factors

There are multiple inter-related risk factors. Overall, only 15% of women with breast cancer have an identifiable risk factor apart from *age* and *gender*, which are of course the major factors. Male breast cancer does occur but is much rarer, accounting for about 1 per 300 breast cancers.

Family History

Between 4 and 10% of breast cancers are due to an inherited trait. Overall, if a first-degree relative has breast cancer, then a woman has

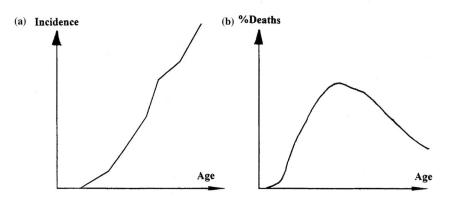

Figure 10.1. (a) Incidence of breast cancer versus age. **(b)** Percentage of deaths attributable to breast cancer versus age.

double the normal risk. This risk is increased if the relative had breast cancer at an early age (<50) or had bilateral breast cancer at any age. The pattern is probably an autosomal dominant trait with limited penetrance. In other words, you may inherit the gene from your father or mother, yet you or your mother may never get breast cancer. The commonest breast cancer genes to have been identified are BRCA1 and BRCA2 genes (on the long arms of chromosome 17 and 13, respectively). BRCA1 affects 2% of Ashkenazi Jews. BRAC1, but not BRAC2, is commoner in patients with a family history of breast and ovarian cancer. Women with either of these genes have a 40–80% lifetime risk of developing breast cancer.

Exposure to Oestrogens

In general, the greater the number of menstrual cycles and the later those cycles are interrupted by a pregnancy, the greater the risk. Thus, a late menarche, an early menopause (or ovariectomy), pregnancy at a young age and increased parity protect against breast cancer. Pregnancy after the age of 35 is associated with an increased risk compared to nulliparity.

The Oral Contraceptive Pill

Use of the oral contraceptive pill (OCP) for greater than 4 years in younger women before their first pregnancy increases the risk of premenopausal breast cancer. Women who use the OCP for short periods to space pregnancies are at no increased risk.

Hormone Replacement Therapy

The 'Million Women Study' has demonstrated that oestrogen-only hormone replacement therapy (HRT) carries a small increase of risk. Women on oestrogen–progesterone HRT have double the risk of breast cancer and this risk increases from when HRT is started. There is currently considerable doubt about whether it should be prescribed to prevent osteoporosis or heart disease. Use of HRT by women aged 50–64 in the UK in the past decade has resulted in an estimated 20,000 extra breast cancers.

Previous Benign Breast Disease

Fibroadenomas and most types of benign breast disease are not a risk factor. Atypical epithelial hyperplasia on breast biopsy, particularly with a positive family history does, however, increase the risk of breast cancer.

Other Factors

Breast cancer has a low incidence in the Far East and Eastern Europe. Obesity increases risk in postmenopausal women. The source of oestrogens in these women is the peripheral aromatisation of androgens produced by the adrenal glands. High socioeconomic group, a diet high in saturated fats and high alcohol intake are also linked with an increased risk of breast cancer. Smoking does not seem to be a risk factor and finally lactation probably protects against breast cancer.

Management and the Clinic

The ideal breast clinic has a multidisciplinary team (MDT) which includes at least one consultant breast surgeon, a consultant oncologist, a breast care nurse, two radiologists, a histopathologist who has experience of cytology and an MDT coordinator. All cases of breast cancer should be reviewed at a weekly meeting of the team and a management plan discussed for each case.

Patients are referred to the clinic via two routes — from the GP or from the screening programme. GPs decide whether a woman needs to be seen urgently. Any woman presenting with a breast lump undergoes *triple assessment*.

Triple Assessment

1. A careful history and examination
2. Mammography and ultrasound
3. Fine needle aspiration cytology (FNA) or core biopsy

The results of the FNA or core biopsy are available later in the day in some clinics or at least should be available within 2–3 days. The radiology results are ready the same day and the majority of women leave the clinic after a discussion with the surgeon, radiologist and breast care nurse about the likely diagnosis and with a provisional plan of management.

In your *history* you must ask about all of the above risk factors for breast cancer and then obtain a history of the lump (see page 176). Do not forget to ask about menarche, parity and age at birth of children, menstrual cycle and regularity, age of menopause, use of medication including OCP and HRT, family history, etc.

Benign breast disease tends to be related to the menstrual cycle, and the woman may have had previous cysts drained by a surgeon. It is worth noting that cysts can appear overnight, and it is not uncommon for breast cancers to go unnoticed and present as though they appeared suddenly. Cancers are usually painless and have unremitting growth. Cysts and fibroadenomas are also usually painless, so you really cannot tell the difference without investigations. Lumpy breast tissue (fibrocystic disease), periductal mastitis, benign cystic disease and fibroadenomas in adolescents are usually tender. If the complaint is of nipple discharge then ask whether it occurs spontaneously or only on squeezing and note the viscosity and colour of the fluid. A spontaneous watery orange fluid from a single duct is probably an intraduct papilloma (benign). Bright red blood is also probably a papilloma, but it maybe ductal carcinoma *in situ* (DCIS). Thick white or green discharge from multiple ducts is not a serious condition. Bilateral milky discharge (galactorrhea) may be due to a pituitary prolactinoma (but this is as rare as hens' teeth).

Fine Needle Aspiration

If there is a lump then an FNA is performed. A 10 ml syringe is attached to a green needle and inserted into the lump. A cyst will disappear as it is aspirated, giving an immediate diagnosis and a happy patient. A solid lump may be lumpy breast tissue, a fibroadenoma or breast cancer. The contents of the needle are expressed onto a slide, smeared with another slide, labelled with the patients name and hospital number, air dried or fixed (depends on the local practice) and sent to the pathologist for interpretation. The slide is stained with haematoxylin and eosin and assigned a cytology code (1–5) — C1, insufficient material to make a diagnosis (usually fat cells only were seen); C2, benign cells seen; C3, uncertain about the diagnosis; C4, probably breast cancer; and C5, breast cancer.

Mammography

This is performed in the radiology department and may be painful, so warn the patient. You should witness a mammogram before the finals. The breast is compressed between two plates. The upper is made of clear Perspex and the one below contains the X-ray plate. The X-rays are directed through the compressed breast onto the X-ray plate. Craniocaudal and oblique views are obtained. Breast cancer is characteristically a white asymmetrical spiculated lesion containing microcalcification. DCIS may be just a cluster of microcalcification. The X-rays should be juxtaposed on the viewing box to assess symmetry. Ask a radiologist to show you how it is done. Mammography misses about 7% of breast cancers, rising to about 12% in premenopausal women who may have dense impenetrable breast tissue. Lobular carcinoma is the classical type of breast cancer missed on mammography.

Ultrasound

This is used in conjunction with mammography and increases the accuracy of radiological diagnosis of a lump. However, it does not usually 'see' microcalcification; it is time-consuming and requires great skill. It is not useful as a screening method for breast cancer but excellent for picking up cysts.

Core Biopsy

If the FNA is C1 or C3 and radiology and clinical examination suspect breast cancer, then there are two choices in the next stage of diagnosis: either the lump is excised or a core biopsy is performed. This allows a histological diagnosis to be made on the lump and discriminates between invasive and *in situ* cancer. The patient returns to the clinic after a few days for the result. A bleb of local anaesthetic is injected into the skin overlying the lump, followed by deeper infiltration. The skin is then punctured with a scalpel blade and the core biopsy needle pushed into the lump. Most needles have an automatic firing mechanism or are attached to a 'gun' resulting in a core of tissue within the sheath of the needle.

Core biopsy and FNA may be guided using ultrasound, mammography or a stereotactic machine integrated to digital mammography (Mammomat).

Clinical Staging

Once the diagnosis of breast cancer has been confirmed by radiology and cytology or histology, the patient is clinically staged. This is used to decide on the initial treatment. Early breast cancer is clinical Stages 1 and 2; advanced breast cancer is Stage 3 and Stage 4. The International Union against Cancer (UICC) Tumour Node Metastases (TNM) system is complicated and often revised. It is not used for the practical management of breast cancer, but is used in research, and unfortunately you are expected to know its principles for the exam.

TNM Staging System (Stage)

T_1 — Tumour <2 cm (1)
T_2 — Tumour 2–5 cm (1)
T_3 — Tumour >5 cm (2/3)
T_4 — Direct extension to skin or chest wall (3)
N_0 — No palpable lymph nodes (LNs) (1)
N_1 — Mobile LNs on same side (1/2)
N_2 — Fixed LN's on same side (3)
N_3 — Supraclavicular or infraclavicular LNs or arm lymphoedema (3)
M_0 — No evidence of distant metastases (1/2/3)
M_1 — Distant metastases present (4)

The presence of nodes in the axilla can be confounding. If nodes are palpable then they will not contain metastases on histological examination in

25% of cases, and likewise, 25% of nodes containing metastases will not be palpable. An accurate prognosis is important in deciding the treatment of the patient after surgery. Clinical staging, based on clinical findings, is not accurate and, therefore, is revised once further information, such as histology, becomes available.

Clinical Stages 1 and 2 are suitably treated by surgery. In later stages (Stage 3, Stage 4, locally advanced cancers or metastatic spread) surgery should be avoided. Fortunately, only 6% of presentations have Stage 4 disease.

The majority of patients have Stage 1 or 2 and arrangements are made to admit and resect the cancer. Patients with Stages 3 and 4 require further investigations, which would include a core biopsy of the primary cancer if not already performed for the sake of diagnosis, CAT scan of lungs and liver, bone scan and a full blood count. Investigations for metastatic disease in presumed Stage 1 or 2 disease are not performed. If the patient does not have symptoms or signs of metastatic disease then these tests can wait and should not delay admission. The treatment of advanced breast cancer is discussed later.

TREATMENT OF BREAST CANCER

This has been simplified by the results of large randomised controlled trials (RCTs) and the development of meta-analysis. In an RCT patients are randomly allocated to two or more treatments. The process of randomisation ensures that all variables (known and unknown) controlling the outcome of treatment are nullified apart from the treatment under study. Meta-analysis summates the outcome of trials with similar treatments and effectively improves the confidence in the outcome statistics. There are three outcome events in breast cancer; death from any cause, death from breast cancer and recurrence of the cancer. Combinations of these events may be reported, for example, recurrence-free survival.

The modalities of treatment are surgery, radiotherapy, endocrine therapy, cytotoxic chemotherapy and psychotherapy.

The treatment is usually discussed at the first visit to the clinic when a provisional diagnosis of breast cancer has been made. In most cases this explanation should be simplified. The dominant thought of the patient is whether a mastectomy is necessary and whether there is some effective treatment. The clinician needs to have a full knowledge of breast cancer and of the social circumstances of the patient, understand how to break bad news and judge the effect of his words on the patient. At the second visit within 3 days the patient should bring a friend, spouse or relative and a more detailed discussion can take place. The breast care nurse should be involved from the first visit and will provide support and education to the patient during the period of treatment and follow-up.

Clinical trials have shown that radical surgery, for example, mastectomy, axillary clearance and postoperative radiotherapy compared to wide local excision (WLE), limited axillary surgery and radiotherapy to the residual ipsilateral breast do not influence survival. Chemotherapy, either endocrine or cytotoxic, reduces the risk of recurrence and death by about 20%. These empirical trials have led to the hypothesis that recurrence and death are due to the growth of microscopic metastases (i.e. these are undetectable micrometastases) which are present in the majority of patients with Stage 1 or 2 breast cancer (so-called early breast cancer). Therefore, systemic therapy is necessary to alter survival. Surgery and local radiotherapy may still have an effect on survival, but this has not been tested in large trials. (It would be unethical to have a no-treatment group.) It is the magnitude of local treatment that has been tested. Therefore, the treatment of breast cancer can be categorised into the treatment of the primary breast cancer, treatment of the axilla and chemotherapy.

Treatment of the Breast

About 80% of patients are treated by WLE of the breast cancer followed by 50 Grays of external beam radiotherapy given 5 days a week for 5 weeks to the remaining ipsilateral breast. The majority of patients have microscopic multifocal disease in the affected breast. A booster dose of 10 Grays is given to the tumour bed in the sixth week. Radiotherapy reduces the risk of local recurrence in the breast from about 30% to about 7% over a follow-up period of 10 years. Simple mastectomy is performed if the lump is too large to remove without a good cosmetic result, if the nipple is involved, if the disease is obviously multifocal or if the patient chooses a mastectomy (which is now a rare event). Radiotherapy is not usually necessary after mastectomy. It compromises the subsequent reconstruction of the breast. Radical mastectomy involves mastectomy plus removal of the pectoralis muscles and is never performed in the UK nowadays. You may still see patients in the finals who have had this operation.

If the lump is impalpable (usually picked up by screening mammography) then stereotactic localisation is performed under mammographic control. A needle is placed into the area of microcalcification. The patient goes to theatre and has the area containing the needle and a surrounding margin excised. While the patient is still on the operating table the sample goes back (with the needle in it) to mammography, and is X-rayed to ensure that the entire area of calcification has been excised.

Occasionally a *frozen section* is needed. In this case the lump is removed and taken to the laboratory while the patient is still on the operating table, and the lump is frozen, sectioned and looked at under the microscope. The pathologist then rings the surgeon in theatre to report the result. If invasive breast cancer is confirmed, then the surgeon goes on to treat the axilla in the same operation. This would be used, for example, if a definitive diagnosis has not been established preoperatively. For example, radiology may fail to show a lobular carcinoma but FNAC has been reported as C4 or C5; or radiology suggests a breast cancer but it has not been confirmed by FNAC or core biopsy. Frozen section is never used to decide on the need to proceed to mastectomy. It is no longer an acceptable practice. The surgeon should always perform the operation defined on the consent form and no more.

Treatment of the Axilla

The number of lymph nodes in the axilla varies from 10 to 30. The presence of involved axillary lymph nodes is the single best predictor of survival from breast cancer (Figure 10.2). Treating the axilla does not probably affect survival. The hypothesis is that the cells of the primary breast cancer invade the local lymphatics and the local blood vessels with equal force. The number of local lymph nodes containing tumour reflects the probability of widespread micrometastases which have spread by the

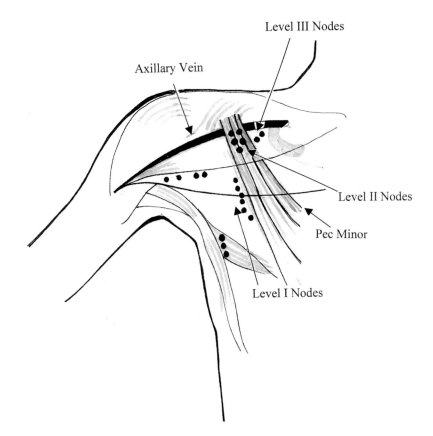

Figure 10.2. The axillary lymph nodes.

haematogenous route. The aim of treating the axilla is two-fold: first to prevent uncontrollable growth of cancer in the axilla and second to establish the prognosis (the risk of recurrence and death) of the patient.

There are two methods to determine whether nodes contain tumour. The first is to remove a critical number of nodes and submit them to histology or to excise the sentinel node, submit this for histology and perform a second operation on patients with tumour in this node. The sentinel node is the first node to be involved and can be detected by injecting blue dye 10 min before attempting to excise the node or by injecting radioactive material which emits gamma rays and using a gamma counter to detect the node with the highest count during the operation. Sentinel node biopsy is still unproven and is currently the subject of an RCT (almanac trial). The critical number of nodes is still uncertain. Axillary sampling involves removing the lower part of the axillary fat pad whereas axillary clearance involves removing the nodes up to the axillary vein (Level 1), medial border of pectoralis minor (Level 2) or border of the first rib (Level 3). The more extensive the node removal, the greater the risk of damage to the sensory nerves of the axilla (intercostobrachial nerves) and the development of lymphoedema of the breast, hand, forearm and/or arm.

The obvious advantage of sentinel node biopsy is that about 30–40% of patients will avoid axillary clearance and the morbidity associated with it. Axillary sampling and sentinel node biopsy (if the detected node is false negative) may leave the tumour behind and finally, if a patient has nodes involved at Level 3, then their prognosis is so poor that it is unlikely that they will survive for long enough to develop uncontrollable axillary disease. Thus, the extent of axillary surgery remains uncertain for an individual patient. In general, radiotherapy should not be given to the axilla after axillary clearance at any level because the risk of lymphoedema is greatly increased.

Pathology of Breast Cancer

Surgery provides the means to grade the breast cancer, count the number of lymph nodes involved with metastases, measure the true diameter of the primary and perform histochemistry using monoclonal antibodies against oestrogen and progesterone receptors and C-ERB-2 (Her2/Neu) antigen. Breast cancer is either *in situ* or invasive. The latter by definition has not breached the basement membrane of the duct and is potentially curable.

Carcinomas *In situ*

The commonest form of noninvasive cancer is DCIS, accounting for about 20% of screen-detected and 3% of symptomatic cancers. Untreated DCIS may progress to invasive breast cancer. About 20–30% of these patients will develop invasive breast cancer in 10 years. The introduction of the national screening programme has resulted in a marked increase in the incidence of this type of cancer. Lobular carcinoma *in situ* (LCIS) is the other type of noninvasive cancer. It is rarer and tends to be multifocal. The natural history of LCIS is uncertain.

Invasive Cancer

Invasive breast cancer is either a special named type (e.g. lobular, tubular, medullary, mucinous, papillary) or 'not otherwise specified' (NOS). Special types tend to have a better prognosis than NOS. About 80% of invasive breast cancer is NOS, so this is categorised into three grades based on the Bloom Richardson method, where the number of mitoses, the tubule formation and the degree of nuclear pleomorphism are scored and the total score used to assign the cases as Grade 1 (good prognosis), Grade 2 or Grade 3 (worst prognosis). The maximum tumour diameter is measured and finally the number of lymph nodes with and without metastases counted. Addition of these prognostic variables gives a reasonable assessment of the risk of recurrence and death. The number of involved nodes carries greater weight in this regression equation than the grading or tumour size. *Paget's disease of the nipple* is a unilateral red, eczematous lesion of the nipple and areola that may ulcerate and bleed. Histology of the skin shows infiltrating malignant cells. There is usually an underlying invasive or DCIS breast cancer. Treatment is usually mastectomy.

An accurate assessment of the prognosis allows us to assess the potential benefit of adjuvant chemotherapy. Overall, chemotherapy will reduce the risk of recurrence and death by 20%. Thus, if the risk of death in 5 years is 50% then 10 patients will be alive at 5 years as a result of treatment; if the risk is 10% then two patients will be alive as a result of treatment. This means that a proportion of patients will receive chemotherapy with no benefit. These are patients unresponsive to treatment and those who do not need the treatment because they would not have recurred. The potential benefit of chemotherapy has to be weighed against the toxicity of the treatment.

Systemic Chemotherapy

The majority of patients (>90%) now receive chemotherapy. This may be cytoxic chemotherapy or endocrine therapy or a combination of both. The type of chemotherapy given is based on the results of controlled trials which show the following. Adjuvant chemotherapy is more effective in women younger than 50 years of age than for older women. Combination chemotherapy and particularly that containing anthracylines are more effective than single-agent chemotherapy. Six cycles of cytotoxic chemotherapy given about once per month are sufficient. Adjuvant endocrine therapy has very little effect if the primary breast cancer does not contain oestrogen receptors. The optimal duration of Tamoxifen therapy is 5 years. Tamoxifen and Arimidex reduce the incidence of new or contralateral breast cancer. Ovarian ablation by oophorectomy or Zoladex effectively reduces the risk of recurrence and death from breast cancer in premenopausal women.

The combination of Tamoxifen and cytotoxic therapy is more effective than chemotherapy alone or Tamoxifen alone for patients with hormone-receptor-positive tumours.

If the primary tumour contains oestrogen receptors (ER) and progesterone receptors (PR) (produced by an intact ER pathway in the cancer cell) then Tamoxifen, 20 mg daily, is given for 5 years. Tamoxifen is an antagonist on the endometrium and increases the risk of endometrial cancer. At 5 years the risk of breast cancer recurrence is low and balanced by the risk of endometrial cancer. About 30% of women on Tamoxifen suffer menopausal symptoms (hot flushes, vaginal dryness and pruritis, loss of libido). The commonest cytotoxic chemotherapy regime given at the moment is FEC (5-fluorouracil, Epirubicin and cyclophosphamide) as six cycles for over about 6 months. The side effects include exhaustion, nausea, vomiting, hair loss, suppression of the bone marrow and infertility. There are other drugs available for the treatment of breast cancer. These include the Taxanes, Herceptin (a humanised monoclonal antibody which binds to the HER2/neu oncoprotein) and many others which are in various stages of development.

Based on the empirical results enumerated above, a premenopausal woman of 40 with a 2.5 cm Grade 3 NOS ductal carcinoma and two out of eight axillary nodes involved with tumour which is ER positive and HER2/neu negative would have a 5-year survival rate of about 70%. She would be advised to have FEC and Tamoxifen and asked whether she wishes to enter a clinical trial involving a treatment which compared this regime against this regime and the addition of one of the new drugs. She might accept this advice or wish to consider less toxic regimes. These discussions are complicated and may require at least two meetings with the oncologist and the breast care nurse. A postmenopausal woman of 65 with a Grade 2 breast cancer and zero out of six nodes involved would be treated with Tamoxifen or Arimidex for 5 years.

Treatment of Advanced Breast Cancer

Advanced breast cancer includes locally advanced breast cancer (Stage 3), metastatic breast cancer at presentation (Stage 4) and recurrent breast cancer. The investigation and treatment of these three separate groups of patients are very similar and depend on understanding the spread of the disease.

Like any other cancer, spread is by *direct extension* — to the muscle and chest wall, resulting in fixity, and to the skin, resulting in ulceration which may bleed and become infected; via *lymphatics* — of the breast leading to blockage of the lymphatics and oedema of the overlying skin, which becomes pitted by the adherence of the sweat ducts and hair follicles, leading to the appearance of peau d'orange and lymphoedema of the arm (direct extension from involved axillary nodes may cause axillary vein thrombosis and infiltration of the brachial plexus); *blood spread* — especially to the bones (resulting in bone pain and hypercalcaemia), lungs (dyspnoea and pleural effusion) and liver (abdominal pain and compromised liver function); and *transcoelomic spread* — for example, pleural seedings leading to a malignant pleural effusion. A bone scan, CAT scan of lungs and liver and full blood count and biochemistry will detect the majority of these potential problems.

It is essential to know the ER status of the tumour. A patient with a Stage 3 breast cancer and no evidence of metastases may be treated with endocrine therapy or cytotoxic chemotherapy. This so-called neo-adjuvant therapy often results in shrinkage of the primary tumour allowing surgical resection, which may be followed with more chemotherapy and radiotherapy. Local recurrence of a previously treated breast cancer (WLE) may be suitable for mastectomy if there are no metastases. Unfortunately, local recurrence in the breast or in the scar of a previous mastectomy within 5 years is often a sign of widespread metastatic disease.

If metastases are discovered then only 15% of patients will survive for 5 years; life expectancy (50% mortality) is 2–3 years. Treatment is therefore palliative. If the woman has no symptoms then there is a reasonable argument not to treat. Bone metastases are often painful and cause hypercalcaemia and pathological fractures. Hypercalcaemia is a medical emergency and is treated with hydration (IV saline), diuretics and bisphosphonates (e.g. pamidronate). Metastases in the lower long bones and in patients with pathological fractures of these bones require orthopaedic fixation. Painful fractures of the vertebral bodies may cause spinal cord compression and require urgent decompression and fixation. Bone pain in any site should be treated with bisphosphonates and radiotherapy. Patients with only bone metastases may have a good prognosis and should be treated with the expectation of a good response to chemotherapy. Patients with lung and/or liver metastases have a poorer prognosis, but again may respond to escalating chemotherapy using the newer agents. However, there will come a time when control of the tumour is lost and hospice care is all that remains. Judging when this is the case is difficult.

Treatment of DCIS (Usually Asymptomatic and Picked up by Screening Mammography)

Breast

WLE, may be under stereotactic guidance, and if the margins are clear and the tumour is small and not of an aggressive grade, then radiotherapy. If the margins are not clear, re-excise and treat as above. If the DCIS is extensive, involving large areas of the breast, or is multifocal, then the usual treatment is mastectomy with immediate reconstruction of the breast. Sentinel node biopsy should probably be undertaken for most cases of extensive DCIS, particularly if it is high grade and therefore liable to harbour microscopic areas of invasive carcinoma.

SCREENING FOR BREAST CANCER

Mortality from breast cancer may be reduced by 30% in women who attend screening by mammography. Breast self-examination does not affect the outcome of breast cancer. In 1986 the Forest Report was published. It took account of the Swedish screening programmes and made recommendations for the use of screening in the UK. Women between 50 and 65 are invited every 3 years for a single oblique mammogram (most centres now perform two-view mammography).

About 60 cancers per 10,000 attendees are picked up in the British screening programme. For the finals you need to be able to talk about any screening programme (generalised topic), namely, that the disease is a significant cause of mortality, that there is an effective treatment and that the test is simple, cheap, acceptable to the population and unambiguous in its interpretation, with high specificity and sensitivity.

Regarding breast cancer, you should think about the following points:

- The test (mammography) is expensive, requiring highly trained radiologists, and at best detects only 93% of breast cancers.
- Many women who are recalled are put through unnecessary investigations and worries (about two-thirds of women recalled are subsequently shown to have no cancer).
- Screen-detected cancers are more likely to be *in situ* than symptomatic cancers — are we, therefore, treating women who would never go on to develop invasive cancer?
- How frequently should women have a screening mammogram? In the UK we invite women every 3 years, because this is cost-effective. However, studies from other countries suggest that 2 years or less is more appropriate for picking up interval cancers (cancers presenting between screenings).

- How many views — one or two? Will two views detect more cancers? There are no convincing data to confirm this. Remember, women would receive double the radiation exposure.
- Should we stop screening at age 65? After all, the incidence of breast cancer continues to rise with increasing age.

Breast Reconstruction after Mastectomy

Reconstructive surgery should be available to any woman who requests it. It should be part of the preoperative counseling at the time that mastectomy is discussed. It can be carried out either at the time of mastectomy or later after a course of chemotherapy or years later if the woman wishes. The type of reconstruction depends on the patient and the surgeon. The Beckers prosthesis is a tissue expander which is placed under pectoralis major muscle. It consists of an inner bag of silicone and an outer sheath which can be inflated with saline through a port which is placed subcutaneously on the ribs inferior to the breast. The sheath is overinflated to cause tissue expansion and deflated after about 2 months so that the breast droops naturally (ptosis). The port is removed. The other technique is to create a myocutaneous flap which is placed in the defect created by the mastectomy. The flap is taken from latissimus dorsi and swung through the axilla into the defect or may be taken as a free flap from the lower part of rectus abdominis with the inferior epigastric artery anastomosed to the axillary artery or a branch thereof. The muscle of the flap is tacked onto the pectoralis major muscle and a silastic prosthesis is placed within this muscle pocket. The nipple is reconstructed in a subsequent operation. The aim of reconstruction is to create symmetry, so augmentation or reduction of the opposite breast may be necessary.

BENIGN BREAST DISEASE

Breast tissue naturally undergoes cyclical change during the menstrual cycle. Under the influence of oestrogen and progesterone during the luteal phase there is epithelial proliferation, increased tissue pressure and vascularity. This results in lumpy breast tissue which is tender and may be painful. Lumpy breast tissue may be focal and persistent. It forms the major differential diagnosis for breast cancer.

In most cases (>90%) triple assessment and review of the patient will define the diagnosis, but in the rare case of persistent lumpiness or C3 cytology, core biopsy or open operative biopsy may be necessary to rule out a diagnosis of breast cancer.

The histology of lumpy breast tissue may show epithelial hyperplasia, sclerosing adenosis, apocrine metaplasia and other pathological changes. It is only epithelial hyperplasia with pleomorphism of the cells and nuclei which is a risk factor for the development of breast cancer.

Benign discrete lumps in the breast are fibroadenoma, which consists of overgrowth of the collagenous mesenchyme which surrounds each terminal lobuloalveolar unit (TLAU) and usually presents before the age of 30; benign cystic disease of the breast, which usually presents in the 5–10 years prior to menopause, when the terminal ducts undergo apoptosis and leave an isolated TLAU which continues to produce fluid and fat necrosis, which is a brisk inflammatory response after an injury to the breast. Fibroadenomas can be treated conservatively or excised as a day case procedure. They occasionally grow to a great size (giant fibroadenoma). There are other rare conditions such as phylloides tumour, lymphoma, metastatic disease from other sites and chronic infections such as TB, but these are very small type differentials.

Breast Pain

Breast pain is either cyclical, occuring in the week prior to menses, or unrelated to the menstrual cycle. The former is common and usually lasts for four to five cycles, easing each time during or shortly after menses. It can be treated by blocking the effect of oestrogens on the breast using Tamoxifen or Danazol. However, these drugs have side effects and most women feel this overtreatment. Evening primrose oil may help but must be taken for at least 2 months. Noncyclical breast pain is a completely different condition. Characteristically, the women has suffered severe pain in the left breast with sudden lancing pains into the nipple for about a week. This is often associated with pain in the axilla and radiation down the arm. In about 15% of cases it is associated with back pain. After a week the pain settles into a chronic ache and she finds it painful lying on the side in bed or when she hugs her children. On examination there is marked tenderness at the parasternal border of Rib 3 or 4 and similar tenderness at the midaxillary on pressing the same rib. The cause of this condition, which affects the left side of the chest in 90% of cases, is a complete mystery. I suspect that it is related to the branches of the spinal nerve. It is called Tietze's syndrome or atypical breast pain and remains one of the great medical mysteries. The treatment is Ibuprofen as required.

Breast Infection

This most commonly affects women of childbearing age and can be divided into those related to lactation and those not related to lactation.

Lactational infection usually occurs during breast feeding. It presents with pain, swelling and tenderness. The usual organism is staph aureus, and antibiotics should be started (usually flucloxacillin). If an abscess develops, then this can be treated by repeated aspiration and antibiotics so that the woman can continue breast feeding. If the abscess persists, then breast feeding should be stopped with conversion of the baby to a bottle.

Nonlactational infection can affect the periareolar region and is often called periductal mastitis. Complications from this condition are commoner in women who smoke. The major ducts under the areola become dilated (duct ectasia), there may be a lymphocytic infiltrate in the interstitial tissues and the major complication is rupture of one or more of the ducts. This results in the development of a periareolar collection of pus-like fluid, which is usually sterile. In most cases the fluid is absorbed and the duct heals, but in other cases the collection ruptures through the skin or a surgeon is tempted to surgically drain the collection and a mammillary fistula is established. These are difficult to treat successfully. Excision of the whole major duct system may be necessary.

Discharge from the Nipple

Nipple discharges can be of many colours (blood-stained discharges are the most sinister) and can come from either a single duct or multiple ducts. Physiological nipple discharge is common and can range in colour from white to green or black. Other nonmalignant causes of discharge include a duct papilloma.

A duct papilloma may present with a blood-stained discharge from a single duct and the differential diagnosis includes an underlying carcinoma, which must therefore be excluded. A careful history should be taken and an examination performed. It is important to note whether a single duct or multiple ducts are involved. The secretion can be sent off for culture and cytology if there is enough of it. Some form of imaging of the breast is necessary in order to exclude an underlying cancer. If all the tests are normal and the discharge is from multiple ducts and not blood-stained, no treatment apart from reassurance is necessary. If the patient remains anxious or the discharge affects her lifestyle, or if a single duct is involved and is persistently blood-stained, then the affected duct can be removed by microdochectomy. In this procedure a probe is passed into the affected duct, which is excised and sent to histology.

11

LUMPS IN THE HEAD, NECK AND SKIN

Nigel Jones

Questions on lumps in the head, neck or skin are common in the finals, particularly in the short case section of the exam. Students often find these difficult, because they have not prepared separate techniques for examining the different types of lumps. It is easy to forget things under pressure, so you should prepare ways of assessing the common lumps in advance. Do not forget to look and feel inside the mouth and examine facial nerve function when you suspect a parotid lump, and remember to examine draining lymph node groups if there is any chance that a lump could be malignant. Remember also that common things occur commonly and that, as well as lumps specific to the head and neck, lumps such as sebaceous cysts, lipomas, neurofibromas and skin tumours on the head, neck or face are also common short cases in finals.

When any lump is examined you should think of the following list of features: site, size, shape, colour, contour (edge), consistency, compressibility (fluctuance), temperature, tenderness, tethering, transilluminance, pulsatility and spread (this means to examine the regional lymph nodes). This is easy to remember by: SSS, CCCC, TTTT and PS. When describing a lump you do not need to note each of these features — just the ones relevant to the particular lump. For example, a breast lump may be described as 'a 3 cm irregular, firm lump in the upper outer quadrant of the left breast, with no associated lymphadenopathy'.

LUMPS IN THE HEAD AND NECK

Triangles of the Neck

Conventionally, lumps in the neck are described in relation to certain anatomically defined landmarks. Lumps in the neck anterior to the anterior border of the sternocleidomastoid muscle are within the anterior triangle of the neck (its boundaries are the sternocleidomastoid, the midline and the lower border of the mandible). Lumps posterior to the anterior border of the sternomastoid are within the posterior triangle of the neck (boundaries — sternocleidomastoid, trapezius and the clavicle). The base of the posterior triangle is more commonly referred to as the supraclavicular fossa. Lumps under the jaw are in the submandibular region. Therefore, if you are shown a lump in the neck, decide into which triangle it fits and you may almost have the diagnosis already (Figure 11.1). Remember that lymph nodes can occur in any of the areas (including the parotid) and can be multiple or single, while lumps in the midline are invariably of the thyroid gland or are thyroglossal cysts.

Branchial Cysts

Branchial cysts are relatively rare in practice but are common in examinations! They are believed to represent retained elements of the second branchial cleft which have failed to disappear during embryological development. However, they are not present at birth but appear subsequently, usually in young adult life. They are lined by squamous epithelium and are often surrounded by lymphoid tissue. They contain so-called 'glary' fluid containing cholesterol crystals. On examination a branchial cyst will usually be a swelling emerging from the anterior border of the sternomastoid muscle at the junction of its upper and middle thirds. These should usually be excised because secondary infection can occur and lead to recurring bouts of infection.

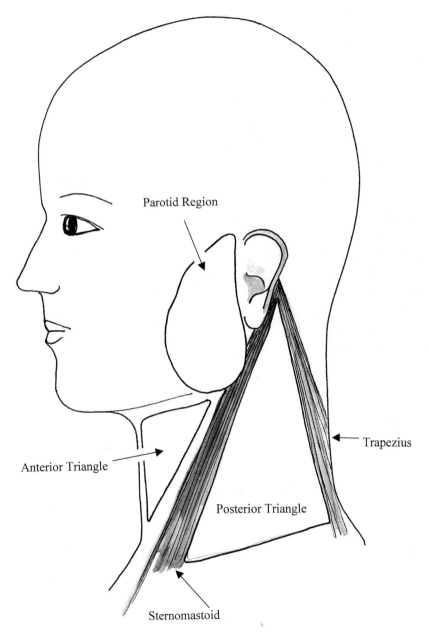

Figure 11.1. The triangles of the neck.

Branchial Sinus or Fistula

This presents as a small opening in the lower third of the neck at the anterior border of the sternomastoid. Treatment is by excision, which may be difficult because the track can extend back to the lateral pharyngeal wall through the fork of the carotid artery.

Cystic Hygroma

This is a lump which usually presents in infancy. It is usually found in the lower part of the posterior triangle but can also extend into the axilla. If missed at birth it can present in childhood. It is also known as a cavernous lymphangioma, because histologically it consists of multiple lymph-filled spaces. Clinically, it is soft and poorly compressible. It increases in size when the child cries or coughs and is said to be brilliantly translucent when transilluminated. You are unlikely to see a case in the finals, but it is commonly asked about. Treatment is by excision but recurrence is possible.

Dermoids

These are congenital inclusions found at sites of embryological fusion, such as the angles of the eyebrow and under the tongue. They are often in the midline. They are not common but may be asked about. Treatment is by excision.

Pharyngeal Pouch

(These are usually not palpable: see section on oesophageal disorders.)

Carotid Body Tumours

Carotid body tumours, also called chemodectomas, arise from the cells of the carotid body found at the carotid bifurcation. They usually present as asymptomatic lumps in the neck and can be bilateral. Patients are usually middle-aged or elderly. Most of these tumours are benign, although about 10% may be malignant and 5% may metastasize. Clinically, they should be suspected when a lump in front of the sternomastoid muscle has a strongly transmitted pulsation. Investigations include imaging with CT, power Doppler ultrasound and MRI. On angiography the characteristic appearance is of splaying apart of the carotid bifurcation (the goblet sign).

Treatment consists of excision by a surgeon used to dealing with the carotid artery.

Thyroid Gland

Lumps in the thyroid are very common in the clinical section of the finals, although the management of thyrotoxicosis and myxoedema per se is usually considered under 'medicine'. In the short cases listen very carefully to what the examiner asks you to do. If asked to 'examine the thyroid' you should start with the hands, etc. If asked to 'examine the neck' you should just examine the neck and only then do a more general examination of the thyroid, including hands and eyes if you think the lump is in the thyroid gland.

First, inspect the neck from the front, looking for masses. If a mass is seen, ascertain if it moves up on swallowing. This is best done by asking the patient to take a mouthful of water. A glass of water next to a patient in the finals is often a clue that it is a thyroid patient. If there is no glass of water, always ask the examiners for one. Next, feel the neck. This is usually best done by standing behind the patient, but first check that the trachea is central by placing a finger in the suprasternal notch. From behind palpate the thyroid. If a lump is present decide on its size and whether it is solitary, multiple or a diffuse enlargement of the whole gland. Again, ask the patient to take a mouthful of water and see if the lump moves upwards on swallowing. Now feel for cervical lymphadenopathy and other neck lumps. Then, go around to the front again, look into the mouth for any lingual thyroid (at the back of the tongue) and percuss over the sternum for dullness (which may indicate retrosternal extension) and listen for a bruit (present in the thyrotoxic patient when the thyroid is very vascular). If you suspect thyroid disease, then the hands are inspected for temperature, tremor, pulse rate (tachycardic or AF). There are five eye signs that go with Graves' disease (exopthalmos, lid retraction, lid lag, opthalmoplegia and chemosis).

If the thyroid feels normal, examine for lymphadenopathy or any other lumps. If you cannot feel any lumps and there are no skin lesions, then check the neck pulses, listen for bruits and test sensation and neck movements. If you are asked to examine 'the neck' of a patient, it is perfectly reasonable to examine as above and then say: 'This lady has a 4 × 4 cm lump just to the left of the midline that moves upwards on swallowing. This is consistent with a lump in the left lobe of the thyroid gland. The lump is firm, with a smooth contour. I could not feel any other lumps or any associated lymphadenopathy. The trachea is central. There is no retrosternal extension detectable clinically and I could not hear a bruit on auscultation. I would now like to examine this patient for signs of thyroid disease'. The examiner will then either tell you to go on or, more likely, ask you what you would look for.

Goitre

The word 'goitre' means any swelling of the thyroid gland. The pathology books can make the causes of goitre very complicated, but from a clinical perspective the situation is more straightforward. First, ascertain whether the swelling appears to involve the whole thyroid gland or whether it is a swelling in just part of the thyroid gland. This can be attempted on clinical examination, but in practice nowadays many goitres will require an ultrasound scan to fully decide this. Ultrasound also provides the opportunity for fine needle aspiration cytology of a solid lesion or aspiration of a cyst.

Causes of Goitre

1. *Diffusely swollen thyroid*
   - Graves disease (thyrotoxicosis in a younger person)
   - Hashimoto's thyroiditis (an autoimmune condition)

- Iodine deficiency/puberty/pregnancy or ingestion of goitrogens (rare)
- Multinodular colloid goitre with nodules too small to feel
- Rarely De Quervain's thyroiditis (also called subacute thyroiditis — usually a self-limiting condition)

2. *Multiple nodules in the gland*
   - Multinodular colloid goitre (the commonest thyroid swelling to be seen in the finals)
   - Multiple cysts
   - Multiple adenomas

3. *Solitary nodule in the gland*
   - Cyst
   - Tumour (benign or malignant, primary or rarely secondary)
   - Dominant single nodule in multinodular goitre

Multinodular Colloid Goitre

This is thought likely to be an autoimmune condition. It is more common in middle-aged women and there may be a family history. The goitre may be asymptomatic; however, it may be a cosmetic worry to the patient or it may actually be causing symptoms, usually by pressure on adjacent structures, i.e. dysphagia (pressure on the oesophagus) and stridor (pressure on the trachea). In the longer term it may lose its capacity to function, resulting in hypothyroidism. If it is asymptomatic, no intervention is likely to be required other than reassurance and tests to exclude a carcinoma. If it is causing symptoms, then usually a thyroidectomy will be performed. For benign colloid goitre the choice lies between a subtotal or total thyroidectomy. In the former a small amount of thyroid is preserved in relation to the superior thyroid artery to protect the parathyroid glands and recurrent laryngeal nerves and also to retain some thyroid tissue to produce thyroxine and prevent hypothyroidism.

Solitary Thyroid Nodules

Clinical examination and ultrasound can determine whether the goitre consists of a single nodule or multiple nodules. However, the mainstay of diagnosis is by fine needle aspiration for cytology which can be carried out in out-patients. This can also be under ultrasound guidance if lumps are small or close to the carotid arteries.this is very good at making a diagnosis, although it cannot differentiate between follicular adenomas and follicular carcinomas. As discussed above, multiple nodules are usually benign, whereas solitary nodules may be malignant. Occasionally, a radioisotope scan is performed if the thyroid function tests show hyperthroidism, to look for a toxic nodule.a nodule is said to be 'cold' if it fails to take up radioiodine. Such a cold nodule has a 10% chance of being malignant. Radioisotope scanning has less of a role than it used to have.

Fine needle aspiration (if necessary under ultrasound guidance) should be the first-line investigation of any thyroid lump. However, if the lump is clinically suspicious, a hemithyroidectomy may be performed to get a histological diagnosis.

Thyroid Cysts

May present as a lump or may cause pressure symptoms. Local pain caused by bleeding into the cyst can be troublesome.The important thing is to rule out malignancy. An FNA may be all that is required to show this is a simple cyst. An ultrasound scan will help if the diagnosis is in doubt. Treatment is by aspiration, but the cyst may require excision if cytology dictates or if it recurs.

Thyroid Function Tests

Thyroxine (T4) is the hormone produced by the thyroid. It is converted to the active hormone tri-iodothyronine (T3). The thyroid-stimulating hormone (TSH) is produced by the pituitary and stimulates T4 production. There is a negative feedback mechanism in action.

- T3 and T4 are low and TSH is high in hypothyroidism
- T3 and T4 are high and TSH is low in hyperthyroidism
- T3 and T4 are normal and TSH is low in patients on adequate doses of T4

Before any patient with thyroid disease is operated on, it is essential to know the thyroid status by sending off thyroid function tests (TFTs). Hyperthyroid patients must be controlled preoperatively with antithyroid drugs (usually carbimazole), and betablockers may be used. Lack of control might cause a thyroid crisis. Some surgeons insist on having the vocal cords checked preoperatively to document any abnormalities prior to surgery.

Primary Thyroid Tumours

It must be emphasised that solitary nodules are benign 90% and malignant 10% of the time. Fine needle aspiration cytology usually dictates management.

1. *Adenomas.* These are benign and may be either functioning (causing hyperthyroidism and appearing 'hot' on a thyroid isotope scan) or non-functioning (appearing 'cold' on a thyroid isotope scan). Treatment is usually by hemithyroidectomy and removal of the isthmus.
2. *Papillary carcinoma (70%).* This occurs in younger patients. It has the best prognosis of thyroid cancers. It is often multifocal. Spread to cervical lymph nodes occurs but may not alter the good prognosis.Treatment is usually by hemithyroidectomy for doubtful cytology. If initial cytology gives a confident report then total thyroidectomy is done. Following a hemithyroidectomy, if the lesion is bigger than 1 cm, a completion total thyroidectomy is done. Since the tumour is sensitive to iodine, the patient is usually given radioiodine to target the metastases after a total thyroidectomy, postoperatively, so that it does not get concentrated in the thyroid gland. In a patient treated by hemithyroidectomy alone thyroxine must be given to suppress TSH levels to less than 0.1.
3. *Follicular carcinoma (25%).* This is also found in young adults and is characterised by follicular appearance on histology. It has a good prognosis if appropriately treated, though prognosis is poorer in older patients. When it spreads, metastases are blood borne. It cannot be confidently diagnosed on cytology and so a hemithyroidectomy is the usual initial treatment. In 10% of these cases a carcinoma rather than an adenoma is confirmed. The patient then has a completion

thyroidectomy unless the lesion is 1 cm in size or less. Since the tumour is sensitive to iodine, the patient is usually given radioiodine to target the metastases after a total thyroidectomy, postoperatively, so that it does not get concentrated in the thyroid gland. Thyroxine is given for TSH suppression again to hemithyroidectomy patients.

4. *Medullary cell carcinoma (5%)*. This is a tumour derived from the calcitonin-producing C-cells. It is relatively rare and is part of the MEN-I syndrome. Cytology would pick this tumour up preoperatively and diagnosis would be confirmed by calcitonin measurement. Treatment is by total thyroidectomy. It does not take up radioiodine.

5. *Anaplastic carcinoma (rare)*. This is a highly aggressive and locally invasive tumour and is seen in older patients. The history is of rapid increase in size over about 6 weeks. It is usually incurable, and treatment is usually palliative but may involve a tracheostomy and external beam radiotherapy.

6. *Lymphomas*. Lymphomas, both Hodgkin's and non-Hodgkin's, may arise within the thyroid gland. This is suspected in a big goitre that is rubbery and has recently enlarged. Diagnosis should be made by fine needle aspiration and open biopsy may be needed to classify the lymphoma. Treatment is primarily with chemotherapy which will also treat involved lymph nodes. Surgical excision is less often needed. Lymphoma may develop in a gland affected by Hashimoto's thyroiditis.

COMPLICATIONS OF THYROID SURGERY

A relatively common question in surgical finals relates to the complications of thyroid surgery (1–4) or, alternatively, what you would warn someone about who is going to have thyroid surgery (2–4). The following should be the basics of such an answer:

1. *Acute haemorrhage*. Bleeding into the neck after thyroidectomy can be a life-threatening complication, as it can cause acute airway obstruction. If you are called to a patient in whom this is occurring, first call the on-call anaesthetist who may need to intubate the patient. The clips should be immediately removed but deeper sutures may need cutting

before the haematoma can be evacuated. The patient should be taken to theatre for the wound to be explored and bleeding stopped. This occurs in less than 1 in 100 operations.

2. The *recurrent laryngeal nerve* runs close to the posterior aspect of the thyroid gland and is at risk during thyroidectomy unless it is specifically identified and preserved. Damage may occur when tying the inferior thyroid artery or at the point of insertion into the larynx. Damage to one recurrent laryngeal nerve causes hoarseness of the voice; damage to both causes airway obstruction requiring tracheostomy (because the neutral position of the vocal cord is in the midline).

3. *Damage to the parathyroid glands.* This may be due to poor blood supply or inadvertent excision. This produces hypocalcaemia resulting in tetany. The two physical signs often asked about are Chvostek's sign and Trousseau's sign. Chvostek's sign is when twitching of the facial muscles occurs on tapping over the facial nerve at the posterior aspect of the parotid gland. Trousseau's sign is when carpal spasm is produced by blowing up a blood pressure cuff on the upper arm.

4. *Hypothryoidism*, due to lack of functioning thyroid tissue.

Thyroglossal Cyst

In embryological development the thyroid starts at the foramen caecum at the back of the tongue and descends to its final position, passing close to the hyoid bone. Remnants can be left at any point along this line of descent, including a very rare lingual thyroid (i.e. thyroid tissue at the back of the tongue). Care needs to be taken before excision of a lingual thyroid, in case it is the patient's only functioning thyroid tissue. The classical features of a thyroglossal cyst are that it is in the midline of the neck and rises upwards on protrusion of the tongue. They can become infected. Excision involves excision of the central portion of the hyoid bone and may require dissections as far as the back of the tongue. A thyroglossal fistula can also occur, again usually in the midline, but is not actually congenital; it usually occurs following infection or inadequate surgical removal of a thyroglossal cyst.

Parathyroid Glands

The parathyroids only very rarely produce a palpable neck lump (in fact it is so rare that it should probably never be suggested in the finals). The management of hyperparathyroidism is, however, a common question.

Most cases of hyperparathyroidism are discovered by finding an elevated calcium on routine investigation. Remember that the symptoms of hypercalcaemia are 'bones, stones, psychic moans and abdominal groans' and that hyperparathyroidism can be either of the following:

- *Primary*, i.e. spontaneous (85% due to an adenoma of one gland, 15% due to diffuse hyperplasia of all four glands). In most adenomas parathormone-related protein (PTH-rP) is produced.
- *Secondary*, where hyperparathyroidism is secondary to a low-serum calcium such as is found in chronic renal failure and malabsorption syndromes (the PTH is therefore high, with a low- or normal serum calcium).
- *Tertiary*, where in long-standing secondary hyperparathyroidism the gland has become autonomous (high PTH and normal or high calcium).

The surgical treatment of hyperparathyroidism is exploration of the neck through an incision similar to that used for thyroidectomy and identification of all four parathyroids. If the cause is an adenoma, it is removed. If it is hyperplasia of all four glands, then all four glands are removed.

Salivary Glands

The salivary glands consist of the parotid, the submandibular, the sublingual and other minor salivary glands.

The parotid region is that part of the face in front of the ear and below the zygomatic arch. The gland is delineated into superficial and deep portions by the branches of the facial nerve. This is why you should examine VII nerve function and also why it is so important clinically to recognise that a lump may be in the parotid gland as simple excision could result in a VII nerve palsy. The operation to remove most superficial lesions of the parotid (superficial parotidectomy) involves making a long incision in front of the ear and down onto the neck, and identifying the facial nerve as it enters the parotid gland. The branches of the facial nerve are then followed forward and the superficial part of the parotid gland dissected off them. If a parotid lump is easily palpable when examined bimanually with a finger in the mouth, it may be in the deep portion of the gland and excision is then associated with a much higher risk of damaging the VII nerve. The facial nerve supplies the muscles of facial expression, so test the nerve by asking the patient to smile, show you his teeth and close his eyes.

Acute Parotitis

The parotid gland is surrounded by a tough fibrous capsule, and when it swells, as in acute parotitis, the stretching of the capsule causes severe pain. This condition may be due to viral infection (mumps, coxsackie A and others) or bacterial infection. Bacterial infections usually arise because of obstruction of the duct, usually due to calculus, or because of reduced salivary flow, such as in the postoperative patient or sick dehydrated patient from other causes. This is why mouth care is so important in such patients. Acute bacterial parotitis may result in abscess formation. You are unlikely to see a patient with this in the finals.

Salivary Calculi

Submandibular calculi are the most common type of salivary calculi and may be demonstrated by a plain X-ray or by contrast injection into the salivary duct (called a sialogram). The typical history would be of pain and swelling of the gland in question on eating (due to the production of saliva in an obstructed gland). If the stone is in the submandibular duct in the floor of the mouth, the calculus may be intraorally palpable and easily removed surgically. If it is within the submandibular gland itself, then removal of the whole gland will be required. Parotid calculi are also reasonably common but not usually palpable or easily seen on a plain X-ray. Sialography is usually required to demonstrate them (remember that the duct opens opposite the second upper molar).

Salivary Gland Neoplasms

Salivary neoplasms are common cases in finals. They are usually in the parotid gland (75% of all salivary neoplasms are in the parotid). Most of them are pleiomorphic adenomas.

- *Pleiomorphic adenoma* (mixed salivary tumour). This is the commonest salivary neoplasm. It is called pleiomorphic because histologically it appears to be made up of different types of tissue. Ninety per cent occur within the parotid. They are slow-growing and benign but the tumours have microprocesses which invade locally and make them prone to recur locally if treated by simple enucleation. They need formal excision by superficial parotidectomy.
- *Adenolymphoma (Warthin's tumour)*. This is a benign cystic tumour which contains epithelial lymphoid elements. It occurs in middle and old age and gives rise to a soft, well-defined cystic lump in the parotid.
- *Adenoid-cystic carcinoma*. This is a highly malignant tumour of the parotid gland. It often causes facial nerve palsies, unlike benign parotid tumours, and is usually hard and fixed on examination. It is often incurable.

SKIN LUMPS

Most of the surgically important skin conditions present as 'lumps'. You will be expected to be able to examine and describe them and arrive at a reasonable list of differential diagnoses. For many skin lumps, however, the final diagnosis may only be made after excision biopsy, usually under local anaesthetic.

BENIGN LESIONS

Lipomas

These are very common 'lumps' in the finals. They are benign tumours of adipose tissue. Typically, they consist of a soft swelling not fixed to skin or deeper structures. The edge may be difficult to define in some cases and the swelling may be fluctuant since fat is liquid at body temperature. Dercum's disease is a condition which runs in families where patients have multiple subcutaneous lipomata. Lipomas need removing if they are causing a problem to the patient or are unsightly. Very rarely, a large lipoma can give rise to a liposarcoma.

Neurofibromas

These are benign tumours of nerves which may be multiple and part of von Recklinghausen's neurofibromatosis and associated with café au lait patches. If required, the diagnosis is made by excision biopsy of one of the lesions. They are usually small, firm, smooth, and not fixed to skin or deeper structures.

Sebaceous Cysts

These follow obstruction to the mouth of a sebaceous duct. They are common on the scalp but can occur anywhere except the soles and the palms (which do not have sebaceous glands). Typically they form a round, soft swelling attached to the skin but not deeper structures. A central puctum may be visible and usually clinches the diagnosis. Sebaceous cysts contain cheesy material which smells and may become infected. Less commonly, they may ulcerate or form a sebaceous horn. They are usually simply removed under local anaesthetic.

Benign Naevi (Pigmented Moles)

Surgically, the main importance of benign naevi is in the differential diagnosis of malignant skin lesions, principally malignant melanoma.

Papillomas

Papillomas arise from either squamous or basal layers of the skin. They include:

- Infective warts — due to viral infection.
- Keratin horns.
- Basal cell (seborrhoeic or senile) warts. These occur in elderly patients and are often multiple and may be pigmented flat discs.
- Pedunculated papillomas (skin tags). These are of no medical significance but may need removing if they are catching on clothes or are a worry cosmetically.

Campbell de Morgan Spots

These red spots appear as patients grow older and are of no clinical significance. They need no treatment.

MALIGNANT LESIONS

Melanomas

The incidence of malignant melanoma is rising sharply. Exposure to ultraviolet radiation is thought to be the major aetiological factor (especially sunburn as a child).

Melanomas are highly malignant tumours derived from melanocytes and need to be diagnosed and removed early if a cure is to follow. Fair or red-haired individuals are at the highest risk. The commonest sites are the torso in males and the legs in females (suggesting that sun exposure is a risk factor). Rare sites include the nail bed, the anorectal junction and the choroid in the eye. If you come across a patient in the exam with a glass eye and an enlarged liver, think melanoma!

Any mole which either grows or appears rapidly, changes shape or colour, itches, ulcerates or bleeds should be regarded as suspicious and removed. You should examine the regional lymph nodes. The types include

- Superficial spreading melanomas (about 80%) — these grow slowly and metastasise late, and have a better prognosis.
- Nodular melanomas — these invade deeply and metastasise early, and have a poorer prognosis.

Total excisional biopsy is the method of choice for diagnosis, although in some circumstances (for example, in a huge lesion) a partial biopsy is necessary.

You need to be familiar with two staging systems used for melanomas. The *Breslow thickness* is the depth of the tumour in millimetres and gives a good indication of the prognosis. Another system is *Clark's staging*, which breaks down the depth into five anatomical levels (e.g. Stage I — confined to the epidermis; Stage V — penetrated into the subcutaneous fat). In practice, the two are combined together with the histological grade to give a more accurate stage.

Prognosis

The thickness of the primary tumour is the single most important prognostic factor for patients with no evidence of distant spread. As a rough guide the following table lists the 5-year survival rates based on the depth:

Thickness (mm)	Five-Year Survival (%)
<0.76	96–99
0.76–1.50	87–94
1.51–4.0	66–77
>4.0	<50

Tumours in the BANS areas (back, arms, neck and scalp) tend to do worse than tumours on the periphery. Women seem to survive longer than men, and this may be due in part to their having more tumours on the legs than men. Various histological types (such as those with increased mitoses) and those with satellite lesions (implying that the dermal lymphatics are involved) have a worse prognosis. Ulceration is a poor prognostic indicator.

The surgical margins for resection are still controversial but, as a rough guide, impalpable lesions (thought to be <1 mm) should have a 1 cm margin, whereas thicker palpable lesions (>1.5 mm) should have a 2–3 cm clearance. Survival is independent of the width of excision, but local recurrence may not be. Dissection of the regional lymph nodes is again a controversial subject, but most surgeons would agree that this should only be performed if they are clinically palpable.

Other modalities used include chemotherapy and isolated limb perfusion, although with limited success, and prognosis is not greatly improved. Close follow-up of out-patients is important in order to detect recurrence early.

Basal Cell Carcinomas

Basal cell carcinomas (BCCs) are very common lesions and are often asked about in the finals or seen as short cases. They are low grade malignancies, rarely metastasising, but they can erode into bone or other adjacent structures if they are left to grow large enough. Exposure to sunlight is a risk factor but they do not occur until middle age or later. Ninety per cent are found on the face, usually above a line from the lobe of the ear to the corner of the mouth. Early lesions consist of a raised pearly pink papule with fine telangectasia over it. Later, the lesion ulcerates and is often called a 'rodent ulcer'. Treatment is usually by surgical excision, although cryotherapy or radiotherapy is sometimes used.

Squamous Cell Carcinomas

Squamous cell carcinomas (SCCs) are less common than BCCs, but once again exposure to sunlight is a risk factor. With these and BCCs a cumulative effect of UV light appears to be important, whereas with melanomas short periods of intense exposure (burns) appear to be responsible.

SCCs are more malignant than BCCs and may arise in pre-existing lesions such as leg ulcers (where they are called Marjolin's ulcers). Metastasis is often to regional lymph nodes, which should always be examined. Treatment is by excision, with radiotherapy being used to treat recurrence or involved lymph nodes.

Bowen's Disease

This is characterised by single or multiple brownish plaques, usually well defined and slightly raised and scaly. It is an intraepidermal squamous carcinoma. This often occurs on the legs of elderly women.

Kaposi's Sarcoma

This tumour is increasingly seen because of its association with HIV. It usually consists of raised purplish nodules which may be single or multiple.

12

HERNIAS

Hernias are common cases in surgical finals and are also often asked about in the written papers. Their assessment is usually straightforward if a common sense approach to their examination and management has been developed and practised.

DEFINITIONS

A fairly common question is to ask you to define a hernia. We would suggest the use of the following definition:

> A hernia is the protrusion of a viscus or part of a viscus through the walls of its containing cavity into an abnormal position.

When writing an answer on hernias, remember that they can also occur in sites away from the abdomen, such as when there is herniation of the brain through the foramen magnum with raised intracranial pressure or herniation of a muscle through a fascial defect in the leg. These other types of hernia should be mentioned for a complete written answer, although they should certainly not be more than a small part of any general answer about hernias. In the clinical section of the exam, however, you are very unlikely to see anything other than abdominal hernias. Abdominal hernias may be external (i.e. they emerge to the subcutaneous tissues as with inguinal hernias — so there is a lump to feel) or internal (such as with hiatus hernias, where there is no lump to feel).

There are a number of terms applied to (abdominal) hernias and it is worth defining these:

- *Sac.* The sac is the peritoneal lining of the hernia. Within it are the contents of the hernia (usually intestine or omentum). The sac may be complete or incomplete (i.e. not surrounding all the contents), as is found in a sliding hernia.
- *Neck.* The neck of a hernia is the margin of the defect through which the hernia has emerged.
- *Reducible.* A hernia is reducible when its contents can return to the abdominal cavity either spontaneously or with manipulation.
- *Irreducible.* The hernia cannot be reduced despite pressure or manipulation.
- *Incarcerated.* This term is usually used to describe an irreducible hernia where the irreducibility is due to adhesions within the sac in the absence of obstruction or strangulation. Some textbooks, however, define it as meaning a hernia which is irreducible because of faeces within the large bowel. Perhaps because of this confusion about the true definition of this term, it is best simply to refer to a hernia as being irreducible but not obstructed or strangulated.
- *Obstructed.* The bowel within the hernia is obstructed. The patient may have the four cardinal signs of obstruction (pain, vomiting, distention and constipation).
- *Strangulated.* The blood supply to the contents of the hernia is occluded by pressure at the neck of the hernia. If the bowel is within the sac, the viability of the bowel is impaired. Usually, the veins are occluded first and then further swelling leads to arterial occlusion, which precedes gangrene developing. If the hernia contains only omentum, then this too can strangulate, but in this case bowel obstruction does not occur.
- *Sliding hernia.* A sliding hernia is one which contains a partially extraperitoneal structure, such as the caecum on the right or the sigmoid colon on the left. Therefore, the sac does not completely surround all the contents of the hernia. The importance of this is that particular care must be taken when excising the sac, to avoid damaging the bowel.
- *Richter's hernia* (see Figure 12.1). This is where just part of the bowel wall is caught in the sac, and may become strangulated.

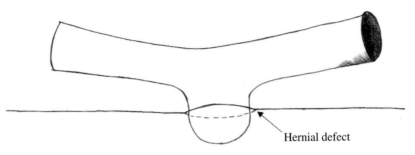

Hernial defect

Figure 12.1. Richter's hernia.

Because only part of the bowel wall is in the sac, the patient is not usually obstructed.

- *Herniotomy.* This term is used to describe ligation and excision of the hernia sac.
- *Herniorrhaphy.* This term is used for actual repair of the hernial defect.

HERNIAL DEFECT

The natural progression of a groin hernia could therefore be that the patient notices a lump in the groin that is reducible, and this may go on for years. Then, one day, the lump becomes irreducible, implying that it had become incarcerated. The patient may be well at this point. The lump may then become painful and the overlying skin reddened, implying strangulation (he may or may not have symptoms of obstruction, depending on whether there is bowel within it). At this point this becomes a surgical emergency and the patient requires an urgent operation to relieve the ischaemia.

CLASSIFICATION OF HERNIAS

Hernias require a defect in the wall of their normal cavity for their formation. This defect may be of two types:

- Congenital
- Acquired

Congenital

The commonest types of congenital hernias are inguinal and umbilical hernias appearing in childhood.

Infantile inguinal hernias are usually seen in males. In males, when the testes develop and descend *in utero* they pass down and through the abdominal wall into the scrotum, forming what will subsequently develop into the inguinal canal. As this happens a finger-like projection of peritoneum, called the processus vaginalis, is carried down with the testicle. This usually obliterates, but if it remains patent fluid or abdominal contents may enter down it, forming either a hydrocoele (fluid around the testicle) or a hernia (containing bowel or omentum). The treatment is simple operative ligation of the processus vaginalis, i.e. a herniotomy. *Umbilical hernias* are commonly seen in infants and represent failure of complete obliteration of the umbilical opening. They often disappear spontaneously and rarely strangulate. Surgical repair should therefore be reserved for those which persist after the age of five and those with a defect greater than 1 cm in size.

Acquired

To acquire a hernia, a weakness of the abdominal wall has to be produced. The following may be predisposing factors:

- Chronic cough
- Chronic constipation (and straining to pass faeces)
- Straining to void urine (prostatism)
- Severe muscular effort (heavy lifting)
- Obesity
- Weakening with age
- Surgery

GROIN HERNIAS

Groin hernias are the commonest type of hernia encountered in the finals, and indeed they account for about 75% of all hernias. They may be either femoral or inguinal. Inguinal hernias are further divided into direct and indirect. Inguinal hernias are proportionally more common in males than in females, and femoral hernias are proportionally more common in females than in males (possibly because of a wider pelvis and, hence, femoral canal). In both sexes, however, inguinal hernias are more common than femoral hernias in absolute numbers. Hernias may present in three ways:

1. As a lump (which may come and go; classically, the lump would appear on straining or lifting and disappear on lying down or when pressed on by the patient).
2. With pain in the groin.
3. Because of a complication (obstruction or strangulation).

To understand groin hernias properly, some basic anatomical knowledge is required.

Femoral Hernias

Femoral hernias emerge through the femoral canal, which normally contains only fat and lymph nodes. The medial border of the femoral ring (the upper and widest part of the femoral canal) is the sharp-edged lacunar ligament, which makes these hernias more prone to strangulation than inguinal hernias. Anteriorly is the inguinal ligament, posteriorly is the pectineal ligament and laterally is the femoral vein. Consideration of the position of the femoral canal will show why these hernias emerge below and lateral to the pubic tubercle. If identified, all femoral hernias should be repaired because of the risk of strangulation. Elective repair involves excision of the sac (herniotomy) and repair (herniorrhaphy), usually by suturing the inguinal ligament to the pectineal ligament with interrupted nonabsorbable sutures. Emergency repair is similar but usually utilises an incision through the inguinal canal or abdominal wall so that the bowel can be carefully assessed for strangulation and a bowel resection performed if necessary.

Inguinal Hernias

Inguinal hernias emerge into the subcutaneous tissues through the superficial inguinal ring and thus emerge above and medial to the pubic tubercle (see Figure 12.2). They have, however, left the abdominal cavity above and lateral to the pubic tubercle to enter the inguinal canal. This point often confuses finals students, especially as in a thin patient a cough impulse or hernia bulge can be seen or palpated above and lateral to the pubic tubercle beneath the external oblique aponeurosis (i.e. it is within the inguinal canal and has not yet emerged from the superficial inguinal ring).

Inguinal hernias are classified into direct and indirect. Indirect hernias leave the abdominal cavity through the deep inguinal ring along with the structures of the spermatic cord. Some of these may be due to a patent processus vaginalis (see 'infantile hernias') which has not presented until adult life. Direct inguinal hernias enter the inguinal canal 'directly' through a weakness or defect in its posterior wall. Both then emerge through the superficial inguinal ring. Indirect hernias, because of their close association with the spermatic cord, often then extend down into the scrotum. Direct hernias rarely extend into the scrotum. Students are often asked in exams to assess whether a groin hernia is inguinal or femoral. The key to this is the position of the pubic tubercle in relation to the point where the hernia emerges into the subcutaneous tissues. A hernia emerging above and medial to the pubic tubercle is an inguinal hernia, whereas a hernia emerging below and lateral is a femoral hernia. Sometimes a hernia is so large that it may appear anywhere in relation to the pubic tubercle. In this case the key is to reduce the hernia, place your finger on the pubic tubercle and ask the patient to cough and see where the lump emerges from.

Once a diagnosis of an inguinal hernia is made, students may be asked to comment as to whether they feel the hernia is direct or indirect. To our mind this is largely an unfair and pointless exercise, since good studies have shown that even consultant surgeons are often wrong when it comes to this assessment; the only way to be certain is to see which it is at the operation, and anyway it does not alter the surgical approach. However, if asked you must be able to carry out the relevant assessment with skill and

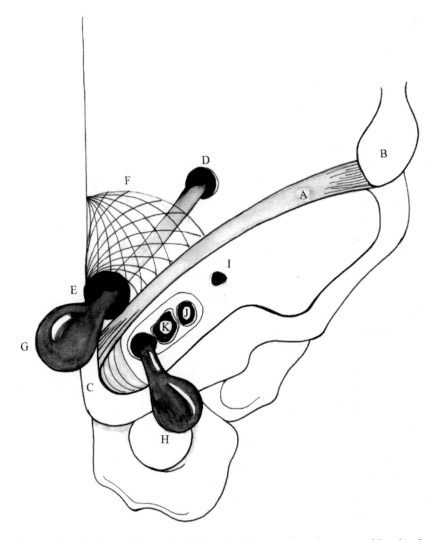

Figure 12.2. Anatomy of the groin. (A) Inguinal ligament inserting onto pubic tubercle, (B) anterior superior iliac spine (ASIS), (C) symphysis pubis, (D) deep inguinal ring, (E) superficial inguinal ring, (F) external oblique aponeurosis, (G) indirect inguinal hernia, (H) femoral hernia, (I) femoral nerve (outside femoral sheath), (J) femoral artery, and (K) femoral vein.

confidence. Your confidence can legitimately be increased by the knowledge that your examiner may not be able to get the correct answer himself. The basis of the test is to reduce the hernia, then apply pressure with a finger over the deep inguinal ring. The patient should then be asked to cough or strain. If the hernia is controlled it is probably indirect, but if it comes out anyway it may be a direct hernia (most of those we say are direct are in fact indirect).

Of some controversy is the actual site of the deep inguinal ring. Most surgical textbooks state that it is about 1.5 cm above the midpoint of the inguinal ligament, which is slightly lateral to the midinguinal point (the site of the femoral artery). However, most anatomy textbooks suggest that the deep inguinal ring is directly above the midinguinal point (i.e. above the femoral pulse), in which case the midpoint of the inguinal ligament becomes redundant as a landmark!

The treatment of an inguinal hernia consists of excision of the sac (herniotomy) and repair of the posterior wall of the inguinal canal and deep inguinal ring (herniorrhaphy). The older operations involve suturing the posterior wall of the inguinal canal with nonabsorbable sutures, but repairs are now being introduced where a nylon mesh is used to close the defect, producing less tension in the sutures and therefore less pain and a lower risk of sutures cutting out leading to a recurrence of the hernia. Such nylon meshes can be inserted either at open operation or by a laparoscopic technique.

Differential Diagnosis of a Lump in the Groin

Occasionally, a lump in the groin will be something other than a hernia. The list of differential diagnoses includes

- Inguinal lymph nodes (often multiple and usually below the inguinal ligament)
- Saphena varix, a dilated varicose vein at the sapheno-femoral junction (disappears on lying flat, and there may be other varicosities in the legs)
- Femoral artery aneurysm (pulsatile)
- Encysted hydrocoele of the cord (can get above it)

- Lipoma of the cord
- An incompletely descended testicle (absence of the testicle on that side)

Remember you cannot get above a hernia and these other lumps will also not usually exhibit the classical features of hernia:

1. Cough impulse
2. Reducibility
3. Bowel sounds heard over the hernia

Although a single enlarged femoral node can sometimes be difficult to distinguish from a strangulated femoral hernia containing omentum, such cases will rarely be seen in the finals. Usually, if care is taken to examine the patient lying down and standing, the diagnosis will become obvious. Remember also to carefully examine both groins (as hernias are often bilateral) and the scrotum as there may be associated epididymal cysts or hydrocoeles to find. This is particularly important for the short case section of the exam, where questions such as 'This patient has a lump in his groin — examine him and tell us what you think' are fairly common.

Here is a summary of how to examine 'a lump in the groin':

1. Introduce yourself and ask the patient if he minds your examining him.
2. Expose the abdomen, groin and legs. Ask the patient to stand, and inspect for any obvious lumps or scars and comment on your findings (if the patient is already lying it is perfectly reasonable to perform the examination in this position; however, you must stand him at the end of the examination, or you may miss small hernias, saphena varices and varicocoeles).
3. Examine the genitalia and both groins. If you can see an obvious lump feel it gently and ascertain the features of the lump. Ask the patient to cough and feel for a cough impulse, listen over it for bowel sounds and ask him if he is able to reduce it. Once it is reduced find the pubic tubercle and place your index finger on it. Ask the patient to cough and observe where the lump appears from in relation to your finger. An inguinal hernia will come out from the inguinal canal above and medial to your finger, whereas a femoral hernia will protrude below and lateral.

If you think this is an inguinal hernia, then state, for example, 'The patient has a 5 cm smooth lump in his right groin. I think this is an inguinal hernia, because I cannot get above it, it is reducible, exhibits a cough reflex and protrudes above and medial to the pubic tubercle'. The examiner might then ask you to tell if it is direct or indirect.

4. If a scrotal swelling is present determine if it has an upper border, remembering that you cannot get above a hernia. Therefore, a lump with no upper border is likely to be an inguinoscrotal hernia. If you can get above it, then it is likely to be either a cord or a testicular lump. Ask yourself two questions: Is it separate from the testis, and does it trans-illuminate? Do not forget to feel the epididymis and the skin of the scrotum as well (see Figure 12.1).

Other Types of Hernia

Incisional Hernias

These can be simply defined as hernias which arise through a previously made incision. They are often broad-necked and, therefore, have a low risk of strangulation. Factors leading to the development of an incisional hernia include obesity, old age, chronic cough or straining due to constipation or prostatism (i.e. things which increase intra-abdominal pressure), postoperative wound infection or haematoma and poor surgical technique when the wound is closed. In high-risk patients even large incisional hernias are often managed conservatively with an abdominal elastic support corset. Repair may be difficult and require the insertion of a nylon mesh to allow closure of the defect without tension.

Umbilical Hernia

In adults the hernia usually emerges adjacent to the umbilicus (unlike the congenital type) and is usually termed 'paraumbilical'.

Richter's Hernia

This is a hernia where only part of the circumference of the bowel is within the sac. It is most often seen with femoral hernias. This is the only type of hernia which can strangulate without obstructing (other than hernia which contains only the omentum). Although rather unusual in practice, it seems remarkably common in exam questions, which is why you need to know about it (see Figure 12.1).

Epigastric Hernia

This hernia arises in the midline through the linea alba. It is usually small and often difficult to feel, especially in overweight patients. It rarely contains bowel but often has extraperitoneal fat. It can cause symptoms out of proportion to its size, however, and patients often undergo unnecessary investigations for other causes of upper abdominal pain before the correct diagnosis is eventually made.

Spigelian Hernia

Again, this is very rare but common in exam questions. It is a hernia which occurs into the posterior rectus sheath at the point where the posterior sheath becomes deficient (i.e. at the arcuate line of Douglas).

Obturator Hernia

This hernia occurs into the obturator foramen and does not usually produce a palpable lump. It is most commonly seen in thin elderly women, and pressure on the obturator nerve gives rise to pain felt on the inner aspect of the thigh. It is usually diagnosed only when obstruction has occurred, often not being suspected prior to laparotomy. The typical presentation would be a thin old lady with distention, vomiting, colicky abdominal pain, absolute constipation and pain in the inner thigh.

13

VASCULAR DISEASE

INTRODUCTION

Vascular patients constitute a significant number of the cases seen in surgical finals, and in addition many written papers will have some questions about vascular surgery. Most cases will be covered within the categories of arterial disease or venous disease, and most patients with venous disease will have varicose veins or venous leg ulcers. Questions about deep venous thrombosis and pulmonary embolism are usually considered part of general medicine. The exception relates to prophylaxis against DVT for surgical patients — this is a very common question. Questions relating to cardiac surgery are not usually considered fair game for surgical finals except in their relation to cardiology, which again comes under general medicine.

Unfortunately many students have not been given the opportunity to work in a vascular unit or vascular firm and they often find this a confusing area when it comes to preparation for the finals. As vascular surgery is a fairly specialised area, students will not be expected to know anything about the minutiae of the specialty. What would be required, however, is a good knowledge of principles in the following areas:

1. How to examine the vascular system
2. Management of the acutely ischaemic leg
3. Management of the chronically ischaemic leg
4. Management of aneurysms
5. Management of carotid artery stenosis
6. Surgical aspects of venous disease.

In addition, make sure you know how to feel the pulses, including the popliteal, dorsalis pedis and posterior tibial pulses, and do not forget to listen for bruits. Also remember the importance of identifying and treating risk factors such as smoking, diabetes and hyperlipidaemia.

ARTERIAL DISEASE

Examination of the Peripheral Arterial System

Examination of the peripheral arterial system should obviously be included as part of a full cardiovascular examination and as part of a full examination of a patient in the long case section of the finals. However, it may be helpful to detail how one would carry out an examination restricted to the peripheral arterial system. First of all, one would inspect the patient for signs of peripheral arterial disease, such as ulcers, gangrenous toes, previous amputations, peripheral cyanosis, etc. In order to do this the patient must be adequately exposed, and usually the examination will be done with the patient supine, with no clothes on except for something to cover the genitalia to preserve his dignity. Do not forget to look for abnormal pulsations that might be caused by abdominal aortic aneurysm. The examination then proceeds with inspection of the hands and feeling of the radial pulses. These should be felt individually on both sides and the two sides then compared. Likewise, the brachial pulses should then be felt and compared. The brachial pulse is best palpated just above the elbow crease on the medial aspect of the upper arm. A surprising number of patients have radial pulses which are difficult to feel, whereas the brachial pulse is usually highly palpable unless there is an arterial occlusion higher up. If there is doubt about the pulses being present or being equal, then it would be appropriate to suggest taking the blood pressure in each arm in order to get a more objective confirmation of this. There should not be more than 15 mm of mercury difference between the blood pressure in the arms unless there is a vascular problem.

The next part of the peripheral arterial examination is checking of the carotid pulses. Remember that the common carotid, which divides into the internal and the external carotid, is within the carotid sheath which lies under the anterior edge of the sternocleidomastoid muscle. The best way to feel the carotid pulse is with the patient's head resting on one pillow; ask him to look in the opposite direction, and then feel under the sternocleidomastoid. It is then important to listen for a bruit over the carotid. The best way to do this is to ask the patient to take a breath and then hold it whilst you listen with the diaphragm of the stethoscope. If you listen whilst he is breathing, you will find it difficult to hear soft bruits because of the noise made by the air moving in and out of the trachea. The process is then repeated for the carotid on the other side of the neck. Do not palpate the two carotids at the same time, as some patients may faint if that is done. If you are examining the cardiovascular system in general, then it would be appropriate at this point to move on to examination of the heart; if not, the next step is to examine the abdomen.

First of all, look for pulsation which might be caused by an aortic aneurysm and then palpate for such an aneurysm. Remember an aneurysm is expansile as well as pulsatile. Then, the abdomen should be auscultated for bruits. Remember that a bruit heard in the upper abdomen may be due to renal artery stenosis. Remember also that the bifurcation of the aorta is at the level of the umbilicus and so aneurysms are usually felt in the upper abdomen.

The next stage of the arterial examination is to check the pulses in the groins and legs. The femoral pulse should be palpated on both sides and one side compared with the other. In coarctation of the aorta there may be radiofemoral delay. This is manifested by feeling the radial and femoral pulses simultaneously and feeling that the femoral pulse wave is occurring fractionally after the radial pulse. Coarctation of the aorta is, however, very uncommon. Such patients are usually young and often present with severe hypertension, so do not be tempted to overdiagnose this condition.

After palpation of the femoral artery, noting also whether it is of normal calibre or aneurysmal, auscultation of the femoral artery should be carried out to listen for bruits.

The next thing to do is to feel for the popliteal arteries. This should be done routinely, as otherwise one may miss a popliteal aneurysm. It is, however, often very difficult to feel the popliteal arteries in many patients, especially if they are overweight. Indeed, it is said that if one feels the popliteal pulse very easily one should suspect immediately that there is a popliteal aneurysm present. It is not therefore a matter of shame for a student to say that he cannot feel the popliteal arteries, but it is important that you do know how to examine them properly. The best way to proceed is as follows.

The patient's leg should be almost straight and you should take great care to try and get him to relax it as much as possible. The principle of the method for feeling the popliteal arteries relates to the fact that there is a triangular bare area on the lower end of the femur between the heads of the gastrocnemius muscle and it is against this bare area that one tries to press up into the popliteal fossa so that the pulsation can be felt between the fingers and the bone. To do this, one needs to have a counterpressure, and this is done by resting the thumbs on the front of the knee and then gently pushing up into the popliteal fossa with the first and second fingers of both hands at the same time.

The next part of the peripheral arterial examination is to feel the foot pulses. There are two pulses which are normally palpated: the dorsalis pedis pulse (which is absent in 10% of normal people) and the posterior tibial pulse. The dorsalis pedis pulse is found on the dorsum of the foot in the groove between the extensor tendons of the big toe and the second toe. The posterior tibial pulse is about a centimetre behind the medial malleolus, just above the level of the ankle joint. Again, these pulses can be difficult to feel and there is no shame in saying that you could not feel them. You must, however, look professional in the way you palpate them, and of course feeling for them in the wrong position looks very bad indeed. The commonest mistake that students make when trying to feel the foot pulse is in fact to press too hard. This results in your being much more aware of the pulse in your own fingers as well as making the pulse in the artery more difficult to palpate. Whilst you are examining the foot pulses it would be appropriate to just look again at the foot in more detail than was done at the start of the examination. The foot should be felt to see whether it is warm, and the two sides compared. Any pallor or cyanosis should be commented on, as well as any areas of ulceration or necrosis. It is often useful to test for capillary return and compare the two sides. This is normally done by pressing on the pulp of one of the toes for a second or two to make it blanch and then seeing how long it takes for the colour to return. Unfortunately, this test may be influenced by the patient having cold peripheries or being generally shut down, but a difference between the two sides is suggestive of arterial disease.

The final clinical test which you need to know about is Buerger's test. This is done by elevating the legs to an angle of about 50°. Ideally, the two legs should be elevated at the same time. They should be kept up for about 2–3 min and the rate at which the skin blanches should be observed. Again, differences between the two sides are often more useful than any absolute change. After this period of elevation the legs are swung over the edge of the bed and kept in a dependent position (ideally, the patient is placed in a standing position). You should then look for the rate at which the veins in the foot refill, again comparing the two sides. Then, look at the rate at which colour returns to the leg. If the blood supply is poor, then after about 2 min the foot develops an intense hyperaemic response called reactive hyperaemia. This is due to vasodilation caused by the accumulation of products of anaerobic metabolism during the period of elevation. In practice, you may not be required to actually do this test in the examination, but you may be asked about it and you should certainly know the principle of the test. If asked if there are any other tests you would do remember to mention the ankle brachial pressure index (ABPI) although you will not be asked to do this in an exam. The ABPI is measured using a blood pressure cuff and hand-held Doppler to take the systolic pressure in the dorsalis pedis and posterior tibial arteries. The highest of these pressures (="ankle pressure") is divided by the systolic pressure in the arm (="brachial pressure") to give the ABPI. Normal is defined as >0.9.

Management of the Acutely Ischaemic Leg

Patients with an acutely ischaemic leg will not be found in the clinical cases section of final exams, but it is a relatively common question in vivas and in written papers as to how one would identify and manage a patient with an acutely ischaemic leg.

A useful way to remember the clinical signs and symptoms is the so-called list of 6 Ps: Pain, Pallor, Pulselessness, Parasthesiae, Paralysis and

Perishing cold. Of these, paralysis and parasthesiae are the two which indicate severe ischaemia threatening the loss of the limb. Remember also that the two commonest causes of acute ischaemia of the leg are an embolus and a thrombosis.

Embolism most commonly comes from the heart, where a thrombus has formed because of atrial fibrillation, heart valve disease or myocardial infarction. More rarely, emboli may be thrown off into the arterial circulation from aneurysms of the thoracic or abdominal aorta. Although it occurs extremely rarely, most students have heard of the socalled *paradoxical embolus*, where a deep venous thrombosis (DVT) thrombus passes into the arterial circulation through a septal defect of the heart, thereby getting into the arterial circulation instead of causing a pulmonary embolus (PE) as it would usually do. Although this is incredibly rare, it is one of those interesting little facts which seem to pepper finals and which therefore you probably need to know about.

Thrombosis is the other main cause of acute ischaemia and usually occurs on top of pre-existing arterial disease. In such patients there may thus be a history of pre-existing claudication and pulses may be absent in the opposite leg as well as in the symptomatic one.

Because of the relatively poor ability of muscle and nerve cells to cope with prolonged ischaemia, acute leg ischaemia needs to be treated as a surgical emergency and revascularisation should be produced within 4–6 h if the limb is to be saved.

An embolus is suggested by the absence of any previous vascular history (i.e. claudication), the presence of normal pulses in the other leg and the presence of atrial fibrillation. There is some debate as to exactly what sequence of events should be preferred, but most surgeons would agree that if it is clearly an embolus, then the patient should be taken without delay to theatre for an emergency embolectomy. This is done by exposing the femoral arteries in the groin. The arteries are then opened after clamps have been applied and a special catheter, called a Fogarty balloon embolectomy catheter, which is basically a long, thin flexible catheter with a balloon on the end, is passed down the artery with the balloon deflated. Once it has been passed as far as possible, the balloon is gently blown up and the catheter is drawn back, pulling out any thromboembolus with it. This catheter was designed by Thomas Fogarty when he was a medical student, and questions about it seem to come up fairly often in surgical finals.

Once the thomboembolus has been removed, the arteriotomy (i.e. incision in the artery) can be closed and the procedure is over. A sample of the embolus is usually sent for histology as well as culture. This is to exclude two of the rarer causes of peripheral emboli, namely an atrial myxoma (a benign tumour arising in the atrium of the heart) and an infected thrombus forming in subacute bacterial endocarditis. The patient should then be started on heparin whilst investigations to identify the source of the embolus are carried out, such as echocardiography. If a thrombosis is suspected rather than an embolus, then it is usually best to try and arrange for the patient to have an arteriogram carried out before going to theatre, as an embolectomy will probably not be sufficient. Arteriograms can be performed either by injection of contrast material into the venous circulation, with films being taken as the contrast subsequently passes into the arterial circulation, or by direct injection into the arterial circulation. The commonest site for the injection for peripheral arteriography is through the femoral artery, when a catheter is then passed up into the aorta before contrast is injected. Many hospitals have facilities to do a procedure called digital subtraction angiography, in which a computer system is used to subtract the images from before and after injection of the contrast so that structures such as the bones and soft tissues are removed, thereby improving the resolution of the image of the arteries. Depending on the precise findings of the angiogram, the leg will often require some form of bypass surgery in order to restore blood flow (as in chronic ischaemia). After successful restoration of flow it is usual to divide the deep fascia of the calf (i.e. a 'fasciotomy') to prevent damage occurring if the muscles swell. Care must also be taken to avoid renal failure caused by myoglobin leaking out from damaged or dead muscle (i.e. 'myoglobinuria'). These are termed reperfusion injuries.

Management of the Chronically Ischaemic Leg

Minor degrees of narrowing of major arteries may be completely asymptomatic. As narrowings progress or as occlusions occur, the degree of symptoms will depend on the anatomical level of the occlusion or stenosis as well as the presence of collateral vessels. For most patients with peripheral vascular disease, the first thing they will notice is pain in the calf muscles when they walk, so-called vascular claudication, and this is due to muscle ischaemia. The pain then disappears on resting. The only condition which commonly mimics this is pain due to lumbar spinal canal stenosis, so-called spinal claudication. In these patients, however, rather than true pain they usually suffer from numbness and pins and needles when they exercise and the symptoms are not usually well localised to the calf muscles as they are with true vascular claudication. As the degree of arterial occlusion worsens, the patient may suffer shorter and shorter distance claudication before eventually getting rest. Unlike the calf pain of claudication, rest pain is usually felt in the foot or toes (rest pain is ischaemia of muscles and also the soft tissues at rest). This typically occurs at night and the usual history is that the patient wakes due to the pain and has to hang the foot out of bed or walk on a cold floor in order to gain some relief. The reason the pain occurs at night is that we lose the effect of gravity helping to supply blood to the feet, and also that the cardiac output drops when we are asleep and the warmth of the bedclothes causes vasodilation to the skin diverting the blood from the soft tissues.

Patients who have severe arterial disease sufficient to give them rest pain are usually classified as having something termed 'critical ischaemia'. Critical ischaemia can be loosely defined as ischaemia which is severe enough to threaten the loss of the limb or part of the limb. It can also be defined with the help of the ABPI. Basically, this involves taking the blood pressure in the foot using a blood pressure cuff on the calf and a Doppler probe in order to pick up the foot pulse signal in either the posterior tibial or the dorsalis pedis pulse. The cuff is blown up until the signal disappears, and this is taken as the systolic pressure in the foot. This systolic pressure is then taken in a similar way in the arm, and the ratio of the two is calculated. The normal ABPI is 1 or slightly greater than 1. In claudication it is usually between 0.5 and 0.9. Below 0.5 the patient may start to suffer with rest pain or, if more severe, perhaps necrosis or gangrene of the toes. Occasionally, a claudicant may have a normal ABPI at rest, but this will be found to drop on exercise when an increased blood requirement to the muscles is limited by the stenosis. Currently, most vascular surgeons would agree that patients with mild claudication are best managed conservatively, with the main advice being to stop smoking and keep walking. In addition, medical problems such as anaemia, hypertension, hyperlipidaemia, diabetes and heart failure should be corrected. Overweight patients should be advised to lose weight. All patients should be on an antiplatelet agent (e.g. aspirin) and a statin. Risk factor management will be similar to that for cardiac patients. For more severe claudication or where there is thought to be a high risk of an iliac artery lesion, an angiogram should be arranged to see if there is an angioplastiable lesion. Treatment of patients with chronic arterial disease may be carried out either by radiological intervention, i.e. balloon angioplasty, or by surgery. Balloon angioplasty consists in passing a special catheter into the narrowed area of the artery in a way similar to that in which an angiogram is carried out. The balloon on the end of the catheter can then be blown up to a high pressure to stretch open the narrowing. Angioplasty is a good technique in that it does not involve an anaesthetic and can be done with relatively little risk to the patient. It is particularly useful for narrowings or short occlusions of the iliac arteries but is less good for disease below the inguinal ligament. Usually, only when there is either critical ischaemia or severe claudication, which is making the patient's life intolerable, should surgery be considered. In general terms, there are only a small number of vascular surgical procedures which are commonly carried out and specific details will not be required for surgical finals. Occlusion in the aorta or iliac artery is usually treated by an aorta-bifemoral bypass graft, in which an artificial graft, usually made of Dacron, is taken from the aorta above the blockage down to the femoral arteries in the groin. In patients who are considered too unwell to undergo this fairly major procedure, the femoral arteries can be revascularised by taking a graft from the axillary arteries just beneath the clavicle and running this down the sides of the thorax and abdomen under the skin into the groin arteries. In a patient with one good femoral pulse but a blocked iliac artery on the opposite side, a similar result can be achieved by taking a graft from the good common femoral artery across the subcutaneous tissue suprapubically into the ischaemic leg. This is termed a 'crossover graft'.

For blockages further down the leg either a femoral-popliteal or a femoral-distal procedure may be performed ('distal' in this context means 'distal to the popliteal artery', i.e. to one of the three tibial vessels — posterior tibial, anterior tibial and common peroneal). The preferred choice of graft for these bypasses is usually the long saphenous vein, which may be either used with its valves destroyed by a special valve-cutting instrument or reversed so that the valves do not interfere with the blood flow. Only if a suitable vein is not available do vascular surgeons resort to using an artificial graft material for grafts below the inguinal ligament. The commonest artificial material used below the inguinal ligament is polytetrafluraethylene (PTFE).

In broad terms, the further down the leg the graft goes the less likely it is to work, such that for femoral distal bypasses only about 50% of them are still working after 1 year.

Aneurysms

The word 'aneurysm' comes from the Greek word for 'widening' and is usually applied to abnormal widening of the arteries. Aneurysms can be found at various sites within the arterial circulation (e.g. aortic, femoral and popliteal). Berry aneurysms are found within the arteries in the circle of Willis and, if they rupture, can cause subarachnoid haemorrhage. These are not usually considered under general surgery, but aneurysms of the peripheral arterial system are.

Causes of Aneurysms

Most aneurysms are so-called atherosclerotic aneurysms. This means that they appear to be caused by atherosclerosis and the patients have the risk factors for this. Other, rarer causes of aneurysms include connective tissue disorders such as Marfan's syndrome and Ehlers–Danlos syndrome. Another, relatively uncommon cause of aneurysms is syphilis. Although rarely seen nowadays, it used to be a common cause of thoracic aneurysm. A false aneurysm occurs when there is a hole in an artery and the wall of the aneurysm is made up of organised blood clot — not an arterial wall. They occur following trauma and procedures involving sticking needles into arteries such as for angiography. Nowadays, many false aneurysms can be treated by direct injection of thrombin which makes them clot. A dissecting aneurysm is most commonly found in the thoracic aorta. A split (dissection) occurs in the wall of the aorta leading to two lumens instead of one being present. With time this can dilate to form an aneurysm. Atherosclerotic aneurysms share some of the risk factors for ordinary peripheral arterial occlusive disease, such as smoking and hypertension. However, there is probably an underlying genetic tendency, as these aneurysms also appear to run in families. They are more common in men and are rarely found before the age of 50 years, suggesting that there may also be an underlying predisposition to form aneurysms on top of specific precipitating risk factors.

Complications of Aneurysms

There are a number of possible complications for all aneurysms:

1. Rupture
2. Thrombosis
3. Distal embolisation
4. Pressure on adjacent structures
5. Fistula into adjacent structures such as vena cava or intestine
6. Infection of the aneurysm thrombus

These complications can all occur to a greater or lesser degree, with arterial aneurysms at different sites.

Abdominal Aortic Aneurysms

Aneurysms of the abdominal aorta affect the segment of aorta below the renal arteries in 90% of cases. Aneurysms that go higher than the renal arteries usually require an incision through both the chest and the abdomen for their repair. These are called 'thoracoabdominal' aneurysms. Whilst nowadays infrarenal aortic aneurysms should have an elective mortality rate of less than 10%, ruptured abdominal aortic aneurysms have a mortality rate of approximately 50%. Clearly it is better to operate before they rupture.

The best screening test for abdominal aneurysms is an ultrasound scan, which is cheap and provides a reliable method of sizing the aneurysm. In patients where surgery is to be considered or where the exact level of the aneurysm in relation to the renal arteries is in doubt, further imaging including a CT scan or an MRI scan may be needed (Figure 13.1). An important point to remember is that most abdominal aortic aneurysms are lined with a thick layer of organised thrombus. This means that the lumen size of the aneurysm is very much smaller that its overall size. An angiogram will therefore not show the true extent of the aneurysm, as it only outlines the lumen of the vessel. Hence, angiograms are not of great help in assessing aortic aneurysms and are usually done only in those patients who also have symptoms suggestive of occlusive arterial disease. Likewise, angiograms are not useful in following up cases where the mainstay is usually still the ultrasound scan.

Infrarenal abdominal aortic aneurysms less than 5.5 cm in maximum diameter are usually managed conservatively. The question is: When do you decide to operate? The crucial factors that come into this decision are the risk of rupture, the operative mortality and the age and general condition of

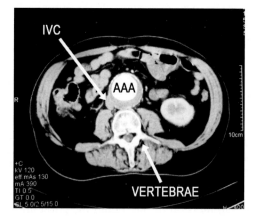

Figure 13.1. Abdominal CT scan of an aortic aneurysm (AAA). Note the layer of thrombus lining the aneurysm sac.

the patient. Therefore, if the risk of rupture is considered to be much greater than the risk of the operation, then surgery is sensible. Aneurysms of greater than 5.5 cm maximum diameter will usually be recommended for surgery if the patient is fit enough. Key points in assessing fitness for surgery include an assessment of cardiac, respiratory or renal problems. Of these, cardiac disease is the most common cause of mortality following aneurysm repair and should be assessed carefully with a full history, focusing specific attention on getting details of the patient's exercise tolerance.

As mentioned above, aortic aneurysms of greater than 5.5 cm diameter will normally be operated on if the patient is considered fit enough. Symptoms such as abdominal or back pain or tenderness when the aneurysm is palpated are thought to represent an increased risk of rupture, and such patients are usually also advised to undergo urgent surgery. Ruptured aneurysms should of course be taken immediately to theatre, with no delay for investigations or resuscitation. Effectively, these patients will not survive unless 'the tap is turned off'.

Surgery is traditionally by 'open' operation where the upper end of the aneurysm, called the 'neck of the aneurysm', is clamped below the renal arteries and then an artificial graft is sewn inside the aneurysm sac either down to the bifurcation of the aorta, i.e. using a straight graft, or onto each iliac artery, i.e. using a bifurcated graft. The graft material often used is Dacron. Nowadays some aneurysms are repaired using less invasive radiological techniques (this is called endovascular aneurysm repair), although currently these are available only in a small number of highly specialized centres.

Popliteal Aneurysms

Popliteal aneurysms are found less commonly than abdominal aortic aneurysms, although 50% of patients with a popliteal aneurysm will also have a coexistent aortic aneurysm. A popliteal aneurysm should be suspected when the popliteal pulse is unusually prominent or easily palpated. Whilst with abdominal aortic aneurysms the major risk is rupture, popliteal aneurysms seem to rupture rarely and the most common complication is acute thrombosis of the aneurysm causing acute ischaemia.

Such an event usually requires emergency surgery with femoropopliteal bypass grafting. If it is identified before thrombosis has occurred, then grafting and tying-off of the aneurysm should be carried out electively in order to prevent the catastrophe from occurring.

Aneurysms at other sites are relatively unusual. Those that involve the thoracic aorta may require extremely major surgery for their repair, with attendant high rates of morbidity and mortality. Nowadays many of these are treated with minimally invasive stenting. Aneurysms of the visceral arteries, such as the renal arteries or splenic arteries, have a tendency to present only after rupture, and also have a relatively high rate of mortality because of this. Femoral aneurysms occur but rarely rupture or require surgery.

It is very unlikely that a student will be asked to see cases other than infrarenal or popliteal aneurysms in surgical finals. One thing to be aware of, however, is the case where there are ectatic (i.e. tortuous) arteries which may feel aneurysmal when palpated from the outside. The commonest situation where this occurs is in the carotid arteries, where an ectatic carotid artery may easily be mistaken for a carotid artery aneurysm. Another situation to be aware of is where a mass lying in front of an artery (such as a pancreatic cancer in front of the abdominal aorta) is felt as a pulsatile mass. This pulsation is, however, transmitted only to the mass. The key to diagnosing a true aneurysm is to demonstrate expansile pulsation whereby the mass can be shown to be truly expanding in size with each pulse when examined using both hands. If in doubt, state you would obtain an ultrasound scan to confirm the presence/absence of an aneurysm and to measure its size.

CAROTID DISEASE

Typically, atherosclerosis of the carotid arteries occurs at the point where the common carotid divides into the internal and external carotid arteries (Figure 13.2). Narrowing or occlusion of the external carotid artery does not usually matter clinically because of the rich collateral arterial network within the head and neck. Stenosis or occlusion of the internal carotid artery is, however, potentially much more serious and can cause either strokes or transient ischaemic attacks. The precise details of the neurology

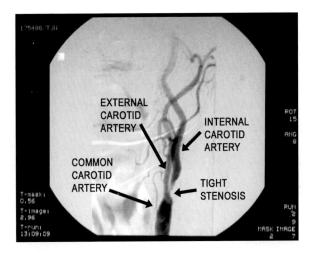

Figure 13.2. A carotid angiogram — Note the tight stenosis at the origin of the internal carotid indicated by the arrow.

related to these events should be sought in medical textbooks. However, in summary, a transient ischaemic attack is described as a neurological deficit which completely reverses within 24 h of its onset. A stroke is obviously a neurological deficit which persists for longer than 24 h. Amaurosis fugax is an ischaemic event usually due to an embolus passing through the retinal arterial circulation and is effectively a type of transient ischaemic attack ('amaurosis fugax' simply means 'fleeting blindness' in Latin).

Clinically, carotid artery stenosis may be diagnosed either because of a finding of a bruit over the carotid artery on examination or, after investigation, because of a transient ischaemic attack or a stroke. The main investigation used to screen for carotid artery stenosis is duplex ultrasound scanning of the carotid artery. In addition, angiography may be used to confirm the severity and type of stenosis. There is now good evidence that symptomatic carotid stenosis of greater than 70–80% should be treated by carotid endarterectomy in patients who are otherwise well. If these patients are treated with medical therapy only (i.e. aspirin), they have a significantly increased risk of stroke. The operation of carotid endarterectomy involves incision over the anterior border of the sternocleidomastoid muscle in the neck and dissection of the common, internal and external carotid arteries.

The common and internal carotid arteries are then opened using a longitudinal incision at the site of the stenosis, and the atheroma is 'cored out' and the artery closed. In some patients it may be necessary to put in a temporary plastic bypass tube in order to maintain blood flow to the brain during this operation. The major complication of the procedure is a perioperative stroke (at the best centres this risk is 5% or less). This is also an area where less invasive techniques such as carotid angioplasty and stenting are being developed. When a carotid stenosis has been found in an otherwise asymptomatic patient, the role of surgery is much less clear, and the benefits are less. It is probably only worthwhile in younger patients with severe stenosis.

VENOUS DISEASE

Varicose Veins

Medical students often find varicose veins a rather daunting case to meet in surgical finals, because they have not prepared a systematic way of examining them and presenting their findings. This is a mistake! At least one varicose vein patient is to be found in most surgical short case exams. These patients are plentiful on most hospital waiting lists and they are usually quite happy to come up to participate in finals, with the offer of getting their operation done rather more quickly than it might otherwise. Usually, the patients who have been selected will have quite obvious and significant varicose veins, and at first sight examination can be daunting in view of the large number of varicosities that they may have.

Probably the best way to consider how to approach a case of varicose veins is first to consider how varicose veins arise. Simplistically, we can think of the deep venous circulation as being at a higher pressure than the superficial venous system. Where the two systems join there are valves which have the purpose of preventing the pressure within the deep system coming out into the superficial system. If these valves go wrong (i.e. become incompetent), then the superficial veins dilate up and appear as varicose veins. The common sites where this may occur in the lower limb are first at the long saphenous femoral vein junction in the groin (this is the commonest site), second at the short saphenous popliteal vein junction in the popliteal fossa behind the knee and third from so-called perforating veins (veins which pass directly from superficial to deep) which become incompetent. Calf perforating veins are usually found on the medial side of the calf. Typically, there are three: one just above the medial malleolus, one a hand's breadth higher and one hand's breadth higher than that. In addition, some patients have a perforator in their medial thigh which is usually connected to the long saphenous vein. The position of perforators may, however, vary. When one is assessing a patient with varicose veins, it is therefore important to try and categorise the varicose veins into three groups:

1. Long saphenous veins
2. Short saphenous vein
3. Veins arising from calf perforators

In addition, the patient may have disease of the deep veins, which may be either obstructed or incompetent, or may have a leg ulcer.

Points in the History

It is important to ascertain what it is about the varicose veins that troubles the patient. He may just be worried about them from a cosmetic point of view. Alternatively, he may be getting aching pains which are usually worse after a period of standing. Some patients find that they get swelling of the ankles, again most often after a period of standing. Varicose veins do sometimes cause cramps and other nonspecific pains in the leg, but one must always be on the look-out for other pathology which might be causing the pain, as many patients will immediately ascribe pain from any cause (arthritis of the knee, for example) to their obvious and visible varicose veins.

Other points in the history which are usually taken include asking for a family history of varicose veins, any previous medical history suggestive of deep venous thrombosis or pulmonary embolism and, most important, whether the patient, who is usually a young woman, is on the oral contraceptive pill as this is something that really should be stopped 6–8 weeks before surgery because of the risk of DVT. Most varicose veins in women seem to worsen after pregnancy, and it is also a good idea to enquire about the number of past pregnancies and whether the woman wishes to have further pregnancies in the future. Some surgeons will suggest delaying treatment if that is the case.

Points on Examination

Never forget that occasionally abdominal or pelvic masses (including pregnancy) or malignancies can present as varicose veins due to pressure on the inferior vena cava or iliac veins. A full examination of the abdomen should therefore be part of examining a patient for varicose veins. In the short case section of the final examination, you may not be expected to do this by the examiner (because of the lack of time), but you should make a point of mentioning, 'I would now wish to do a full abdominal examination.'

Another point not to forget is to examine the arterial pulses in the legs. This is especially important in patients who have a leg ulcer. Varicose veins will usually be best seen with the patient standing up. The legs should be exposed from the groin to the toe. As with all clinical examinations, the inspection should come first. You should particularly be looking for the presence of any signs of current or past leg ulceration. In patients who have had long-standing varicose veins and venous hypertension, you may see the changes of skin pigmentation (the skin is brown in colour due to haemosiderin deposits) or lipodermatosclerosis (there is atrophy and loss of elasticity of the skin and subcutaneous tissues). Because most patients with significant skin changes will have calf perforator disease, and because the calf perforators are found on the medial side of the calf above the medial malleolus, these changes are usually most prominent in the medial lower calf. In addition you should inspect the veins to try and make some preliminary judgment as to whether it seems they are likely to be arising from the long saphenous, short saphenous or perforating system. Remember that the long saphenous vein runs from the groin down the medial aspect of the thigh and calf. The veins below the knee which arise from it will therefore be mostly situated on the medial side of the calf, and in a thinner patient you may see a dilated varicose long saphenous vein running up the thigh. The short saphenous veins arise from the popliteal vein at a variable level within the popliteal fossa and then run down to the lateral side of the calf. By just looking at the legs with the patient standing you may be able to make a good guess as to which of these two patterns the veins fall within. Calf perforating veins, which are incompetent, may produce very few varicosities but, as mentioned earlier, they will often be associated with significant skin changes of pigmentation and lipodermatosclerosis. Therefore, one can usually make a preliminary (educated) guess as to which of the three categories the veins fall into just on inspection (Figure 13.3).

Next comes palpation. Patients with a prominent saphena varix at the saphenofemoral junction may actually have a lump visible in the groin, and this will need to be palpated to make sure it is not due to a lymph node

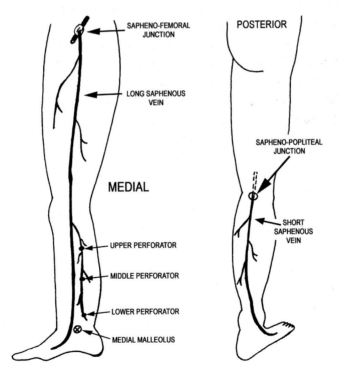

Figure 13.3. Distribution of varicose veins.

or hernia. Otherwise, the mainstay of palpation is the so-called 'tap' test, whereby the veins are tapped down on the calf and palpation over the saphenous vein in the thigh will reveal a transmitted thrill if the veins are in continuity. It is also at the stage of palpation that one should quickly check the femoral, foot and popliteal pulses. Next comes the so-called 'tourniquet' test, or Trendelenberg's test. Perhaps it is this which confuses more medical students than any other aspect of varicose vein examination. This test can be adapted to be as complex or as simple as one would wish. In the days before vascular laboratory tests were widely available and reliable, some surgeons used variations of this test involving more than one tourniquet placed at several levels. This is now rarely done. The principle of the test is that it is possible to compress the superficial veins by a tourniquet applied around the leg. The best way to proceed with the test in the finals is to get the patient to lie down, and elevate the leg and then milk the veins with your hand to emptiness before applying a tourniquet initially as high on the thigh as possible. Most finals will have available suitable tourniquets. The ones used for taking blood from the arm may not be large enough for some patients' legs. The patient is then asked to stand and the veins are inspected to see if they refill rapidly. Remember that all varicose veins will refill slowly as blood passes through the arterial circulation, through the capillary bed and back into the venous system. What one is looking for is a rapid refilling within a few seconds, indicating that the tourniquet has not prevented the superficial reflux. For example, if there is saphenofemoral junction reflux causing varicose veins, a high thigh tourniquet will prevent this rapidly refilling as the patient stands. If, however, there is short saphenous or calf perforator incompetence, the veins will fill rapidly despite a high thigh tourniquet. If the veins are controlled by the tourniquet in the thigh, then they are long saphenous veins due to saphenofemoral reflux. If they are not controlled, the next manoeuvre should be to position the tourniquet just below the knee and repeat the test. If the veins are now prevented from refilling rapidly, then there is either saphenopopliteal reflux or, very occasionally, a thigh perforator that is incompetent. If the veins continue to fill rapidly despite this tourniquet just below the knee, there is almost certainly calf perforator incompetence. Some people do this test using pressure from the fingers instead of a tourniquet. However, adequate pressure is much more difficult to achieve using this technique, and we would not advise it in the finals.

In practice, this is the limit to which the tourniquet test can be taken in the finals. To expect a student to apply the tourniquet at more than these positions is almost unheard of, and in many cases the examiner will be satisfied with simply describing what you would do and not require you to actually do it. Remember also that some patients will have a mixture of the three types of veins, i.e. long saphenous incompetence and calf or perforator incompetence. In such patients the tourniquet test will be difficult to interpret with any certainty.

Leg Ulceration

Ulceration can have many causes, although by far the commonest is venous disease, which accounts for about 80% of ulcers. The following is a list to help you remember the other causes:

1. *Arterial.* Due to either major-vessel disease or small-vessel disease, e.g. vasculitis, rheumatoid arthritis.
2. *Neuropathic.* Most traumatic ulcers have a neuropathic element, e.g. alcoholism, peripheral neuropathy, diabetes, tabes dorsalis and syringomyelia.
3. *Traumatic.*
4. *Systemic disease.* For example, pyoderma gangrenosum.
5. *Neoplastic.*

Venous ulceration may be either superficial venous incompetence or incompetence of the valves of the deep veins. Venous ulceration will usually be found above the medial malleolous in the position where the calf perforators arise. There will usually be the signs of pigmentation and lipodermatosclerosis. About 10% of leg ulceration is caused by arterial disease. These ulcers may be situated anywhere in the leg or foot and may be associated with other signs of peripheral ischaemia, such as gangrenous toes. Five to ten per cent of patients may have a mixture of the two causing their leg ulceration (this is why you must always feel the pulses). The main differential diagnosis is a neuropathic ulcer. Such ulcers are probably due to repetitive trauma to an area, with absent or decreased sensation. When you are assessing an ulcer, therefore, it is important to decide whether it is a vascular problem (major or small vessel) or whether it is neuropathic. A neuropathic ulcer is painless, the surrounding skin is insensitive and the rest of the foot should be warm, with a good blood supply.

Treatment of Leg Ulceration

Once the cause of the leg ulceration has been investigated, initial treatment may be directed towards underlying causative factors, such as arterial ischaemia, vasculitis, etc. However, the majority of leg ulcers are due to venous disease; it is the management of this which is most likely to be asked about in surgical finals and which the student needs to know in some detail.

The principles underlying treatment for leg ulceration can be summarised as follows:

• Dressing of the ulcer
• Pressure bandaging
• Elevation

Systemic antibiotics should be reserved for patients who have a cellulitis surrounding the ulcer. Ulcers are always affected to some degree by colonising skin organisms, and antibiotic treatment does nothing for the rate of ulcer healing and may just breed resistant organisms. A very dirty or sloughy ulcer may require treatment with antiseptic or desloughing dressings initially, i.e. dressings which may contain agents such as iodine or streptokinase. Such agents may, however, impair the rate of epithelial regrowth of an ulcer. After the ulcer becomes clean, simple dressings which maintain a moist environment over the ulcer should be used in order to promote epithelial regrowth. Elastic bandaging or graduated compression stockings (these have a higher pressure at the ankle than they do higher in the leg) should also be applied and, in addition, the patient should be asked to elevate his leg as much as possible. The use of compression bandaging and elevation is to reduce venous hypertension. In severe cases it may be necessary to admit the patient to hospital for elevation and bed rest in order to promote ulcer healing. In some cases where there is a large ulcer with a clean granulating bed, it may be appropriate to consider the use of skin grafting in order to reduce the length of time required for the ulcer to heal. Finally, an assessment of the venous system should be made, and if there is significant superficial venous incompetence (i.e. long saphenous, short saphenous or calf perforating veins), then consideration should be given to treating this surgically. Unfortunately, when deep venous valve incompetence is present (usually following previous deep venous thrombosis), there is currently no good surgical procedure to improve deep venous function. For such patients the mainstay of treatment is to try and get the ulcer healed using the above methods and then to maintain healing by fitting a good quality elastic graduated compression stocking. Patients who have their ulcers successfully healed should be encouraged to wear such stockings on a life-long basis.

DEEP VENOUS THROMBOSIS AND PULMONARY EMBOLISM

Management of DVT and PE is usually considered part of the medical finals. However, PE is the commonest preventable cause of death in surgical patients, and it is appropriate to be asked about it in surgical exams, especially in relation to prophylaxis.

At an early stage the only signs of a DVT may be an increase in warmth and dilatation of the superficial veins. As the thrombosis progresses, the leg will swell. At a later stage the leg may be extremely swollen, with impairment of skin circulation (phlegmasia caerulea dolens or phlegmasia alba dolens), and occasionally this may lead to venous gangrene. PE may present in different ways. Massive PE will produce cardiorespiratory arrest and may initially be misdiagnosed as a primary cardiac problem. A PE should always be suspected in a patient suffering a collapse or cardiac arrest within the first 2 weeks of their surgical procedure. Less major degrees of PE may produce lesser degrees of collapse, or perhaps dyspnoea or pleuritic chest pain.

The treatment of DVT is anticoagulation, usually with heparin at first, followed by Warfarin. Nowadays the majority of patients can be managed as out-patients with once-a-day injections of low molecular weight heparin whilst awaiting adequate Warfarinisation. If a patient continues to have pulmonary emboli despite adequate anticoagulation, then he should be considered for insertion of a venacaval umbrella filter.

Prophylaxis against DVT in Surgical Patients

Patients having anything other than minor surgery should have prophylaxis against DVT. This is particularly so if they have any risk factors, such as age, obesity, cigarette smoking, the contraceptive pill or a previous history of DVT or PE. The commonest type of prophylaxis employed is subcutaneous low molecular weight heparin, It is also common practice to use TED stockings (thromboembolic deterrent stockings), and many units have intermittent pneumatic compression devices which work by blowing up a series of cuffs on the leg and keeping the venous pump flowing even when the patient is immobile or in theatre.

Lymphoedema

This is an abnormal collection of interstitial lymph fluid either due to a congential absence of the lymphatics (primary) or secondary to blockage of the lymphatics.

Primary lymphoedema can be present at birth (congenital lymphoedema), but more often it presents in the teens as lymphoedema praecox (Milroy's syndrome). This usually affects young females who present with progressive swelling (nonpitting) of one or both legs. Less often, it can present late at around the age of 30–40 years and is then called lymphoedema tarda ('tarda' is 'late' in Latin).

Secondary lymphoedema can be caused by anything that damages or obstructs the lymphatics. The term FIIT is helpful in remembering the causes:

Fibrosis, e.g. following radiotherapy
Infiltration, e.g. by tumour, especially prostatic in men and lymphoma in women (in certain parts of the world infestation with filariasis is a common cause for lymphoedema)

Infection, e.g. TB

Traumatic, e.g. after block dissection of lymphatics

Treatment of lymphoedema is usually nonoperative. This involves elevation and external compression stockings, and early intervention if infection develops. There are now lymphoedema nurses who use various compression devices and massage techniques that are very good at reducing the swelling in such patients.

There are no curative surgical procedures available and only the most severe cases come to surgery, which usually involves debulking procedures to improve mobility.

14

UROLOGY

Jonathan Glass

Questions on urology feature quite often in essays and short answers, such as 'Discuss the investigations for painless haematuria' or 'Discuss the management of benign prostatic hypertrophy'. There will be a good chance that you will get a urological problem as a long case, since such patients are usually not too ill before or after their operation to assist with the exams. If you have never seen an irrigation bag and three-way catheter before, you may be caught out. In the short case section you may see a lump in the scrotum, but urology does not feature high on clinical signs. It may also appear in OSCE's and EMQ's (see Chapter 17).

CATHETERS AND CATHETERIZATION

The most commonly used catheter is the Foley catheter (named after Fredrick Foley in the 1930s). Such catheters have inflatable balloons at the bladder end to hold them in position. They can be two-way (one lumen for the urine and one to allow the balloon to be blown up) or three-way (with an extra lumen to allow irrigation fluid to be passed into the bladder). The balloon can be inflated by injecting about 10 ml of saline into the side port of the catheter.

Catheters can be made from different materials, such as latex, plastic or silicone (silastic or long-term in-dwelling catheters). The *external circumference* of the catheter (in millimetres) is sized by the Charriere (Ch), also called the French (Fr) gauge system (to calculate the diameter, divide by π!). Ten French is small and 22 Fr is large. The usual size used for males is size Fr 14 or 16. The catheters have standard lengths, male catheters being about twice as long as female catheters.

Male Urethral Catheterization

Retract the foreskin if the penis is not circumcised, use the aseptic technique (clean the area with antiseptic, one hand holding the penis and the other holding the cotton wool with forceps, and the region is draped), instil anaesthetic gel into the urethra and introduce the catheter fully into the urethra (the penis is usually held vertically or at 45°); once urine drains, inflate the balloon and connect the catheter to either a free drainage bag or an hourly measuring urine bag. Never inflate the balloon unless you are sure you are in the bladder with urine seen passing through the catheter. Return the foreskin to prevent a paraphimosis. Note the residual volume of urine and send the specimen of urine for bacteriology. The complications of urethral catheterization include local trauma, introduction of infection, urethritis and stricture formation. Some centres advocate the need for routine antibiotic cover for this procedure (usually one dose of gentamycin 80 mg IM); others feel this is unnecessary. In certain situations antibiotics are essential, for example, if the patient had a metal prosthesis such as a hip replacement or if the patient had a heart murmur, since infection in these patients could be disastrous.

Suprapubic Catheters

Suprapubic catheters (SPCs) are used when urethral catheterization is not possible (e.g. urethral stricture) or is inappropriate, such as when urethral trauma is suspected (pelvic injury with a high-riding prostate). There are many types of SPCs, and they can either be specially manufactured SPCs or inserted using a special introducer such as the Add-a-Cath; a normal Foley catheter can be used. The Add-a-Cath has a plastic sheath around a sharp-ended trocar. The catheter is inserted into the bladder in the midline about 5 cm above the symphysis pubis. Prior to inserting a SPC there must be no doubt that the bladder is palpable. Urine should be aspirated through a green needle on a syringe prior to attempting SPC insertion. If there is any doubt, an ultrasound should be performed. The plastic sheath around the introducer can be zipped down and torn off to allow the whole sheath to be removed once the catheter is in the bladder. The only way to understand this properly is to ask a urologist to show you the actual catheter.

Haematuria

Haematuria can be a finding on urine analysis (microscopic haematuria), or the patient complains of passing red urine (macroscopic or frank haematuria). Over 35% of patients with frank haematuria have a urological malignancy. Indeed, if you ever see a patient with frank haematuria you should immediately be thinking about renal cell carcinoma or bladder cancer. Haematuria can be due to general or localized causes. The local causes can be bleeding anywhere along the urinary tract — the kidneys, ureters, bladder, prostate or urethra. At any of these sites the bleeding may be due to infections (TB, schistosomiasis or UTI), stones, trauma or, most importantly, tumours, etc. Renal diseases such as glomerulonephritis also cause haematuria. The general causes include bleeding disorders, leukaemias, the use of anticoagulants, haemoglobinopathies and sickle cell disease. These are relatively rare. In your history you should elicit the following points:

1. Is the blood definitely in the urine and not from the vagina or rectum?
2. Is it true haematuria? There are many other causes of red urine, including drugs (rifampicin, nitrofurantoin), foods such as beetroot and systemic disease such as porphyrias or rhabdomyolysis.
3. Is the haematuria associated with loin pain or pain on passing urine? Pain usually implies stones or infections, whereas painless haematuria should set alarm bells ringing for more sinister causes. Pain may simply tell you which side is the site of any pathology.
4. The nature of the bleeding — is it microscopic or macroscopic? Are there any clots in it? Is the bleeding at the beginning of the stream in

an otherwise clear stream (suggestive of a urethral or prostatic lesion) or is it throughout the stream (suggestive of a lesion in the bladder, ureters or kidneys)? Bleeding only at the end of the stream is unusual, although it does occur classically with schistosomiasis.

Examination of such patients should include an assessment of their general health. Look for signs of anaemia, feel for a renal mass and conduct a digital rectal examination to assess the prostate.

Investigations

1. *Urine tests.* A midstream urine (MSU) should be dipsticked and sent for microscopy and culture. The urine should also be sent off for cytological analysis to identify transitional cell carcinoma.
2. *Haematological tests.* Send a full blood count to see if the patient is anaemic and carry out U & Es to assess renal function.
3. *Radiological tests.* An ultrasound of the renal tract can detect tumours in the renal parenchyma and bladder lesions and is the initial radiological investigation. If a renal mass is seen, then a CT scan is performed. A plain abdominal X-ray which includes the region of the kidneys, ureters and bladder (known as a KUB) is taken (a normal plain abdominal radiograph cuts out part of the bladder). The soft tissue of the renal tract is not seen well on a plain film, so an intravenous urogram (IVU) is performed, where images of the kidneys, ureters and bladder are obtained after the patient has been given an injection of a contrast medium that is excreted by the kidneys. This is particularly good for looking at the collecting system of the kidneys and the ureters, but not good for looking at lesions in the bladder.
4. *Special investigations.* Cystoscopy means a look inside the bladder. This is usually performed under local anaesthesia using a flexible (fibreoptic) cystoscope, but sometimes rigid cystoscopy is needed (for example, when the haematuria persists at the time of the cystoscopy and rigid cystoscopy allows a washout to be performed). Other special investigations include early morning urine samples (EMUs) for TB culture and, very rarely, angiography to exclude arteriovenous malformations. For

macroscopic haematuria and persistent microscopic haematuria, an ultrasound and cystoscopy should always be performed. If these are normal, then an IVU should be requested, particularly in patients over 50 years.

If you ever had to write an essay on haematuria you could talk about the above and obviously discuss the causes in detail using an aetiological and pathological sieve. Remember, frank haematuria means cancer until proven otherwise.

BLADDER OUTFLOW OBSTRUCTION

Bladder outflow obstruction (BOO) is most commonly caused by benign prostatic hyperplasia (BPH) or prostate cancer. Only these two causes will be discussed in detail. Other causes include bladder neck obstruction (which affects young to middle-aged men and is due to bladder neck dysfunction, treated by bladder neck incision or drugs) and urethral stricture (which is due to urethral trauma, catheterisation, previous transurethral surgery or sexually transmitted diseases such as gonorrhoea and chlamydia, and is treated by urethrotomy and dilators). Bladder calculi can sometimes cause BOO. Lower urinary tract symptoms can be divided into obstructive and irritative symptoms:

Obstructive symptoms
- Hesitancy (as a higher bladder pressure is needed to initiate micturition to overcome the obstruction)
- Poor stream
- Intermittent flow and terminal dribbling
- Incomplete emptying [feeling like you need to go again straight away (*pis en deux*), also associated with bladder diverticulae]

Irritative symptoms
- Frequency
- Urgency (and urge incontinence)
- Nocturia (needing to get up more than once at night)

The aetiology of the irritative symptoms is poorly understood. These symptoms may be secondary to BPH but can also be a feature of intravesical pathology, such as bladder cancer, urinary infections and stones.

The complications of BOO include urinary tract infection as a result of urinary stasis, formation of bladder calculi, hydronephrosis and subsequent renal impairment, and acute (painful) and chronic (painless) urinary retention.

BENIGN PROSTATIC HYPERPLASIA

The prostate is a capsulated fibromuscular gland, which measures approximately 4 cm × 3 cm × 2 cm and normally weighs about 15 g. As the male gets older the gland enlarges, especially in the transitional zone (in contrast to cancer, which affects the peripheral part of the gland). The symptoms are those listed under BOO.

The abdomen should be examined to exclude urinary retention. On rectal examination the normal prostate has a smooth surface and there is a palpable midline sulcus. In BPH the normal findings are present but the gland is enlarged. The size and consistency should be noted.

Investigations

• Urine should be dipsticked and sent for microscopy and culture. Send U & Es to assess renal function. Prostate specific antigen (PSA) is a protein produced by prostatic acinar cells (both normal and cancerous, although cancerous cells produce about 10 times as much). The level of PSA in the blood increases as the prostate increases in size (both BPH and cancer). The PSA also increases with age. The normal PSA is <4 but the normal value varies with age. The higher the PSA the greater the chance of cancer being present (however, it can be raised markedly with BPH). If the PSA is high or clinically the prostate is suspicious, then a transrectal ultrasound and biopsy of the prostate can be performed. Patients should be carefully counseled before having their PSA tested.

- A urine flow test is performed. This involves passing urine onto a flow meter and generates a graph of urinary volume (ml) against time (s). An ultrasound of the urinary tract is usually performed to assess the residual bladder volume and to look for upper tract dilatation, which may result if the obstruction is severe.
- More invasive investigations might include a cystoscopy if a urethral stricture or bladder calculus is suspected or if irritative symptoms predominate. Urodynamic (bladder pressure) studies can be performed for complex cases.
- A voiding diary is helpful in seeing how much bother the symptoms cause the patient.

Management

If the symptoms are mild and do not bother the patient, then a policy of watchful waiting may be adopted, with a review in the clinic to see if the symptoms have changed. Approximately 65% of patients will either not improve or get worse.

As long as there is no evidence of complications of BOO, such as hydronephrosis, recurrent UTIs or urinary retention, treatment is a choice between surgical and medical options, depending on symptom severity and patient preference.

Medical treatment involves the use of $\alpha1$ adrenoreceptor blockers such as Tamsulosin, Prazosin, Alfuzosin and Terazosin, which relax the prostatic smooth muscle increasing urinary flow and help with the obstructive symptoms. Side effects from these drugs are rare but they can cause postural hypotension. 5-α-reductase inhibitors such as Finasteride (which block the conversion of testosterone to the more active dihydotestosterone, the hormone important in developing BPH) have been used but are of doubtful efficacy.

Surgical treatment involves removing the obstructing part of the prostate. Transurethral resection of the prostate (TURP) is the most frequently performed operation for this condition [and the second most common operation (after cataract surgery) performed on men over 60].

The patient is placed in a lithotomy position and a resectoscope, passed through the urethra, is used under direct vision to remove the prostate piece by piece using cutting diathermy, the chippings being sent to histology.

Diathermy is also used to stop any bleeding. A three-way catheter is inserted postoperatively to irrigate the bladder until the fluid is no longer heavily blood-stained. This stops any clots forming and blocking the catheter. The procedure can be performed with a LASER.

Complications of TURP include general and specific, early and late, etc.

- *Early*. Septic shock, bleeding and transurethral syndrome.

  Transurethral (TUR) syndrome is uncommon and is like water intoxication, thought to be due to absorption of hypotonic irrigation fluids during the TUR (saline cannot be used, because it limits the use of diathermy). It usually occurs during a particularly long and difficult TURP with significant bleeding. The problems include electrolyte imbalances (especially hyponatraemia), haemolysis, fluid overload, and if brain oedema occurs the patient can become confused and can fit and lose consciousness. Treatment is difficult but essentially involves fluid restriction, diuretics and close observation.

- *Late*. Secondary haemorrhage, urethral strictures, impotence, recurrent prostatic regrowth and recurrent symptoms. It is essential, when consenting the patient, that he knows that between 65 and 85% will develop retrograde ejaculation (sperm flows into the bladder on orgasm and hence he becomes infertile). Some urologists believe that impotence might occur in up to 3–5% of patients postoperatively, although this is debatable. TURP is the gold standard treatment of BPH. As so many men develop BPH, a day case procedure is being sought which will be as effective as TURP. Newer methods for treating BPH include microwave therapy, laser prostatectomy, radiofrequency ablation and prostatic stents (find out which technique is used at your hospital). Open prostatectomy (retropubic or transvesical) is only performed nowadays for very large prostates where the gland is larger than 100 g and TURP would take too long, leading to a high risk of TUR syndrome developing.

UROLOGICAL CANCERS

Carcinoma of the Prostate

The presentation of prostate cancer has changed dramatically in the past 10–15 years particularly since PSA measurement has become available. Whereas previously 70% of cases of prostatic cancer presented late with advanced disease (such as bony metastases), nowadays a high percentage of cases are found in the early stages due to PSA testing of men with BPH or asymptomatic men having a routine health check.

The symptoms can be those of BPH and it can be difficult to differentiate between carcinoma of the prostate (CaP) and BPH. CaP can be diagnosed histologically after TURP for what was thought to be benign disease when the prostatic chippings are seen under the microscope. It is an adenocarcinoma arising in the peripheral zone of the gland (which is also the functional part of the gland). The aetiology is unknown.

On rectal examination the prostate may feel enlarged and 'craggy' or a hard nodule may be palpable. The normal midline sulcus may be lost. Investigations depend on the patient's age and his symptoms. If the PSA is raised or clinically the prostate is suspicious, a transrectal ultrasound and biopsy of the prostate should be performed. If a malignancy is diagnosed, the staging procedures include a bone scan and CT scan or an MRI scan of the abdomen and pelvis, and a set of liver function tests. If the patient has symptoms of BOO, then as well as investigating the prostate cancer it is also necessary to perform an ultrasound and urine flow tests, as you would when assessing BPH.

The stages of prostatic carcinoma (via the TNM system; outline of the T component of staging) are as follows:

T0 — no primary tumour identifiable
T1 — tumour identified incidentally at TURP or with raised PSA
T2 — palpable tumour without extracapsular extension
T3 — spread beyond capsule; mobile tumour
T4 — fixed or locally invasive tumour

Treatment

In early prostate cancer treatment with curative intent can be offered. Radical prostatectomy (open or laparoscopic), radical radiotherapy or brachytherapy (the placement of radioactive seeds within the prostate) is performed in men under 70 years with a life expectancy of at least 10 years, but such treatment remains controversial and the best method of treating early prostate cancer is not established. Many of these treatments have significant complications including impotence and incontinence. Many patients nowadays would have read about the different treatments available (usually on the Internet) and may have an opinion about what treatment they would like.

Prostate cancer is driven by androgens, so in patients with metastatic or locally advanced disease the main aim of treatment is to decrease androgen activity. This is achieved by medical or surgical castration. Medical castration can be achieved by LHRH agonists such as Goserelin (Zoladex), which is administered as a three-monthly subcutaneous injection, or oral antiandrogens such as flutamide or cyproterone. The patients are followed up in the clinic and PSA measurements are used to assess response. Mean survival once metastases are present is a little over 2 1/2 years. TURP can be performed if obstructive symptoms are present, although some of the obstructive symptoms may resolve with hormone treatment.

There is no national screening for prostate cancer. There are several problems regarding prostate cancer screening. The disease is very common, but in many it would not have affected the patient during his life (more than 50% of men over 75 have microfoci at postmortem). An ideal test needs to be found and the best way of treating early prostate cancer needs to be identified. A method of identifying which patients with early prostate cancer will go on to develop metastases is also needed. Until some of these problems are resolved, screening for prostate cancer is inappropriate.

Carcinoma of the Bladder

In Britain almost all bladder cancers (98%) are transitional cell carcinomas (TCC), the remainder being squamous cell carcinomas or adenocarcinomas. In countries with endemic schistosomiasis, squamous cell carcinoma is more common. The aetiology of TCC is unknown, although occupational exposure to chemicals such as aromatic amines and analine dyes has been implicated as carcinogenic. TCC was the first disease for which industrial compensation was awarded. Smoking increases the risk four-fold (nitrosamines are found in cigarette smoke!). Squamous cell carcinomas are associated with calculi and infections such as schistosomiasis. Adenocarcinomas are associated with persistent urachal remnants (an embryological remnant of the communication between the umbilicus and the bladder).

Carcinoma of the bladder affects males more than females and usually presents with painless haematuria (about 15% present with recurrent UTIs). Urine cytology may identify abnormal cells in the urine, but the diagnosis is usually made by cystoscopy. When seeing a patient with haematuria, always think of cancer first.

Staging is by the TNM system (outline of the T component of staging):

Ta — confined to mucosa.
T1 — tumour invading lamina propria.
T2 — muscle is involved
T3 — perivesical fat is involved
T4 — invasion beyond the bladder into adjacent organs or fixed to the pelvic side wall.

The pathologist also grades them histologically into Grades I–III. Grade I means well differentiated and Grade III poorly differentiated.

Superficial Bladder Cancers

These can be low-grade or high-grade Ta or T1 tumours. The low-grade superficial tumours are usually exophytic papillary TCCs and about 15% will progress to invasive cancers over 10 years. Treatment is by cystoscopy and endoscopic resection or diathermy. If no obvious lesion is seen on cystoscopy, multiple biopsies should be taken to exclude carcinoma *in situ* (CIS). High-grade (G3) T1 tumours are aggressive and thus need aggressive treatment. Following resection and diathermy there is evidence to suggest benefit from intravesical chemotherapy (e.g. mitomycin) to reduce recurrences. The patients are usually followed up every few months by regular cystoscopies to watch for recurrences. CIS behaves like a high-grade TCC and therefore also requires aggressive treatment. Intravesical immunotherapy with BCG can be used to prevent progression of CIS.

Invasive Bladder Cancers

T2 and T3 tumours are treated by either radical radiotherapy or radical cystectomy and formation of an ileal conduit or neobladder out of the small bowel (usually a length of ileum). An ileal conduit results in a stoma. Formation of a neobladder is highly complex surgery with a high complication rate and is reserved for patients who are young, well motivated and with a high chance of cure from the cystectomy. T4 disease is treated symptomatically. This may sometimes include cystectomy for intractable bladder symptoms.

RENAL TUMOURS

Cysts are very common in the kidney and are completely benign. Malignant tumours can be primary or secondary, although secondaries in the kidney are unusual. The primary tumours which usually affect those over 50 years old can arise from the kidney substance itself, and are called renal cell carcinomas, or from the lining of the collecting system (in the pelvis or ureters), and are called transitional cell cancers. Other tumours include Wilm's tumour (which affects children) and lymphomas.

Renal cell carcinomas (RCCs) account for more than 80% of renal tumours. These are renal adenocarcinomas (in the past it was thought that they arose from the adrenal rests within the kidney, and hence their old-fashioned name was 'hypernephroma'). They actually arise in the renal tubules and are also known as clear cell carcinomas, since the cells appear clear (they are large, with lots of lipid in the cytoplasm). The aetiology is unknown but there is an increased incidence in tobacco smokers. As RCCs grow they become encapsulated by a rim of normal kidney tissue. They can present with haematuria (invasion into the renal pelvis) or with pain (due to pressure effects on local structures and nerves). The classic presentation of an RCC is therefore the triad of pain, haematuria and a renal mass, although this triad is rare and usually the patient has only one or two of these symptoms. RCCs can grow along the renal vein and up the inferior vena cava, and metastases are therefore usually blood-borne and commonly go to the lungs (cannonball metastases), bone (pathological fractures), brain, etc. They may present with symptoms due to the production of hormones such as erythropoeitin (polycythaemia) or parathyroid hormone-like substance (hypercalcaemia). Although very popular in the older textbooks, these presentations are in fact quite rare. Nowadays about 50% of RCCs are found incidentally in patients having an ultrasound scan or CT scan for unrelated symptoms.

On examination a mass may be palpable in the loin. How do you differentiate a kidney from a spleen? The kidney is ballotable (place one hand on the abdomen and the other in the renal angle, raise the hand in the renal angle and keep the other hand still; if you feel a mass touch your upper hand you have balloted a kidney), it moves vertically down on inspiration and it is resonant to percussion (due to the overlying colon). The spleen, on the other hand, has a notch and moves towards the right iliac fossa on inspiration and is dull to percussion.

If an RCC obstructs the renal vein a varicocoele can result on the left. If you see a varicocoele in the left scrotum, think of an RCC, since the testicular vein on the left drains into the renal vein (it enters the IVC directly on the right). Only 1% of renal tumours, however, present with a varicocoele.

Diagnosis is usually made on ultrasound, showing a solid mass arising from the kidney. A CT scan is necessary for staging the disease. The other kidney must be checked not only to make sure it is present and functioning, but also because the disease may be bilateral. Treatment is usually by radical nephrectomy (kidney, surrounding fat within Gerota's fascia with or without the adrenal gland). Partial nephrectomy can be considered if the tumour is small ($<4\,cm$) or if the patient has a single kidney or poor renal function. Intra-arterial embolisation may be employed to reduce the vascularity of the tumour preoperatively. RCCs have proved themselves to be resistant to chemotherapy and radiotherapy. There is some evidence supporting the use of immunotherapy with interferons in advanced disease but the benefits of these therapies are marginal.

Pelviureteric tumours. These are the same as the TCCs of the bladder, although they account for less than 20% of renal tumours (whereas TCC accounts for almost all of the bladder tumours). They usually present with haematuria. Diagnosis is made by IVU showing a filling defect. Treatment is usually nephrectomy plus removal of the ureter on that side (nephro-ureterectomy). Follow-up must include regular cystoscopies to look for tumours in the bladder. (Fifty per cent of patients will subsequently develop bladder tumours.)

A Wilm's tumour (nephroblastoma) contains a bizarre variety of cell and tissue components derived from the mesoderm (for example, as well as kidney substance they may contain fat, cartilage and bone). This is the commonest intra-abdominal tumour in under-10s, with a peak incidence in 2–3-year-olds. It usually presents with a mass, and diagnosis is by ultrasound, CT or MRI. About 10% are bilateral. It is an aggressive, rapidly growing tumour that metastasises often to the lungs. Treatment is usually radical nephrectomy. Chemotherapy is sometimes given postoperatively, depending on the stage. If the tumour is caught early enough, survival is high.

TESTICULAR TUMOURS

Accounting for less than 2% of male malignancies, these are uncommon (despite being the commonest solid tumours in young men). The incidence is about 7 per 100,000 men. Almost all are malignant (95%). Testicular tumours can be divided into germ cell and non-germ-cell tumours. Almost all are germ cell tumours. The germ cell tumours can be divided into seminomas (40%), nonseminomatous germ cell tumours (NSGCT) (10%) (also called teratomas) and mixed (40%). Rarely, choriocarcinomas and yolk sac tumours are seen (these are types of NSGCT).

For finals the most important testicular tumours to know about are the seminomas and teratomas. The peak incidence is 20–40 years. Two per cent are bilateral and there is a significantly increased risk in men with undescended testes.

Non-germ-cell tumours include Leydig cell and Sertoli cell tumours and lymphomas. The Leydig cell and Sertoli cell tumours are very rare; however, they can produce oestrogens and androgens, resulting in over-virilisation or feminisation. Lymphomas can occur in the testicle in men in the fifth and sixth decades.

Seminomas arise in the epithelium of the seminiferous tubules, tend to grow slowly and metastasise to regional and para-aortic lymph nodes (remember that the lymphatics usually follow the venous drainage and the testicular veins drain towards the IVC and not to the groin). Placental alkaline phosphatase can be raised in metastatic seminomas. NSGCTs arise from all three germ cell layers, can be more aggressive and carry a poorer prognosis than seminomas. They are subdivided histologically, depending on whether the tumour is well differentiated, moderately differentiated or undifferentiated. The more undifferentiated carry a poorer prognosis. They metastasise via the blood and the lymphatics and most of them secrete αHCG and αFP, which can be used as tumour markers.

Staging of Testicular Tumours

Stage I — Tumour confined to testis
Stage II — Involvement of lymph nodes below diaphragm
Stage III — Lymph nodes above diaphragm involved
Stage IV — Extralymphatic spread

The tumours usually present as a painless testicular mass, although they can present with a secondary hydrocoele or a painful lump (10% present with pain). They may be misdiagnosed initially as an epididymo-orchitis. On examination you should look for evidence of lymphatic spread (abdominal, supraclaviular and chest).

A common exam question concerns how to examine a scrotum. You should always ask yourself four questions: Can I get above it (you should be able to get above a testicular lesion, but not a hernia), is the lump in the testis or is it separate, does it transilluminate and is the testis tender? A hard mass in the testis, which you can get above and which does not transilluminate, is likely to represent a testicular tumour.

An ultrasound can be performed to see if a scrotal lump is connected with the testis and if it is solid or cystic. A solid lump suggests malignancy. Serum αFP (never raised in seminomas) and βHCG should be sent, as should placental alkaline phosphatase. To stage the disease a CT scan of the chest, abdomen and pelvis is performed. Treatment starts by an orchidectomy via a groin incision. The reason for the groin incision is three-fold: to allow the cord to be clamped before mobilising the testicle, to prevent seeding of the scrotal skin and to allow the incision to be within the radiotherapy field. The testis is then brought out and examined. If the lump appears malignant (or a frozen section is performed to confirm the diagnosis histologically), then it is excised together with the spermatic cord. Further treatment depends on the tumour type, and its stage and grade. Tumour markers should again be sent off at 1 week, since if they are still high after surgery, it indicates the presence of residual disease.

Seminomas are very radiosensitive. Radiotherapy is usually given both to the groin and to the abdominal lymph nodes. Stage IV tumours are usually given chemotherapy initially, although they are rare (as seminomas usually present earlier than teratomas). Teratomas are less sensitive to radiotherapy, and combination chemotherapy (for example actinomycin, bleomycin, methotrexate and cisplatin) is usually given at the start.

The prognosis for Stage I seminomas and teratomas is extremely good (96–100% 5-year survival) and for Stage IV disease 5-year survival is 55–75%, depending on the tumour and the tumour bulk. Any recurrence following initial treatment is likely to occur within the first 18–24 months and close surveillance is therefore very important over this period, with repeat CT scanning and tumour markers, initially every 6 weeks and then every 3 months.

OTHER CONDITIONS OF THE TESTES

Hydrocoele

This is the presence of fluid around the testis between the tunica vaginalis and the tunica albuginea (Figure 14.1). The condition can be primary or

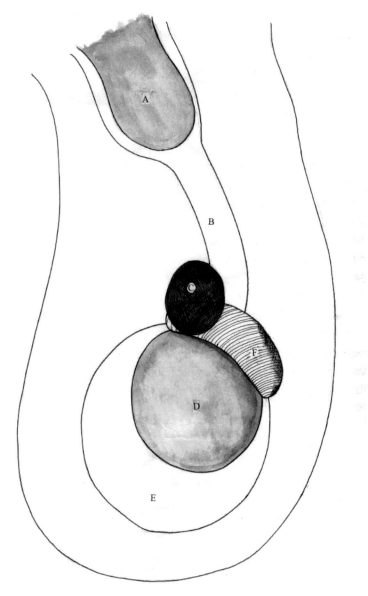

Figure 14.1. Testicular lumps. (A) Indirect inguinal hernia, (B) spermatic cord, (c) epididymal cyst, (D) testis, (E) hydrocoele, and (F) epididymis.

secondary. Primary (idiopathic) hydrocoeles (the vast majority) develop slowly and can become large and tense. They are commonest in the over-40 age group, although they can occur in children. If you recall your embryology, the testis descends from the abdomen taking a layer of peritoneum with it called the processus vaginalis. Normally, the processus closes removing the communication between the abdomen and the scrotum; however, if it remains patent peritoneal fluid can fill the sac, causing an infantile hydrocoele (if bowel contents enter the sac, then this is an infantile hernia; treatment of the infant hydrocoele is the same as that for an infantile hernia, that is, to close off the processus vaginalis). Primary hydrocoeles develop in adults in the absence of a patent processus, the tunica vaginalis producing excessive fluid for unknown reasons. Secondary hydrocoeles are usually secondary to trauma, infection or malignancy. In contrast they develop rapidly, are not tense and may contain blood.

On examination you can get above the swelling (which has a smooth surface), the testis is usually impalpable and it transilluminates brilliantly. An ultrasound should be performed to look at the testis. A small hydrocoele may not need treatment if the patient is not bothered by it. Larger hydrocoeles can be tapped but the fluid (which is straw coloured) will invariably return. Definitive surgical treatment involves either plicating the tunica vaginalis (Lord's repair) or inverting the sac (Jaboulay's repair).

Epididymo-orchitis

This is inflammation of the testis and epididymis due to infection. The young are more susceptible to viral infections (e.g. mumps), the old to bacterial infections (e.g. *Escherichia coli* following a UTI) and the sexually active to chlamydial and gonococcal infection. The typical presentation is acute onset of severe testicular pain. The patient may feel unwell with fever, have a urethral discharge and symptoms of a UTI. Pain may be referred to the right iliac fossa. On examination the testis is tender, red and warm. You can often feel a markedly swollen epididymis separate from the testicle. If you place your hand under the scrotum and elevate it, it sometimes relieves the pain of epididymo-orchitis, but not of torsion.

Testicular Torsion

This can affect any age but is most common between the ages of 12 and 27; it can occur, rarely, in neonates. There is a higher incidence in undescended testes. It is a urological emergency, as the testis will infarct within hours if the torsion is not treated. The testis twists within the tunica vaginalis and the blood supply is compromised. It usually presents with severe pain of very sudden onset and there are invariably no symptoms of a UTI. In contrast, a patient with epididymo-orchitis usually has a longer history of symptoms and may have urethritis with burning pain on micturition. On examination, if the testis lies horizontally or is retracted compared to the other side this could be indicative of a torsion.

An MSU should be dipstixed and sent urgently for microscopy, as this may help in cases where infection is likely. However, if you are in any doubt, then surgical exploration is essential. If you explore it and it is an infection, no harm is done, but if you treat a torsion conservatively the testicle will die. When you are exploring a testicle for torsion, the patient must always be warned of the possibility of orchidectomy if the testicle has infarcted. At the time of surgery both testicles are fixed (with a suture) to the scrotal wall to ensure that they cannot twist in the future. Doppler ultrasound is quite good at showing the integrity of the arterial blood flow to the testis, but should not delay surgical exploration.

RENAL COLIC

Stones may form at any level of the urinary tract. Symptoms depend on the site of stone impaction. The pain is due to the peristalsis and dilatation proximal to the obstruction. The size of the stone is not correlated with the amount of pain, as a large staghorn calculus of the renal pelvis may be painless and a tiny stone in the ureter may be agonising. The classic story is sudden onset of severe pain that makes the patient writhe about in agony, unable to get comfortable (in contrast with the pain of peritonism, where the patient lies still). The patient is sweaty, nauseous and may vomit. A stone in the ureter usually causes pain which starts in the loin and radiates down into the groin. There may also be pain in the scrotum or labia. A stone in the midureter may mimic appendicitis on the right and diverticulitis on the left. Most urinary tract calculi are calcium stones (80%) complexed with oxalate (35%), phosphate (3%) or mixed oxalate and phosphate crystals (40%). Others include struvite (magnesium ammonium phosphate), cystine, urate and xanthine.

They usually form when there is a high concentration of solutes in the urine, especially in dehydration. Most stone formers excrete excessive amounts of calcium in their urine, termed hypercalciuric. There may be a familial tendency and calcium stones may rarely be associated with hyperparathyroidism, renal tubular acidosis and medullary sponge kidney. Triple phosphate (struvite) stones are associated with urinary tract infections, especially *proteus*, which breaks down urea to form ammonia resulting in alkaline urine, which precipitates these stones. In contrast, acid urine tends to precipitate the calcium oxalate and urate containing stones. Ninety per cent of renal stones are radioopaque (urate stones are translucent), in contrast to gallstones, where 90% are radiolucent. Examination is usually normal, although the patient may have tenderness in the renal angle especially on percussion, which indicates retroperitoneal inflammation. A urine dipstix should reveal haematuria (in 90% of cases) and this should be confirmed by microscopy. If the urine shows no blood, you should be thinking of alternative diagnoses. NB: Renal colic is not a diagnosis, it is a simply a symptom of ureteric obstruction which may be caused by a stone but could be due to an aortic aneurysm, TCC of the ureter, retroperitoneal lymph nodes, etc. Other causes of pain, mimicking ureteric colic include an abdominal aortic aneurysm, appendicitis, pyelonephritis, diverticulitis and gynaecological causes. Analgesia should be given once the diagnosis is suspected. The pain from ureteric colic is usually alleviated by nonsteroidal anti-inflammatory agents but may require opiates. Usually an IVU is performed, usually by the casualty doctor. A baseline KUB X-ray is taken first. You should know the normal course of the ureters. They start at the renal pelvis, which lies at the level of L1 or L2 (look for the 12th rib, which is joined to T12, and go down one vertebra). They travel down from here along the line of the transverse processes towards the sacroiliac joint (where they cross over the iliac vessels). At this point they travel backwards towards the ischial spines and then forwards into the bladder. The common sites for obstruction to occur are the pelviureteric junction, the SIJ, where the ureter crosses over the iliac vessels and the vesicoureteric junction (VUJ). Remember that phleboliths (calcification in veins) are common in this region, but they are usually multiple, more rounded and have a radiolucent centre. A venflon is inserted and the radio-opaque contrast is injected into the arm. A film is taken after 5 min and another postmicturition. If there is any abnormality on the IVU, then a delayed film after about 1 h is usually taken. Further films should be taken until contrast is seen down to the level of obstruction. Request films at 1, 2, 4, 8 and 24 h if necessary. In the normal kidney, contrast is seen flowing towards the bladder. The ureter is a hollow tube that peristalses six times a minute. Students often get confused, because they see some contrast in the ureter and then see what looks like a stricture and think this must be a block. Actually, this simply represents a wave of peristalsis and is normal. If there is a block what you see is a standing column of contrast above the stone. The renal pelvis may be dilated and there may be blunting of the calyces. If there is complete obstruction on one side you may see a dense nephrogram (the kidney outline is visibly radio-opaque), with no contrast entering the ureter.

Nowadays instead of an IVU an unenhanced CT scan may be used to image the renal tract when stone disease is expected. This is safe in patients who are allergic to iodine. (The contrast used for the IVU contains contrast.) Diabetics on metformin have to stop taking their medication 24 h prior to having an IVU. Asthmatics may require steroid cover for contrast imaging.

If the patient is known to be pregnant, asthmatic or atopic, then an IVU might be contraindicated. In pregnancy an ultrasound may be performed. If the pain resolves and the kidney is not obstructed on IVU, the patient should be allowed to go home with oral analgesia and an appointment for the urology clinic. If the pain persists or the kidney is obstructed, then admission should be arranged. If the affected kidney is obstructed and there is evidence of sepsis, then this is a urological emergency, as damage to the kidney can occur if it is not drained urgently. Antibiotics should be started and urgent arrangements made to insert a nephrostomy tube to drain the kidney percutaneously.

Routine bloods should be sent to assess renal function; screening for calcium, urate and phosphate levels may be helpful in the case of recurrent episodes. The urine may be sieved to catch the stone as it passes and a 24 h urine collection may be analysed, as this may give information on ways to avoid a recurrence in the future. Ninety per cent of stones less than 4 mm in size pass spontaneously and about half of stones up to 7 mm pass spontaneously. Conservative management is therefore the first line in such patients. The urine is sieved and the patients are given analgesia and encouraged to drink a lot. Stones greater than 7 mm do not tend to pass and intervention is likely to be needed.

The treatment of renal and ureteric stones depends on the size and position of the stone. Extracorporeal shock wave lithotripsy (ESWL) is the treatment of choice for most renal and ureteric stones. In the middle third of the ureter it is often difficult to visualise the stone, due to the overlying iliac bone or sacrum; however, ESWL can still sometimes be used by adjusting the position of the patient.

ESWL can be performed on a day case or out-patient basis. Lithotripters generate a shock wave, using either electromagnetic or piezoelectrical energy to shatter the stone, under X-ray or ultrasound control. Other techniques for removing a stone include ureteroscopy, where the stone is visualised by passing a fine endoscope up the ureter and then fragmented with a pneumatic instrument (called a lithoclast) or with a laser.

If the stone is in the renal pelvis and is too large for lithotripsy, then percutaenous removal may be necessary. Under ultrasound or fluoroscopic guidance a needle is inserted into the calyx of the kidney. A guide wire is passed down the needle into the renal pelvis or ureter, and the needle is then removed. A series of dilators are inserted over the guide wire to create a track to the renal pelvis. The stone is then fragmented under direct vision and the fragments are removed (percutaneous nephrolithotomy).

In summary, ESWL is used for stones less than 2 cm in size in the kidney. If the stone is larger than 2 cm or if there is calyceal obstruction, then percutaneous removal may be necessary. For stones in the upper third or middle third of the ureter, ESWL or ureteroscopy is performed, ureteroscopy usually when ESWL has failed. For stones in the lower third of the ureter, ureteroscopy is usually the treatment of choice. In difficult cases, for example, an impacted ureteric stone, open surgery or laparoscopic surgery is occasionally indicated.

PAEDIATRIC UROLOGY

At birth adhesions are present between the glans and the foreskin and the prepuce normally becomes retractile by the age of 2 years. Sometimes the parents notice the prepuce 'ballooning' up when the child micturates, due to urine collecting in the space between foreskin and glans, before escaping through the narrow opening. This is normal and the parents should be reassured. A phimosis a narrowing of the opening of the foreskin, can also result secondary to infection and, in an adult, may cause painful intercourse. It is usually treated by circumcision. (A *paraphimosis* is a swelling of the glans as a result of a tight foreskin being retracted and not replaced. This can occur after catheterisation or erection. The tight foreskin blocks the venous return and the glans becomes oedematous and swollen. This is usually treated by reducing the oedema with compression, squeezing the foreskin and glans. The glans is then pressed in whilst flipping the foreskin forwards to its normal position.)

Hypospadias

This is an abnormal position of the urethral opening, due to failure of development. The urethra can open anywhere on the ventral (undersurface) surface of the penis. Repair is usually carried out by paediatric surgeons.

Undescended testes

The testis drops into the scrotum in 28–34 weeks of foetal development. In 80% of cases the undescended testis is palpable in the inguinal canal. If the testis is palpable in the inguinal canal or at the top of the scrotum, orchidopexy is performed (the testis is fixed in the scrotum, usually by mobilising the testis and placing it between the dartos muscle and the skin). This should be done by the age of 18 months, to prevent damage to the testis (spontaneous descent is rare after 1 year). After 2 years of age, the testis is likely to be damaged and may become incapable of spermatogenesis.

Complete absence of the testis is uncommon (check notes to see if present at birth check), and if it is not palpable it should be assumed to be intra-abdominal and an MRI or laparoscopy may be needed to locate it. If an undescended testicle presents after puberty, many urologists would advocate location and removal of the testicle because of the risk of malignant change.

15

ORTHOPAEDICS

Andrew Hilton

Orthopaedic trainees specialise in both Trauma and Elective Orthopaedics and in this chapter we have tried to cover all the really important subjects that you need to know for the finals examination. As much as possible we have tried to discuss principles rather than list every type of injury and fracture, and these principles can be applied to many different types of situation.

You should know how to examine the hand, hip, knee and shoulder with fluency and should practise these examinations on patients and on friends before the exam, so that they become second nature. Orthopaedic surgeons have in the past been stereotyped as using four-letter words and so it may come as no surprise that the orthopaedic examination can be summarised by the words: LOOK, FEEL, MOVE and X-RAY.

It is really difficult to learn specialised examination tests from a book and so we urge you to ask an orthopaedic consultant or registrar to demonstrate the examinations to you as well.

Remember, you have two limbs and so you should always examine the normal side first and then use this as a comparison for the abnormal or painful side. Also, in order to be seen to be thorough you should always offer to examine the joint above and below the one you are asked to do.

Always ask the patient if they mind you examining them and whether they have any pain (in a similar way to checking your mirrors in a driving test, make sure the examiners note that you have done so). Also, observe their face for pain during the examination, because hurting your patient is one of the biggest errors you can make in the exam.

EXAMINATION OF THE HIP

Quick Notes on the Hip

- Pain arising from the hip joint is commonly felt in the groin or anterior thigh and can be referred down to the knee. If the pain is predominantly in the back of the hip, it is usually referred from the lumbar spine. It is true to say that pains are usually referred distally, and so a knee pain may be coming from the hip and a hip pain may be coming from the back, etc.

Students often get worried about the correct order in which to examine a joint. The fact is that no order is necessarily correct and often the order of examination will differ, depending on the circumstances. To examine the hips properly, both legs need to be exposed (i.e. undress the patient to their underwear).

On *inspection* look at the *attitude* (or *posture*) of the limbs; for example, is one leg shortened or externally rotated compared to the other. Look for any obvious scars (do not forget to check the buttocks as a scar centred over the greater trochanter extending over the buttock could indicate previous hip replacement), swelling or wasting of the quadriceps, glutei or hamstrings. Inspect the legs for signs of venous or arterial disease (this will be important if an operation is being considered) and examine for any leg length discrepancy.

You should differentiate between real shortening (loss of bone length) and apparent shortening (due to a deformity of the pelvis or pelvic obliquity). First, try to position the pelvis so that the anterior superior iliac spines (ASIS) are at the same horizontal level.

On *palpation* measure the distance from the ASIS to the medial malleolus on each side (true length) and the distance from a fixed point such as the xiphisternum (or umbilicus) to the medial malleolus (apparent length). The apparent will differ from the true length if the pelvis is tilted (pelvic obliquity). Feel the bony contours, including the greater trochanter, the ASIS, the iliac crests and the pubic rami. Note that tenderness over the greater trochanter can also be trochanteric bursitis.

Test *movement* passively and actively. Normal ranges for the hip are flexion (0–130), extension (usually in a prone position, 0–10), abduction (0–45), adduction (0–30), external rotation (0–45) and internal rotation (0–20). Rotation can be tested with the hips flexed (i.e. knees bent to 90°) or the hips extended. In flexion, put one hand on the knee and the other on the foot — remember that external rotation brings the foot medially. To test adduction the limb is crossed over the opposite limb. Power should be recorded for each muscle group using the MRC grading system. One problem with the hip is that limitation of movement can be obscured by movement of the pelvis and hence a gross limitation of extension can be masked by arching the back into excessive lordosis. Therefore, when describing the range of motion always comment on any fixed flexion deformities first. You can use *Thomas's test* to check for this — fully flex the two hips simultaneously to obliterate the lumbar lordosis (you can place one hand under the lower back to confirm this). Whilst holding one leg in this position, ask the patient to straighten the other leg as fully as possible. The angle between the thigh and the bed is the fixed flexion deformity. Repeat the test on the other side. The commonest cause of a fixed flexion deformity is osteoarthritis.

The function and stability of the hip can be assessed by *Trendelenburg's test*. Ask the patient to stand on one leg by bending at the knee (as if they are doing an impression of a pirate with a wooden leg!). The normal pelvis tilts upwards very slightly on the unsupported side by contraction of the abductors on the weight-bearing side. A positive Trendelenburg sign occurs when the pelvis droops on the unsupported side — remember '*sound side sags*'. A positive test is found with any condition that affects the lever arm, such as weakness of the abductors, dislocation or fracture of the hip and any condition causing pain.

You must always examine the patients *gait*. If the patient is dependent on a walking stick or caliper, then you can ask them to use it. Gait involves all the joints of the lower limb, and it is therefore difficult sometimes to discern the exact cause of an abnormal gait. If the patient limps because of pain, then this is called *antalgic gait,* whereby the weight-bearing (stance) phase on the affected side is shorter, as the patient tries to avoid putting weight onto it. The commonest cause is osteoarthritis (OA). If one leg is shorter than the other, this is described as a short-legged gait but the stance phase is not reduced (unless there are coexisting short-legged and antalgic elements).

In the finals, at the end of the exam you are usually asked if there is anything else you would like to do, and it is probably acceptable to say *'I would also like to examine the leg pulses and neurological system'* at that point rather than do it routinely, as time is short and you want to give an impression of succinctness. Incidentally, if you see a case in the finals where the leg is deformed with muscular wasting and sensation is entirely normal, always look around the room for a caliper or cast brace, as polio cases often feature in finals (despite the fact that we see almost no new cases in this country!).

EXAMINATION OF THE KNEE

ΠΟ
Quick Notes on the Knee

- There are three components to the knee joint: the medial and lateral compartments (each between the femoral condyle and tibial plateau) and the patellofemoral compartment. The joint surfaces are lined by hyaline articular cartilage (which becomes worn in osteoarthritis). In addition, there are the two C-shaped fibrocartilaginous menisci lining the medial and lateral compartments. There are two ligaments running in opposite directions at the centre of the knee, which help make it stable, called the cruciate ligaments. The anterior cruciate stops the tibia moving anteriorly relative to the femur, whereas the posterior cruciate stops the tibia moving backwards relative to the femur. The capsule encloses the knee joint and is strengthened on the medial and lateral sides by the medial and lateral collateral ligaments.

As mentioned above, gait can be tested at the beginning or at the end of the examination — it does not really matter, as long as you remember it. With the patient standing, look at the alignment checking for valgus (*knock knees* — deviation of the distal part away from the midline) or varus deformities at the knees. *Look* at the foot arches to see if they are flattened (pes planus) or high arched (pes cavus), which can contribute to knee pathology. Are the patellae symmetrical? Look and measure for quadriceps wasting (which implies lack of use). This ideally should be done at 10 cm from the upper pole of the patella, as this correlates with vastus medialis wasting, which is the first muscle to go with disuse. Look for any visible scars or obvious effusions to the knees (even a small effusion may be noted by the absence of the normal hollow on either side of the patella).

Feel the skin temperature. This is helpful in the knee as the joint is superficial (unlike the hip), always comparing with the opposite side. To test for an effusion you can use the patella tap or stroke test. To perform the *patella tap*, compress the suprapatellar pouch with one hand and press down gently on the patella with the fingers of your opposite hand. You should be able to bounce the patella up and down on the fluid, always comparing to the other side. If there is only a small effusion a better test is the *stroke test*, where you empty the medial compartment by massaging the fluid into the lateral side of the knee. Then, apply gentle pressure over the lateral side, just above the patella, and watch the gutter on the medial side. It will balloon up with the fluid you have pushed over if there is an effusion.

Ask the patient to lift their leg into the air (with the knee extended). If the leg is lifted straight, then the quadriceps must be working normally. If there is a lag (meaning that the knee bends slightly as it is raised) then this either means that the quadriceps are weak or that there is a fixed flexion deformity. Place the flat of your palm under the ankle and ask the patient to let you take the full weight of the leg. If by doing so the leg straightens fully then you know there is no fixed flexion, whereas if it remains bent then there must be a fixed flexion deformity (the commonest cause being capsular fibrosis in OA).

Put your other hand over the knee cap (a right-handed examiner, examining the right leg, would hold the ankle with the right hand and the knee cap with the left hand) and feel for crepitus as the knee is flexed and extended (crepitus can signify irregular articular surfaces, often called chondromalacia patella). Now bend the knee to 90° and place the foot down. Palpate along the joint line of the knee (remember in this position the joint line is angled downwards at about a 45° slant, and so your thumb must feel the joint line which has a spongy consistency (unlike bone). Feel along the medial joint line and lateral joint line. Tenderness at any point usually indicates meniscal pathology (but could indicate a problem with any of the structures below your finger, i.e. skin, capsule, ligaments or bone).

The popliteal fossa should be examined for a popliteal cyst and a pulsatile popliteal aneurysm. A popliteal cyst is a nontender fluctuant lump that follows either synovial rupture or herniation. If there is underlying joint pathology such as OA, then it is called a Baker's cyst. Do not confuse a popliteal cyst or aneurysm (which are in the midline) or with an enlarged semimembranous bursa, which is on the medial side between semimembranous and the medial head of gastrocnemius and is often more prominent in a straight knee.

There are a lot of special tests for the patello femoral joint which you normally carry out if the symptoms are suggestive of patellofemoral pathology. You should test the side-to-side movements of the patella (the patella apprehension test is for patellae that have dislocated in the past — when the patella is pushed laterally, the patient becomes anxious, feeling like it is going to dislocate).

To test for tears of the *collateral ligaments*, flex the knee slightly (about 20°) and apply valgus and varus stress to the knee joint to see if there is any laxity. The knee has to be bent slightly because in full extension it normally 'locks'. Note that if the knee opens up to valgus or varus stress in full extension, then you should be concerned over a very serious injury and complete rupture of the ligaments. If the ligaments are tender to palpation but the knee feels stable to varus and valgus testing, this usually indicates a partial rather than a complete tear.

Diagnosis of meniscal pathology should be made from the history and a finding of positive joint line tenderness. *McMurray's test* assists the diagnosis of a meniscal tear, although the test often causes pain and can potentially propogate a tear. To be fair, this test causes a lot of confusion and so is best avoided. You will not fail an exam for not knowing specific tests, although you could fail if you hurt a patient by doing complex tests inappropriately.

To test the *cruciate ligaments*, have the patient lie flat; bend both knees so that the hip is at 45° and the knees at 90°. Look from the side for any sag of the tibia in relation to the femur. This implies a tear of the posterior cruciate. Now anchor the foot by sitting on it and grab the leg just below the knee with both hands and push backwards (*posterior draw test* — for a posterior cruciate tear) and then pull forward (*anterior draw test* — for a tear of the anterior cruciate). When moving the tibia, bear in mind that it is at right angles to the femur and so the direction you are pushing or pulling must be in the line of the femur. If the tibia moves forward more on one side compared to the other leg, then this is likely to be a positive draw test, implying a rupture of the anterior cruciate ligament. Beware if there was a posterior sag, since you may simply be correcting this rather than testing the anterior cruciate.

A modification of this test is the *Lachman test*, where the knee is flexed only to 30°, one hand grasps the thigh and the other hand grasps the tibia just below the knee. As the thigh is held still the tibia is pulled anteriorly, again testing the anterior cruciate. You need big hands for this test, although it is said to be a more sensitive test than the anterior draw.

One final test for the anterior cruciate rupture is the *pivot shift test*, which reproduces the instability that the patient experiences when their leg gives way. The knee is flexed fully and the foot internally rotated. A slight valgus strain is applied to the knee as it is slowly extended. Again, this test can be very painful for the patient and often has to be performed under anaesthesia. In an exam it would be better to avoid it, but to mention that it is a test one could perform when assessing the ACL.

A positive test is represented by a click as the tibia shifts anteriorly, falling into place when the knee is extended. In the authors' experience these tests are all best learnt by direct demonstration rather than from a textbook.

EXAMINATION OF THE SHOULDER

Quick Notes on the Shoulder

* Pain in the region of the shoulder may be referred from the cervical spine, the chest and the mediastinum, and from irritation of the diaphragm.

- The shoulder is the most mobile of all joints and is thus one of the most unstable.
- The rotator cuff has four muscles (supraspinatus, infraspinatus, teres minor and subscapularis) that surround the joint holding the humeral head in against the glenoid providing some stability, although there is a deficiency inferiorly which is the site of potential weakness.
- Abduction at the glenohumeral joint is only about 50° after which the greater tuberosity impinges on the acromion process. To accomplish any further abduction you need to externally rotate the humerus. In addition, the scapula needs to rotate. Given that the abductors of the arm all originate from the mobile scapula, there needs to be dynamic coordination of all of the muscles involved in stabilising and mobilising the scapulae as the arm moves.
- Serratus anterior holds the scapulae against the chest wall and is supplied by the long thoracic nerve of Bell. Damage to this nerve can lead to *winging* of the scapulae.

Expose the whole torso and observe for bruises, redness and scars. *Look* from the front and then ask the patient to turn around and observe any asymmetry of the shoulders or scapulae from behind. Look for wasting of the deltoid, pectoral muscles, rhomboids and trapezius and any prominence of the acromioclavicular joint (ACJ). Do not forget to inspect the axilla.

Feel the temperature and for any localised bony tenderness (sternoclavicular joint, the clavicle, spine of scapula, acromion process, ACJ, humeral head and greater and lesser tuberosities).

Movement is again active and passive. Ask the patient to abduct both arms above their head. Watch their face for grimacing and note which part of the arc of movement is painful. Pain at the beginning to midrange of movement is usually due to rotator cuff pathology, such as inflammation or a tear of the supraspinatus. Pain at the end of abduction may be due to acromioclavicular OA. Observe movement at the glenohumeral joint and of the scapula on both sides. Test also flexion, extension, rotation and adduction (the arm moves in front of the body). Active rotation is best tested by asking the patient to touch the back of their neck with both hands (external rotation in abduction) and the small of their back (internal rotation). Now passively repeat all of these movements.

Passive rotation is tested with the elbow flexed to 90° and touching the side of the body. In this position, bringing the hand across the body is internal rotation and away from the body, external rotation. Record the power of each muscle group and test for any neurovascular deficit.

Test for winging of the scapulae by asking the patient to place their hands out in front of them pressing against a wall. If the serratus anterior is paralysed, the scapula will protrude like a wing.

There are many special tests for the shoulder; however, you probably just need to know the above for finals purposes. A very rare inherited disorder is craniocleidodysostosis, where there is absence of the clavicles and the patient can bring both shoulders to the midline. This is the sort of rare but interesting case that sometimes turns up at finals, so it is probably worth a mention.

EXAMINATION OF THE HANDS

Quick Notes on the Hands

- The thumb, the index finger and the middle finger are the most important for the functioning of the hand (touch, grip, precise movements), whereas the ring finger and the little finger are more important for grip strength.
- Distal interphalangeal joints = DIPJs, proximal interphalangeal joints = PIPJs and metarcarpophalangeal joints = MCPJs.
- Refer to the fingers as thumb, index, middle, ring and little fingers and not 1, 2, 3, 4 and 5.
- The DIPJs are flexed by the flexor digitorum profundus (inserting into the base of the distal phalanx) and the PIPJs are flexed by the flexor digitorum superficialis (which splits around the profundus and inserts into the base of the middle phalanx).
- The flexor digitorum profundus (FDP) is innervated by both the median and the ulna nerves, usually the median nerve supplying the

part that flexes the index and middle fingers, with the ulna nerve supplying the part that flexes the ring and little fingers.

- The Palmar interrossei ADduct the fingers (PAD), whereas the Dorsal interrossei ABduct or spread the fingers (DAB).
- The interrossei and lumbricals are responsible for flexion at the MCPJs (whilst the PIPJs and DIPJs are extended).
- All of the intrinsic muscles of the hand are supplied by T1 as the ulnar nerve (except the LOAF muscles (see under 'carpal tunnel syndrome'), which are supplied by the median nerve).
- Primary OA tends to affect the DIPJs, whereas RA tends to affect the MCPJs and PIPJs, sparing the DIPJs.

Hands are very commonly seen in finals (usually as a rheumatology case). You may still see a rheumatoid hand as a surgical case, although you are more likely to see a nerve injury, Dupuytren's, trigger finger or a ganglion. As hand examination is covered well in the rheumatology books, you will simply find a summary of the examination here.

Introduce yourself and ask the patient whether they mind you examining their hands and whether they are painful. If a pillow is available place it under the hands for comfort.

Inspect the hands, look at the dorsum and then ask the patient to turn their hands over so that you can look at the palms. Observe any scars, palmar erythema, muscle wasting, nail changes or obvious deformities such as Dupuytren's contracture, mallet finger, Boutonniere, swan neck, Z thumb deformities, Heberden's nodes (which are nodular swellings at the DIPJs, seen in osteoarthritis) and Bouchard's nodes (similar swellings seen at the PIPJs).

Feel the temperature and palpate all of the individual joints (especially the MCPJs), feeling for any synovial or capsular thickening or swelling (indicative of active synovitis). Feel the palm of the hand for thickenings or nodules of the palmar fascia suggestive of early Dupuytrens. Ask the patient to make a fist and then to touch the thumb to the tip of each finger (opposition). Then, test finger abduction and adduction. Test the strength of each of these muscle groups by asking them to grasp your finger in a grip and to stop you pulling your fingers out from between their opposed thumb and little finger. Test resisted abduction by asking them to keep their fingers spread against resistance and resisted adduction by asking them to grip a piece of paper between their adducted fingers as you pull it out.

Test sensation in the median (the tip of the index finger), radial (the dorsum of the base of the thumb) and ulna (the tip of the little finger) nerve distributions. As for testing the nerve function in more detail, see the section on nerve injuries at the end of the chapter. Finally, test function by asking the patient to do up a shirt button, hold an object such as a key or a pen, etc.

If when the fingers are extended (from a grip) one of the fingers stays flexed, consider *Dupuytrens* and *trigger finger*. Dupuytrens usually affects the ring and little finger (see below). Ask the patient if they can straighten the finger themselves. In Duputrens they will tell you they cannot.

If they can straighten it (usually with a snap), this is likely to be a *trigger finger*. Trigger finger is usually caused by thickening of the fibrous tendon sheath, perhaps due to repetitive trauma. Feel along the palm (volar) aspect of the hand (at the level of the MCPs) and you may feel a thickening of the sheath which rolls under your finger as the patient flexes and extends their finger. This is also the location for a small ganglion, sometimes referred to as a *pearl ganglion*, because of its size and consistency, and is worth a mention.

FRACTURE CLASSIFICATION AND MANAGEMENT

A fracture is a break in the continuity of a bone. It should be thought of as a soft tissue injury around a broken bone, since often more problems can arise from the soft tissue damage than from the fracture itself.

Fractures can be open or closed, intra or extra-articular, and displaced or undisplaced. *Open fractures* (used to be called 'compound') are fractures where the surface wound communicates with the fracture and there is thus potential for contamination through the wound (the wound does not necessarily have to be skin and may be an internal body surface, such as the rectum). In *closed fractures* the skin remains intact. You cannot tell from an X-ray whether a fracture is open or closed.

Types of Fracture

Types of fracture pattern include *transverse, oblique, spiral, multifragmen-tary* (i.e. more than two fragments — used to be called comminuted), *avulsion* (a bony fragment being torn off by a tendon or ligament), *compression* (or *crush*, which occurs when cancellous bone is crumpled, such as in the calcaneum after a fall from a height or in the vertebral bodies, especially in the presence of osteoporosis) and *stress fractures* (these occur after repeated stresses that cause the bone to fatigue, often seen in the lower limbs of athletes) (Figure 15.1). Two other types you need to know about are greenstick and pathological fractures.

Greenstick fractures are seen in children, whose bones are softer and more pliable and tend to bend rather than break. The cortex on one side

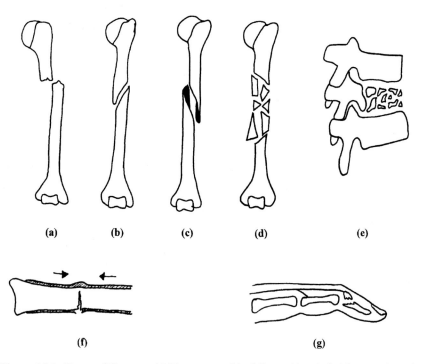

(a)   (b)   (c)   (d)   (e)

(f)   (g)

Figure 15.1. Types of fracture. **(a)** Transverse, **(b)** oblique, **(c)** spiral, **(d)** comminuted, **(e)** crush, **(f)** greenstick, and **(g)** avulsion.

tends to buckle (imagine bending a young green twig — hence the name greenstick).

Pathological fractures are fractures occurring in a bone that has already been weakened by disease, and may occur at normal physiological stresses. There are many causes, including generalised bone diseases or metastatic deposits in the bone. One could think of pathological fractures as being of two types: one where a fracture occurs in a patient with generalised bone disease, such as a crushed vertebra or a fractured neck of femur in an osteoporotic lady; the other type occurs in patients with normal bone structure, but the fracture is in a localised area of abnormal bone, such as through a metastatic deposit.

Osteoporosis is the commonest cause of pathological fracture, especially in the spine and femoral neck. Although most books tend to classify osteoporotic fractures as pathological, in practice we do not tend to refer to them as being pathological, otherwise most of the fractures in the geriatric age group would be 'pathological', and this term is therefore usually reserved for those involving malignancies.

Displacement of Fractures

When a bone breaks, the fragments often displace due to the force of the injury and also due to gravity and the pull of muscles attached to the fragments. There are many terms used to describe displacement, such as impaction, angulation, opposition and rotation. Impaction implies that the fragments are driven into one another, causing shortening. Angulation (or alignment) means that one fragment is angulated in relation to the other, which if left alone may lead to deformity of the limb. Angulation is described in degrees. Whenever describing displacement always refer to the distal fragment relative to the proximal fragment (Figure 15.2).

Dislocations. This is a *complete loss* of congruity between the articulating surfaces of a joint. The term implies disruption to the capsule and soft tissues around the joint. Dislocations should be relocated as soon as possible to prevent long-term complications.

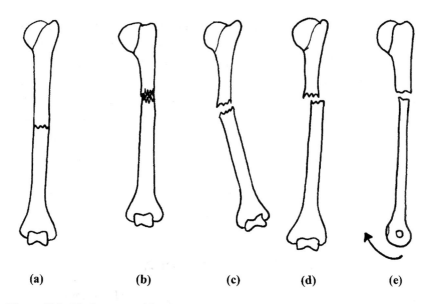

Figure 15.2. Displacement of fractures. **(a)** Undisplaced, **(b)** impacted, **(c)** angulated (25°), **(d)** lateral displacement (i.e. 50% opposed), and **(e)** rotation (note how there is a mismatch between the widths of the proximal & distal fragments).

Subluxation. This is *partial loss* of contact between two joint surfaces, as is seen, for example, at the acromioclavicular joint. Both dislocations and subluxations can be associated with fractures, and they are then termed 'fracture dislocations' or 'fracture subluxations'.

Fracture Healing

There are five stages to the healing of a fracture. There is *bleeding* into the fracture and an *inflammatory* reaction is set up, the cells *proliferate* and early bone and cartilage is formed (callus), which then *consolidates* (as woven bone is transformed into stronger lamellar bone). The bone then *remodels* to the normal stresses it is placed under, and over a period of months to years the bone returns to its normal shape. The rate of repair depends on many factors, including which bone is affected, the position and blood supply of the fragments, the age and general health of the patient and the method of restriction of the fracture (e.g. plaster Vs surgery).

As a rough guide, however, the long bones of a healthy adult's upper limb take about 6 weeks to begin the consolidation process and so we usually treat upper limb fractures in plaster for about 6 weeks. In the lower limb fractures take longer to heal and so if plaster is being used we usually wait 12 weeks before it is removed. It is worth noting, however, that a fracture of the tibia or femur can actually take a lot longer than that to gain full strength (up to 6 months or more). Most ankle fractures, involving the malleoli, are treated like upper limb fractures with plaster on for about 6 weeks.

Children heal much quicker than adults and the younger the patient the quicker the time to healing.

DESCRIBING A FRACTURE ON AN X-RAY

X-rays must be orthogonal, meaning that you should always have two views taken at 90° to each other (usually an AP and a lateral X-ray), and as a rule they should include both the joint above and the joint below the fracture. The part you want to look at should always be at the centre of the radiograph. In addition, if an X-ray is taken of a long bone, such as the femur, the entire bone should ideally be on one X-ray.

If you are given one view of an X-ray in an exam, you should always ask the examiner for another view and an X-ray of the joint above and below. Not only is this the correct way to assess X-rays but it also buys you time to analyse what you are seeing and shows the examiner that you are competent. If there is a red dot on the film or some writing on it (such as the words 'standing film'), always state this, as it usually is there for a reason. The red dot is an informal system devised by radiographers to indicate that they think there is an abnormality.

When you are asked to describe a fracture on an X-ray, always begin with the date and patient details, followed by the part of the body (e.g. the limb), the affected bone or bones, the type of fracture (open, closed, intra-articular or extra-articular) and its displacement.

Example: These are AP and lateral X-rays of the right forearm of Mrs Jane Smith, taken on the 5 March. They show an oblique extra-articular fracture of the distal radius, which is impacted and therefore shortened, and there is about 10° of radial and dorsal angulation of the distal fragment. There is also an associated undisplaced fracture of the ulnar styloid. This injury is known as Colles' fracture.

If asked about management of a fracture, even if you do not know much about this type of fracture, simply describe it on the X-ray and discuss management in terms of the following four Rs.

MANAGEMENT OF FRACTURES

1. Resuscitation
2. Reduction
3. Restriction (maintenance of reduction)
4. Rehabilitation

Resuscitation

Following the ATLS® guidelines (see Chapter 4), one should deal with associated life-threatening injuries first. The airway, breathing and circulation take priority over the fracture. In the case of any major trauma, the standard trauma series of X-rays should be performed as part of the ATLS® primary survey. These include a C-spine, a chest and a pelvic X-ray. The fracture is usually assessed in the secondary survey.

There are obviously some exceptions to this, including active bleeding from an unstable pelvic fracture or an open fracture, in which case they are addressed under C for Circulation in the primary survey. In a bleeding open wound, a sterile pressure dressing is applied and for a pelvic fracture either external splintage or external fixation must be used.

It is vital that you assess the neurovascular status and remember the importance of assessing the condition of the skin and soft tissues. Always ensure that you are not dealing with a dislocation by examining the joints on either side of the fracture. All findings must be documented and all this should be done before any X-rays of the limb are taken.

Open fractures require urgent attention. The life-threatening injuries are dealt with first in the same way, but because of the risk of infection and neurovascular compromise, open fractures need to be booked for theatre as an emergency (within 6 h).

Any gross contaminants in the wound should be removed. Antibiotics should be started (broad spectrum) and a tetanus booster given if needed (a toxoid booster lasts 10 years). A photograph should be taken for reference so that the wound does not need to be inspected repeatedly, and then the wound should be covered with an antiseptic-soaked dressing. The limb is usually immobilised using a splint to prevent pain and further contamination whilst awaiting theatre. If there is gross deformity, manipulation under sedation may be needed before it can be splinted. The neurovascular status must be checked both before and after this is carried out. The patient is booked for examination under anaesthesia (EUA) and debridement.

In theatre, the wound is thoroughly washed out and any contaminated or dead tissue is debrided. The fracture is assessed and stabilised (usually by internal or external fixation). If the wound is large and primary closure is unlikely to be achieved, then a plastic surgeon should ideally be present in theatre, as it may be possible to perform a skin graft or flap procedure (alternatively, the wound can be left open and reinspected at about 48 h for delayed primary closure or a skin grafting procedure).

Remember the saying 'In open fractures — save life, save limb and stabilise fracture'.

Other fractures that need urgent treatment include fracture dislocations and those fractures with vascular or neurological compromise.

Reduction

Not all fractures require reduction, either because there is no displacement or because the displacement is unlikely to affect the final result (e.g. rib fractures). The decision on whether to reduce comes down to a balance between function and acceptable appearance.

Anatomical reduction is ideal and, in particular, if any articular surfaces are involved then these must be reduced anatomically.

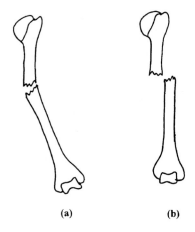

(a)   (b)

Figure 15.3. Alignment of a fracture. **(a)** Well opposed but angulated and **(b)** well aligned but poorly opposed [more acceptable than (a)].

If a fracture is left displaced, it could heal in an unacceptable position, with resultant deformity. Alignment of the fracture is more important than opposition (Figure 15.3).

Methods of Reduction

1. *Manipulation* (or closed reduction). This is usually under local, regional or general anaesthetic. The distal fragment is pulled in the line of the bone to disimpact the fragments and the deformity may need to be exaggerated before the bones can be repositioned manually.
2. *Traction.* This is used when the contraction forces of large muscles need to be overcome, in particular for fractures of the femur. There are two types of traction, skin or skeletal. With skin traction, adhesive tape and bandaging is applied to the skin. With skeletal traction, a pin is placed through a bone distal to the fracture. In either case the limb is pulled, usually via a pulley system, in the direction of a weight applied at the end of the bed.
3. *Open reduction.* This is used only after failure of the above methods. In certain fractures however, this is the first choice. These include

displaced intra-articular fractures [and it is then referred to as open reduction and internal fixation (ORIF)]. It has the advantage of allowing an accurate reduction but carries the risks and complications of surgery.

Restriction (Maintenance of Reduction)

Once the fracture is reduced, it must be held in that position to allow it to heal. Some fractures are liable to displace after having been reduced and these are called *unstable* fractures. These need to be kept in position by some form of restriction.

Other fractures are inherently *stable*, due to splintage from the adjacent soft tissues surrounding the fracture, and these fractures tend to stay in the reduced position. Logic suggests that you do not need to support *stable* fractures, although in practice they are often splinted (for example, in a plaster cast) because of the risk that they may be knocked and may displace again (and also to reduce the pain and rest the affected part).

Methods of Restriction

1. *Nonrigid methods of support.* Slings and elastic supports (e.g. Tubigrip).
2. *Plaster fixation.* The commonest is plaster of Paris. Newer types of fibreglass are lighter and stronger, although more expensive. All plasters can soften if they become wet, and the position of the fragments can be lost.

   Due to the risk of compartment syndrome (see below) during the first 24–48 h after a fracture a back slab (half a cast) is usually applied. This allows for accommodation of any early swelling and can be *completed* by application of a further few layers of plaster after a few days. If a full plaster is applied, then it must be split.
3. *Functional bracing (cast bracing).* Here, the joints are left free to move, but the shafts of the bone are supported in cast segments usually joined by hinges to allow movement only in one plane. This is most

widely used for femoral or tibial fractures. It is usual to wait until the fracture has begun to unite before functional bracing is applied. So in the lower limb fractures tend to be placed in a plaster cast for 6 weeks and are then converted into a functional brace. In the elderly with peri-articular injuries, functional bracing is sometimes the first line of treatment.

4. *Continuous traction.* Skin or skeletal traction can be maintained for several weeks. In adults it does not tend to be used much nowadays, due to the problems of prolonged bed rest and also for social and economic reasons. One common example of traction used nowadays is the collar and cuff for certain shoulder fractures, where the weight of the arm is used as the force of distraction. Another is Gallows traction, used in children less than 2 years old with femoral fractures.

5. *An external fixator (ex-fix).* The bony fragments are held in position by pins inserted through the skin and into the bone. The pins are then joined together with some external mechanical support. This method is especially useful in the management of open fractures where internal fixation with permanent metalwork may in some cases be inadvisable due to the higher risk of infection. Any patient with an ex-fix needs to be educated about pin site hygiene as it is not uncommon for the pin sites to become infected. In the case of deep infection the pins have to be removed.

6. *Internal fixation.* Pins, plates, screws or large intramedullary nails are used to hold the bony fragments in position. They are usually left in permanently, although they can be removed if necessary once the fracture has united. Sometimes a bone graft (see section on nonunion) is used to aid fracture healing, especially if there are large areas of bone loss. Internal fixation is used when the reduction needs to be as near perfect as possible (such as when a joint surface is involved), and also in the management of certain fractures to aid early mobility of the patient (e.g. hip fractures) or where it will not be possible to maintain an acceptable position by splintage or traction alone (very unstable fractures). Internal fixation is advocated in the management of multiply injured patients involving the lower extremity (especially femoral fractures), where early fixation may reduce complications and aid with nursing care.

Rehabilitation

Just because one part of the body is injured does not mean that the patient has to stay in bed and rest. The remaining limbs should be mobilised to avoid other complications. It is often quoted that immobility leads to a reduction in muscle mass of approximately 50% within 2 weeks.

The rehabilitation of the affected part really depends on the type of fracture. For example, after a hip operation it is important to get the patient up mobilising as soon as possible. The physiotherapists are involved early and help with exercises and mobility. Rehabilitation involves restoring not only the injured part but also the patient as a whole. This means the occupational therapist should help with various splints, mobility aids and home modifications, the social services should be involved to increase resources such as home helps and meals on wheels, etc.

Listed above are *all of the options* for the management of fractures; you will, however, find that two surgeons at different hospitals may differ markedly in the way they treat the same fracture. This is because the decision on how a fracture should be treated depends on many factors, including:

- The nature of the accident and the complexity of the fracture
- The condition of the skin and soft tissues
- Any associated injuries
- The age, general health and personality of the patient
- The facilities available
- The skill of the surgeon

COMPLICATIONS OF FRACTURES

General Complications

Complications of Any Tissue Damage

- Haemorrhage and shock
- Fat embolism and respiratory distress syndrome
- Infection
- Muscle damage and rhabdomyolysis

Complications of Prolonged Bed Rest

- Chest infection and urinary tract infection
- Pressure sores and muscle wasting
- Deep vein thrombosis and pulmonary embolus

Complications of Anaesthesia

- Anaphylaxis
- Damage to teeth
- Aspiration

Complications Specific to the Fracture

Immediate	Haemorrhage
	Neurovascular and visceral damage
Early	Compartment syndrome
	Infection (worse if associated with metalwork)
Late	Problems with union (delayed, non- and malunion)
	Avascular necrosis
	Sudek's atrophy
	Myositis ossificans
	Joint stiffness
	Growth disturbance

Compartment Syndrome

Muscles are divided into separate compartments (osteofascial compartments) by membranes that join the bone to the subcutaneous fascia. Swelling that occurs after a fracture can lead to an increase in the pressure within one of these compartments. As the pressure rises, the capillary blood flow to the tissues decreases. Ischaemia results when the capillary pressure is less than the compartment pressure. After about 6 h irreversible changes begin leading to muscle and nerve necrosis. Once infracted, the muscle is replaced by fibrous tissue which will lead to contractures (Volkman's ischaemic contracture). Compartment syndrome can occur inside a plaster that is too tight.

The patients classically have pain that is out of proportion to clinical findings, paraesthesia and a tight feeling in the affected compartment. The best and earliest sign of compartment syndrome is pain on passive stretching of the muscles of the affected compartment (for the forearm flexor compartment this means stretching the fingers straight). Compartment syndrome should not be confused with an ischaemic limb as the limb is commonly warm and erythematous and not cold and pale.

The common sites for compartment syndrome are the lower limb (especially with tibial fractures) and the forearm. If you are called to see a patient in whom you suspect compartment syndrome, your initial management should be to elevate the limb, remove all of the bandages and split the cast (right the way down to skin, if not split already); if this fails to relieve the pain, then you should remove the plaster. Ask a senior immediately to assess the patient. It is possible to measure the compartment pressures directly, using pressure probes if facilities permit, although these can be unreliable and really it is a clinical diagnosis. If the symptoms progress then treatment involves performing a fasciotomy to relieve the pressure.

Neurological Complications

Actual nerve severance is rare, but stretching over a bony edge in a fracture or dislocation is more common. Nerve injuries can be classified according to the Seddon classification, which has three types — neuropraxia, axonotmesis and neurotmesis.

Examples of nerve palsies include axillary nerve palsy (dislocation of the shoulder), radial nerve palsy (fracture of the shaft of the humerus), ulnar nerve palsy (elbow dislocation), sciatic nerve palsy (dislocated hip) and common peroneal nerve palsy (fracture of the neck of the fibula or knee dislocation). Nerve palsies are usually reversible, although it can sometimes take months before the function returns to normal.

Problems with Union

Delayed Union versus Nonunion

There is no exact time that a fracture should take to heal, but some fractures take longer than would be expected (for a person of that age), and this is called delayed union. If the bone fails to unite, then the fracture eventually goes on to a state of nonunion. There is no exact distinction in terms of the time when you should call it delayed as opposed to nonunion; however, if the bone has failed to unite after several months, it is unlikely to heal without intervention and is described as nonunion. The cause of delayed union and nonunion is unknown but, undoubtedly, poor blood supply, excessive shearing forces between the fragments, infection, interposition of tissue between the fragments, etc., all contribute.

There are two types of nonunion, hypertrophic and atrophic. Each has a characteristic X-ray appearance. Usually, the bone ends look rounded (like elephant feet) and appear dense and sclerotic, and this is called *hypertrophic nonunion*. In some cases a false joint may form (pseudoarthrosis) between the two ends. In these cases there is plenty of new bone formation but for some reason the two ends do not unite (perhaps because of movement or interposed tissues). Less commonly, the bone can look osteopenic, and it is then called *atrophic nonunion*, which is probably due to inadequate blood supply.

In the case of a nonunion the patient may require an operation such as ORIF and/or bone grafting to help the fracture unite (see section on bone grafting below).

Factors Employed to Encourage Bone Healing

The most important thing to get a bone to heal is stability. Another tool is bone grafting. Bone graft has traditionally been taken from the patient's iliac crest. This is a painful procedure and often the wound over the donor site causes greater morbidity to the patient than their main operative site. This type of bone graft has no structural integrity and only acts as a framework on which new bone grows (i.e. a graft extender).

There are now a number of commercially available bone graft substitutes with the intention of reducing donor site morbidity and improving the chances of bony union. These include *demineralised bone matrix, bone morphogenic proteins* (e.g. BMP-2 or OP-1) and *bone graft substitutes.* This is a growing field of orthopaedics; however, as with all advances, many surgeons argue that longer-term results of clinical trials are needed before they are prepared to change their practice.

Malunion

This is where the fracture has healed in an imperfect position, either shortened, angulated or rotated. It may cause an unsightly appearance despite good function, or it may look fine but functionally have a poor result (especially if a joint is involved). Worse still, it may be both.

Avascular Necrosis

Avascular necrosis (AVN) (see page 339) is the death of part of a bone due to a deficient blood supply. Common sites for this to occur include the head of the femur, the scaphoid and the talus after fractures or dislocations where the blood supply is disrupted. The affected bones become soft and deformed, causing pain, stiffness and OA. X-ray changes include sclerosis of the affected bone, which may appear distorted in shape; however, symptoms usually appear before any radiological changes.

Complex Regional Pain Syndrome Type I (Reflex Sympathetic Dystrophy or Sudek's Atrophy)

This is a collection of symptoms, including persistent pain, swelling, redness and sweating, thought to be due to an abnormal sympathetic response to injury. It is usually not noticed until the plaster has been removed, several weeks after the injury. For example, a small proportion of patients following a Colles' fracture have swelling of the hands and fingers, the skin is warm, pink and glazed in appearance, movement is decreased and the wrist and hand are painful to touch. It can also be seen in the lower limb. This problem is underdiagnosed in many cases. Although the condition is usually self-limiting, some patients find it disabling and need the care of the anaesthetic pain specialists. Guanethidine nerve blocks and sympathectomy can help in some cases.

Myositis Ossificans (Post-traumatic Ossification)

This is a condition where calcification forms in soft tissues following injury or surgery. It causes restricted, painful movement. The commonest site for this is the elbow region. The exact cause is unknown but thought to be due to calcification and then ossification of blood that collected during the trauma. The affected area may be excised surgically at a later date if necessary.

Growth Disturbance

X-rays in children are difficult to interpret, as the growth plate is often confused for a fracture. If there is damage to the growth plate (physis — see section on bone tumours for a discussion on the physis), abnormal growth may result. Injuries at the epiphyseal end of long bones of children can be categorised according to the Salter–Harris classification into five types (Figure 15.4). The results of these injuries depend on the injury pattern and the management at the time of injury. Type I tend to do well, whereas Type V do badly.

If a fracture goes through the epiphyseal plate (e.g. Salter–Harris I), provided good reduction is achieved there may be normal growth. Small amounts of displacement are often acceptable in children's fractures, since they tend to remodel (especially in the plane of movement) as the child grows. The worst fractures are the ones where a growth plate injury, such as a crush, is missed at the time of the injury (e.g. Salter–Harris V) and are not picked up until growth is distorted. Many fractures in children can be treated by manipulation under anaesthetic and then immobilisation in

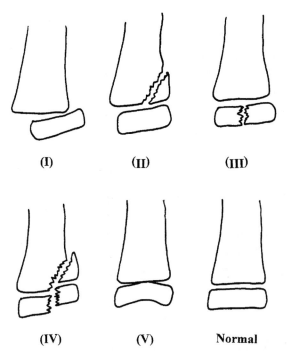

(I)   (II)   (III)

(IV)   (V)   **Normal**

Figure 15.4. Salter–Harris classification of epiphyseal injuries.

plaster. Intra-articular epiphyseal injuries require anatomical reduction and are usually treated by ORIF.

FRACTURES YOU SHOULD KNOW SOMETHING ABOUT

Fractures of the Neck of the Femur

These are often referred to as fractures of the proximal femur. They occur mainly in elderly females, usually with osteoporotic bone, and are therefore by definition pathological fractures. There is usually a history of a fall with the patient being unable to get up afterwards (in some cases the fracture may occur spontaneously and precede the fall).

These fractures have a high mortality (reports vary between 20%–40% at 1 year) no matter what treatment is performed in the initial period. The exact reason for this high mortality is unclear (even if you take into account the age and coexisting medical problems) and is the subject of much research.

The normal finding on examination is to see the leg lying externally rotated and shortened. The iliopsoas muscle attaches to the lesser trochanter of the femur. If the fracture is proximal to this attachment, then the pull of this muscle causes the affected limb to lie shortened and externally rotated. This explains the classic clinical appearance of a fractured neck of femur. All movements may be painful and they usually cannot bear weight.

When clerking the patient you should pay particular attention to four factors:

1. Premorbid mobility
2. Mini mental test score
3. Premorbid independence
4. Comorbidity

When documenting their social circumstances, you should focus on what their mobility had been like prior to the fall: Were they walking independently or did they need a stick or frame, etc.? Do they live alone, in a warden-controlled flat or in a nursing home? How many floors and stairs does their house have and who does their shopping, cleaning and cooking? You should also document the patient's mini mental test score. In general, the prognosis is better if the patient was cognitively intact, mobile and independent previously. This will also give you a guide as to what they will be likely to achieve afterwards.

If the patient has a history of a fall and clinical findings support the diagnosis of a fractured neck of the femur but the X-rays appear normal, then an MRI or a bone scan might be helpful.

Fractured neck of femurs are classified as intra- or extracapsular, depending on whether the fracture is proximal or distal to the capsular insertion (which is along the intertrochanteric line) (Figure 15.5).

The main blood supply to the head of the femur comes from vessels that travel under the capsule and along the neck (a small supply is also derived from nutrient vessels in the shaft and from a vessel that travels in the ligamentum teres). Therefore, if a fracture is intracapsular, the blood supply to

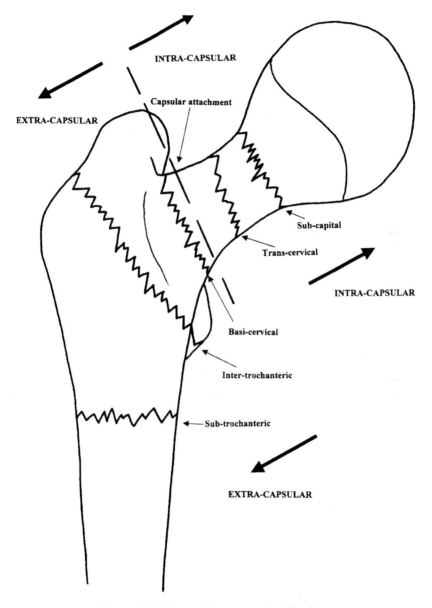

Figure 15.5. Types of fractured neck of the femur.

the head is compromised. It is impossible to tell which fractures will go on to develop avascular necrosis (AVN), but logic tells you that the more displaced the head is, the more likely the vessels will have been torn and hence the higher the chance of AVN. Extracapsular fractures, on the other hand, usually have an intact blood supply and are therefore not at risk of AVN.

Intracapsular Fractures

Intracapsular fractures are described as subcapital or transcervical and are grouped into four types according to the Garden classification (Garden I–IV) (Figure 15.6). Garden I and II are undisplaced and Garden III and IV are displaced.

Undisplaced intracapsular fractures are often impacted and would unite if left alone, although the aim nowadays is usually to mobilise such patients as soon as possible to avoid the complications of prolonged bed rest. Also, about a third of these fractures will go on to displace if not fixed. In most cases, therefore, the fracture is stabilised at operation, usually by the insertion of parallel screws through the neck and into the head to hold it in position.

Displaced intracapsular fractures will not usually unite without reduction and because of the disrupted blood supply to the head of the femur, many such patients go on to develop AVN. The management of these fractures involves an operation to reduce the fracture and hold it in position with screws; however, if you follow the patients up over the next few months many of them will still have pain and require a second operation (due to AVN of the femoral head). For this reason, in the elderly many surgeons would recommend excising the femoral head and replacing it with a prosthesis (hemiarthroplasty, or half-a-hip replacement) at the initial operation.

There are many types of prostheses available. The Thompson and Austin–Moore prostheses have been around for decades. With hemiarthroplasties the false head is large and articulates directly with the patient's acetabulum.

The Austin–Moore (Figure 15.7b) is an example of an uncemented prosthesis, the Thompson or JRI are examples of cemented prostheses. Nowadays bipolar hemi-arthroplasties are available, where a small head is

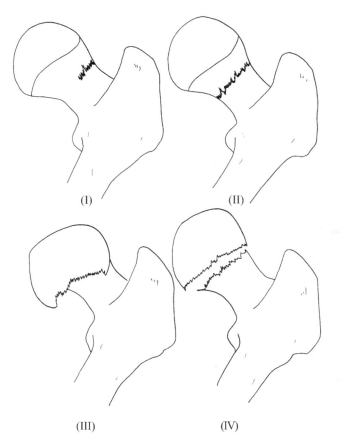

Figure 15.6. The Garden classification of intracapsular fractures.

fitted inside a larger head that sits in the acetabulum. Theoretically, there is reduced wear on the acetabulum due to sharing of the articulation between the small head and the large head and between the large head and the patient's acetabulum.

In the younger patient (aged less than 65) you need to consider the long-term outcome. The disruption to the blood supply is dependent on the severity of the initial trauma, but early reduction may prevent subsequent AVN. Ideally, you want to preserve the patient's own joint for as long as possible. Therefore, all intracapsular fractures in the young should be booked for theatre as an emergency and undergo reduction and have

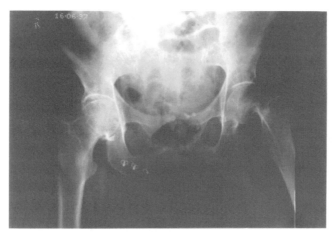

(a)

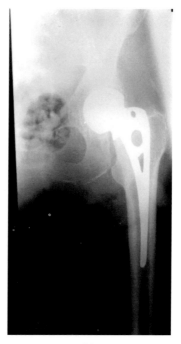

(b)

Figure 15.7. (a) Displaced intracapsular fractured neck of the femur (left).
(b) Austin–Moore hemiarthroplasty (left).

internal fixation (usually with screws). Young patients should be followed up in the out-patient clinic for at least 2 years and if they develop AVN, could be considered for a total hip replacement at a later date.

Extracapsular Fractures

Extracapsular fractures can be described as basicervical, intertrochanteric or subtrochanteric, depending on the relationship to the trochanters.

Extracapsular fractures do not carry the same risk of AVN and if minimally displaced, could be managed nonoperatively. Again, however, most orthopaedic surgeons advocate early mobilisation and it is not possible to mobilise easily if the hip is fractured and unstable, hence we tend to fix these fractures. Fixing these fractures will also help to reduce the amount of pain.

The standard operation nowadays for these fractures is the insertion of a dynamic hip screw (DHS). In this procedure the patient is placed on a special 'fracture' table and the foot is placed into a traction boot. A closed reduction is performed (whereby traction is applied to the leg, under image intensifier control, to reduce the fracture). An incision is made over the greater trochanter and a screw is inserted into the femoral head under image intensifier control. A plate attaches to the DHS and rests along the shaft of the femur, to which it is fixed by screws. The angle between the plate and the screw is 135°, which is the usual angle between the neck and the shaft in most people (note: different angles are available to cover anatomical variants).

These fractures have a natural tendency to collapse and so the screw can slide along the plate to accommodate this. The screw can slide but cannot rotate. The sliding movement of the screw on the plate explains why the hip screw is 'dynamic'. This type of collapse is a good thing as it leads to a more stable construct.

In summary, the management of a patient with a hip fracture involves the following:

1. Obtain a good history and social status for the patient.
2. Insert a cannulae and send off bloods for U & Es, FBC and a group and save.

3. Get an ECG and a chest X-ray and an X-ray of the pelvis and the affected limb.
4. Mark the affected limb in preparation for theatre.
5. Ensure that the surgeon obtains informed consent.
6. If necessary, correct any medical problems (they are usually dehydrated and require fluid resuscitation), optimising them for theatre.
7. If the patient is in severe discomfort skin traction can be applied to reduce the pain.

Extracapsular fractures are reduced and internally fixed (usually with a DHS) (Figure 15.8). Intracapsular fractures if nondisplaced, undergo fixation (screws) and if displaced, undergo a hemiarthroplasty. There is a saying commonly used by medical students that applies to intracapsular fractures classified by Garden: 'One, two, screw, three, four Austin–Moore'. Remember that this applies to patients over 65. All young patients with intracapsular fractures should be given the best chance of survival of the femoral head and should be booked as an emergency to allow the fracture to be accurately reduced and internally fixed.

Some form of DVT prophylaxis must be instituted (e.g. TED stockings, foot pumps, low molecular weight heparin and early mobilisation). Postoperatively, the patients should be examined to ensure that they are comfortable and that there is no evidence of a neurovascular deficit, and they should have a check full blood count and X-ray. Provided the X-rays are satisfactory the patient is usually mobilised after a day or so by the physiotherapists.

Radius and Ulna Shaft

Due to the anatomy, isolated fractures of the shafts of either of these bones are uncommon, and if they are seen one should always suspect an associated dislocation at either the proximal or the distal radioulnar joint. These fracture dislocations are known by their Italian eponyms and are common questions in exams, so they are worth remembering.

A fracture of the ulna shaft with dislocation of the radial head is called a Monteggia fracture (the radial head should normally lie in front of the

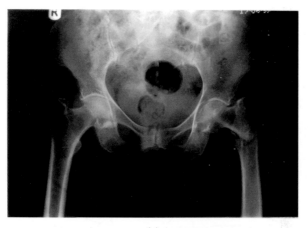

(a)

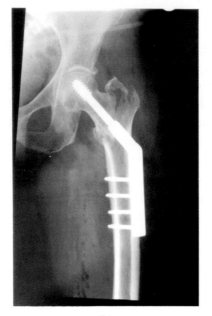

(b)

Figure 15.8. **(a)** Extracapsular fractured neck of the femur (left). **(b)** Dynamic hip screw (DHS) fixation (left).

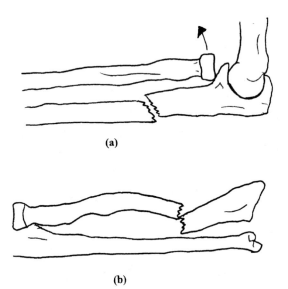

(a)

(b)

Figure 15.9. Types of forearm fractures. **(a)** Monteggia fracture and **(b)** Galeazzi fracture.

capitellum). A Galleazzi fracture is a fracture of the radial shaft with a dislocation of the distal (or inferior) radioulnar joint (Figure 15.9).

These fractures are unstable and are usually treated by ORIF in adults. In children the fracture is usually manipulated under anaesthetic (if displaced) and treated in an above elbow plaster.

If a fracture of the forearm is being treated in plaster, then it should be left in the most stable position. Fractures of the proximal radius and ulna are said to be the most stable in supination, distal fractures are said to be the most stable in pronation, and fractures of the midshaft are said to be the most stable in neutral. For example, a midshaft radial fracture is plastered with the hand in neutral (midpronation). The plaster is extended above the elbow to prevent any supination or pronation.

Fractures of the Distal Radius

Fractures of the distal radius have for some reason been associated with their eponymous names more than any other type of fracture. They can be classified in many ways, although the most commonly observed fracture is that which was described by an Irishman called Abraham Colles in 1814, long before the invention of radiography.

Colles observed a deformity of the wrist, originally mistaken for a dislocated carpus. He showed that it was in fact not a dislocation but a fracture of the distal end of the radius.

The deformity that made people think it was a dislocated carpus has been referred to as a 'dinner fork' deformity, because of how it looks.

These fractures can occur at any age after a fall onto an outstretched hand; however, they are most common in the elderly with osteoporosis. Colles described an extra-articular fracture of the distal radius (within an inch and a half of the joint) with dorsal displacement and radial shift of the distal fragment, and because the fragments are impacted there is also radial shortening. In addition, in rotational injuries the ulna styloid may also get pulled off by its attachment to the triangular fibrocartilaginous disc.

On examination, as with any fracture, the neurovascular function should be documented as the median nerve and the radial artery lie close. If the fracture is displaced, then treatment involves correction of the deformity and this is usually by manipulation. This can be performed under local (haematoma block), regional (Bier's block) or general anaesthetic.

The reduction aims to improve two things: (1) restore the length (the articular surface of the distal radius should be more distal than the ulna) and (2) correct the angulation to allow for optimum function and minimal deformity.

Reduction, as always, is achieved by distraction in the direction opposite to the forces which caused it in the first place. In this case the wrist is left in a neutral or slightly flexed position with some ulna deviation (with the forearm fully pronated). A Colles plaster is applied from the elbow to the metarcarpophalangeal joints, and it encompasses the thumb metarcarpal, again leaving the thumb phalanges free to move. If the fracture is suspected to be rotationally unstable, and in an ideal world, the plaster should be above elbow to prevent supination and pronation. Sadly however, the risk of shoulder stiffness is so great that we tend to leave the plaster below elbow, except in children who will move things as soon as they can and in whom an above elbow plaster is usually applied.

The plaster is usually split for a day or so and then completed when the swelling has subsided (an alternative is to place a back slab on initially, which is completed after a few days). The position of the fracture should always be rechecked once in plaster to ensure no change in position. If the position remains unacceptable or the fragments redisplace or the injury is intra-articular, then surgery may be required. Surgical options include an external fixator, K wires or ORIF with plates and screws.

If treated in plaster this usually remains on for 5 or 6 weeks; meanwhile, movement at the fingers, elbow and shoulder should be encouraged. Once the plaster is removed the wrist will need rehabilitation exercises by physiotherapists.

The complications of a Colles fracture are commonly asked about in the finals. The specific complications include

- Malunion
- Median nerve problems (usually in badly reduced fractures)
- A stiff 'frozen' shoulder (actually adhesive capsulitis and is due to immobilisation)
- Tendon rupture (the tendon of the extensor pollicis longus rubs along the distal radial fragment and can rupture several weeks after the fracture)
- Sudek's atrophy (much less common)
- Carpal tunnel syndrome

Other injuries that can be caused by a fall on to an outstretched hand include fractures or dislocations of the phalanges, scaphoid fractures, radial and ulnar fractures, elbow dislocation or fracture, humeral shaft fracture, shoulder dislocation, rotator cuff tears and shoulder girdle injuries (subluxation of acromioclavicular joint, clavicular fracture, etc.).

Smith's fracture is also called a 'reverse Colles' and is usually caused by a fall on to the back of a flexed wrist. Note that the distal articular surface of the radius is normally tilted in a volar (towards the palm) direction by 11°. In Smith's fracture the distal radial fragment is not only displaced anteriorly (in a volar direction) but also the volar tilt may be greater than the normal 11°.

The fracture can be manipulated to restore the anatomy and placed in an above elbow cast with the wrist slightly extended and the forearm pronated. If conservative treatment is initiated then close follow-up is needed, with regular X-rays in the first few weeks, because these fractures are very unstable and the fragments often slip. If the position is lost then ORIF is required, which usually involves some form of 'buttress plate' to restore the anatomy and prevent the volar displacement.

Barton's fracture is the eponym used for a fracture dislocation where the distal radial fracture is oblique and extends into the wrist joint. A volar Barton's fracture is a variant of Smith's fracture but you can also get a dorsal Barton fracture. You probably just need to have heard of it for the sake of the finals.

Scaphoid Fractures

Diagnosis of a scaphoid fracture is often made from the history and the finding of tenderness in the anatomical snuffbox. Special 'scaphoid' X-ray views should be requested when this injury is suspected. Often the X-ray appearance is normal until about 10 days after the injury. Therefore, if you suspect a scaphoid fracture (because of the history and clinical tenderness) you are obliged to treat it even with a normal X-ray.

The wrist is placed in a plaster. There are two types of plaster one can use, either a scaphoid plaster (which includes the IPJ of the thumb so that the hand is in a beer-glass-holding position) or a Colles plaster (where the thumb is not immobilised). These two types of plaster have been reported as having equally good results.

The patient is advised to return to the fracture clinic after 10 days for a re-X-ray. The fracture may now become apparent due to local decalcification. If the patient is nontender and the X-rays are normal, the plaster can be removed and the patient discharged. If the X-ray is still normal but the patient is still tender, then the plaster should really be replaced for a further 2 weeks. In difficult cases, a bone scan may be helpful in making the diagnosis.

The main concern with this fracture is the risk of AVN. The blood supply to the scaphoid is via small vessels that enter the bone distally and hence the proximal fragment is at risk of becoming avascular (especially if displaced), leaving the patient with pain and stiffness in the wrist.

Scaphoid fractures require a plaster for at least 6 weeks, after which time the wrist is reassessed by X-rays and clinical examination. If a complication such as delayed union or nonunion occurs, then either the arm can be placed in a plaster for a further 6 weeks or ORIF and bone grafting may be considered. ORIF usually involves a single screw across the fracture site.

Supracondylar Fractures of the Humerus

These injuries are most common in children, usually after a fall on to an outstretched hand. The elbow is very swollen and is held in a semi-flexed position. The distal fragment usually displaces backwards and the sharp edge of the proximal humerus may compress or injure the brachial artery which lies just in front of it (Figure 15.10).

The key to management is first to ensure no neurovascular damage results and second to restore the anatomy to prevent long-term malunion.

If the fracture is not displaced then the treatment is to flex the arm fully (checking the radial pulse). The sling provided by the triceps insertion, when the arm is fully flexed, helps to stabilise the fragments. One could apply a collar and cuff with the arm flexed as much as possible or alternatively apply

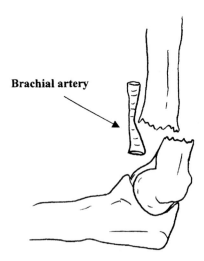

Figure 15.10. Supracondylar fracture of the humerus.

a back slab if necessary for a few days just to prevent the arm from being knocked. The immobilisation is usually about 3 weeks.

If the fracture is angulated with a clinical deformity then the child needs to be admitted and have the fracture manipulated under anaesthesia with image intensifier control. This is urgent if there is any evidence of a neurovascular deficit. Once satisfactory reduction is obtained, the position needs to be held and this is usually achieved by placing a few short K-wires across the fracture. Then, a collar and cuff or a back slab is applied again with the arm fully flexed. If the radial pulse is weak or not present then the arm will need to be straightened a little until it returns.

If the radial pulse is not present or damage to the brachial artery is suspected, an on-table angiogram and/or exploration needs to be done.

Any supracondylar fracture is at risk of compartment syndrome, and so the child needs to be observed very carefully over the next 24 h. Pain on passive extension (stretching the flexor compartment) of the fingers is the earliest warning sign of compartment syndrome. The elbow should be extended slightly to see if this restores the circulation, but if this fails surgical intervention may be needed, otherwise Volkmann's ischaemic contracture can result. This is where the forearm muscles become fibrosed and shortened, leading to a 'claw hand' deformity.

If a supracondylar fracture is missed or the reduction is inadequate, deformity can result. Angular deformities in the coronal plane do not remodel and can result in loss of the carrying angle and cubitus varus. If there is cubitus varus (internal rotation and extension of a healed supracondylar fracture), it is referred to as a 'gunstock deformity', because of its unsightly appearance. Despite the fact that function is usually quite good, these deformities should not really be seen these days with appropriate orthopaedic management.

Dislocated Shoulder

Because the shoulder is the most mobile of all the joints, its stability is sacrificed, especially inferiorly where the rotator cuff is deficient. In addition, in some patients there is underlying laxity of ligaments.

Almost all cases of dislocation of the shoulder are anterior dislocations (95%). Dislocation is usually caused by direct trauma or falling on to the hand where the humerus is driven forward tearing the capsule of the joint. Often the glenoid labrum is pulled off anteriorly, and this is called a Bankart lesion. If the humeral head impacts against the relatively hard anterior glenoid a defect can occur on the superior surface of the humeral head called a Hill Sachs lesion. This occurs in 35–40% of anterior dislocations. A Hill Sachs lesion may destabilise the glenohumeral joint and predispose to further dislocation.

The patient presents in severe pain, reluctant to allow any examination of the shoulder. The normal curved contour of the shoulder may be lost and may appear square. The arm is supported by the opposite hand. It is vital that you examine for any distal neurovascular deficit, especially of the axillary nerve, which can be damaged during the dislocation. The axillary nerve supplies a small egg-shaped patch of skin over the insertion of the deltoid and should be tested and the findings documented both before and after reduction (the axillary nerve also supplies the deltoid but clearly the muscle is difficult to assess whilst the shoulder is dislocated).

X-rays should be an AP and a trans-scapular view (in the line of the body of the scapula) to see in which direction the humeral head has gone in relation to the glenoid, i.e. anterior or posterior.

Reduction is usually performed under sedation in the casualty department. One method has the patient in the supine position with the arm abducted and an assistant applying countertraction to the body (maybe with a towel held around the patient's chest under the axilla). The head can be guided gently back into the socket.

An alternative is to have the patient prone with the arm hanging attached to some weights to apply traction (Kocher's method can slice off the articular cartilage and cause a fracture of the greater tuberosity and so is not recommended). If these methods fail then reduction is usually easy to achieve with some muscle relaxant in theatre.

The arm can then be rested in a sling for about 3–4 weeks, after which physiotherapy rehabilitation can begin. The patient is advised against positions that can increase the likelihood of dislocation, namely abduction and external rotation such as throwing a baseball or when swinging back to serve in tennis.

Recurrent Instability

After an initial dislocation, the shoulder may return to functional stability or it may fall victim to recurrent glenohumeral instability. The older a patient is at the time of initial injury the lower the chances are for developing recurrent instability. Patients under the age of 20 with traumatic dislocations have a substantially higher rate of recurrence (greater than 90%).

While intermediate forms of recurrent instability do occur, the great majority of recurrently unstable shoulders may be thought of as being either atraumatic or traumatic in origin.

Two terms have been described which you may find useful to understand shoulder instability. These are TUBS and AMBRI.

Traumatic Unilateral Dislocations with a Bankart lesion often require Surgery (TUBS). Most dislocations are traumatic and patients presenting with TUBS are usually between the ages of 15 and 30. Surgery usually involves a Bankart repair, whereby the glenoid labrum is reattached to the glenoid, usually by using bone anchors and sutures.

Atraumatic instability is instability that arises without the type of trauma necessary to tear the stabilising soft tissues and is often bilateral. It is called AMBRI because this stands for Atraumatic Multidirectional Bilateral shoulder dislocation (or subluxation) and is best treated by Rehabilitation but occasionally should be considered for an Inferior capsular shift (AMBRI).

Management of shoulder instability requires careful diagnosis based on the history, examination and imaging. Operating on an AMBRI without careful diagnosis beforehand may lead to poor results.

Posterior Dislocation

Posterior dislocation of the shoulder is easily overlooked (and occasionally you will see a patient who sustained a posterior dislocation several days or weeks prior that had been missed). It is caused by direct trauma (and is seen in epileptics). The AP X-ray may give the impression of the humeral head sitting in the glenoid (hence it is missed), although it may appear rounded — the so-called 'light bulb' sign (due to internal rotation, and hence the greater tuberosity is not seen). Reduction is best performed by a specialist.

Femoral and Tibial Fractures

In these injuries, resuscitate the patient and deal with life-threatening injuries first. Blood loss can be great, so cross-match two units in tibial fractures and four units in femoral fractures. A traction splint can be applied for femoral fractures, and a padded board or long leg splint can be used for tibial fractures. Both injuries are at risk of compartment syndrome. In the young most of these fractures are treated surgically. The state-of-the-art treatment for femoral or tibial fractures is to use an intramedullary nail (a long nail placed right down the centre from the top end to hold the fracture). There are alternative treatments, including a plate and screws or an external fixator.

Each method has advantages and disadvantages (for example, the pins of an external fixator go through the muscles in the thigh, limiting rehabilitation), and for the sake of examinations you need to know that all are acceptable options. If the fracture is 'open', management is different (see above). Antibiotics are started, and the patient is taken to theatre for debridement and washout. The fracture is then assessed and stabilised.

There have been studies showing that patients who have their femoral fractures stabilised within 24 h do better in terms of respiratory complications (e.g. chest infection and ARDS) than patients who are left for longer before the operation. One of the main factors in this is that nursing care is made easier, allowing the patients to be sat up once they have been fixed.

Knee Injuries

Knee injuries commonly affect sportsmen and questions on them are likely to come up in exams. Several structures can be damaged in the knee. The collateral ligaments get torn in valgus or varus strains. Twisting injuries can lead to meniscal tears or a rupture of the anterior cruciate ligament (ACL) and there is a triad that can follow a severe rotational injury where the anterior cruciate, the medial meniscus and the medial collateral ligament are all torn ('the unhappy triad of O'Donoghue').

History

The time of presentation will dictate the types of information you should obtain in your history. For example, if assessment is shortly after the injury, the only questions you can ask about will relate to the mechanism of injury and previous injuries to this knee.

If presentation is delayed, for example, until the next day or longer, then you must ask whether the knee swelled up immediately or overnight. If the knee swells immediately, this points to a haemarthrosis, which often occurs with fractures or torn cruciates. Overnight swelling indicates an effusion, which may in turn imply a meniscal tear or another ligamentous injury.

If the patient presents some time after the injury, then an accurate history invariably points to the diagnosis. Symptoms that you should ask about include the four cardinal knee symptoms, namely, pain, locking, swelling and giving way. Locking means that the patient cannot fully extend the knee because of a mechanical obstruction, such as a meniscal tear. Giving way is usually a sign of instability, such as that which can follow a torn anterior cruciate ligament, but may occur because of pain. A history of locking, together with the finding of an effusion and joint line tenderness, usually indicates a meniscal tear.

Management

If a patient presents immediately after the injury with an acutely swollen knee, full examination is often difficult. You will note the extent of the swelling and which areas are tender as well as the range of movement. Testing for menisci or cruciate damage when the knee is acutely swollen can be quite difficult. If the mechanism of injury dictates, then an X-ray can be taken to ensure that there are no fractures. A lateral X-ray might reveal a fluid level indicating a lipohaemarthrosis (mixture of fat and blood in a joint cavity). Even in the absence of an obvious fracture, this should set off alarm bells as it could indicate a torn ACL or an osteochondral injury.

The management of an acutely swollen knee (without fractures) is usually Rest, Ice packs, Compression or splintage, and Elevation (RICE). After a few days, once the swelling has subsided the knee can be re-examined for meniscal, ligamentous or chondral damage.

If a meniscal tear or torn cruciate is suspected, then an MRI scan can be performed to confirm the diagnosis. Some surgeons will take a look into the knee in the absence of an MRI.

Arthroscopy

An arthroscopy means the knee is looked into with a camera. It is imperative that the knee be re-examined under anaesthesia before the arthroscope is inserted into the knee. With the patient asleep and the muscle tone reduced it is far easier to assess the stability.

The arthroscope is inserted through an incision, just lateral to the patella tendon, into the lateral compartment of the knee and a second incision is made into the medial compartment where a probe is inserted. This way the surgeon has the ability to look and feel, touch and pull various structures as part of the examination.

The three joint compartments are inspected — the patellofemoral joint and the medial and lateral compartments. If a meniscal tear is seen it can be trimmed using various instruments and shavers. There are many types of meniscal tears, an example being a 'bucket handle' tear, where the 'bucket handle' can flip in and out of the joint space, causing locking.

In years gone by surgeons used to remove torn menisci but we now know that this predisposes to OA and so the menisci must be preserved as much as possible. Only the outer third of the meniscus has a blood supply and tears in this region are usually repaired using sutures or newer devices. Tears in the inner third have to be trimmed because they are not repairable. When a tear is in the junction of the middle to outer third (referred to as the white–red zone), a difficult decision is made and depending on the age of the patient, the surgeon may attempt a repair.

Apart from the menisci, the other things inspected in an arthoscopy include the articular surfaces, the cruciate ligaments and the various soft tissue pouches to look for loose bodies. The joint is irrigated with several litres of normal saline during an arthroscopy and so infection is rare.

Postoperatively, early mobilisation is encouraged.

Management of a Ruptured Anterior Cruciate Ligament

A torn ACL can lead to instability, especially during twisting and cutting movements that are common in sports. The treatment after rupture of the ACL may be operative or conservative. In both cases, the goal is to reach the best functional level for the patient without risking new injuries or degenerative changes in the knee.

Rehabilitation is an important part of the treatment. By strengthening up the quads and hamstrings and starting proprioceptive exercises it is possible to stabilise the knee without surgery in some cases.

Operative repair involves the use of a tendon (allograft or autograft) or an artificial graft. The results of artificial grafts have so far been poor and nowadays the gold standard involves the use of either the middle third of the patella tendon or the hamstrings tendon (autografts). Allografts are tendons from cadavers and tend to be reserved for revisions or cases where multiple tendons need replacing. The tendon is rerouted through the knee in the same location as the old torn ACL and held using a screw.

In the USA over 50,000 ACL reconstructions take place each year and in the UK about 5000. Long-term results depend on what assessment criteria you are using. Return to a high level of athletic activity has been an indicator of treatment success and indeed if this is the outcome measure, then ACL reconstruction is a very successful operation. If the outcome, however, is prevention of longer-term arthritis, then we really do not know the answer. It is logical to assume that an unstable knee has a higher chance of developing osteoarthritis earlier than the same knee with an intact ACL. The confounding factors include other injuries, such as meniscal tears and damage to the articular surfaces at the time of injury. Also, injuries sustained subsequently will further confound the long-term results of any ACL repair. The definitive answer to the question, "Will an ACL repair prevent me from getting osteoarthritis?" may never be found.

Current postoperative rehabilitation programmes encourage an immediate range of motion. Commonly, the patients are allowed to return to light sporting activities such as running 2–3 months after surgery and to contact sports, including cutting and jumping, after 6 months.

In less active patients a decision may be made to persist with nonoperative management. Approximately, a third of patients can develop sufficient stability without the need for surgery, mainly through muscular training and education. These patients are unlikely to be able to engage in activities that require very stable knees (for example playing football or rugby) without risk of further damage.

In addition, the patient's occupation might influence the decision to operate, since a torn cruciate may not be as important in a person who works behind a desk as it is in a roofer who climbs up ladders.

Osteochondral Injuries

Articular cartilage (hyaline cartilage) covers the articulating surfaces of bones within synovial joints and is crucial for their smooth articulation. It also serves to absorb shock by spreading the applied load to the bony supporting structures below. In most cases articular cartilage is able to carry out its task of strenuous load bearing for a lifetime.

However, cartilage is avascular, aneural and alymphatic and has a very low cell density and hence has limited intrinsic repair potential. If the surface becomes damaged and is left untreated, the initial damage will lead to further matrix disruption and the development of progressive degenerative arthritis. Sadly, up to a quarter of all severe ligament or capsular knee injuries that result in a haemarthrosis are associated with cartilage damage.

If left alone, partial thickness lesions do not heal. However, if the lesion extends deep into the subchondral bone, so that bleeding occurs, some repair does ensue. The repair is due to the flow of stem cells from the marrow to the site. Surgical techniques were developed to replicate this, such as subchondral drilling, microfracture and abrasion arthroplasty; however, these methods have generally revealed the formation of fibrocartilage repair tissue, which lacks the same durability as hyaline cartilage and wears away quicker and thus does not represent a long-term solution. No one knows why fibrocartilage forms instead of hyaline cartilage.

A newer technique involves the use of autologous chondrocytes. This technique [autologous chondrocyte implantation (ACI)] was pioneered by a Swedish group in the 1990s. In brief, cartilage from the margins of the affected knee joint is harvested by arthroscopy, and the cells are cultured and expanded in a laboratory for 4 weeks, after which they are transplanted back into the damaged area. The cells are held in position by a membrane of either artificial collagen or periosteum taken from the upper tibia. The membrane is sutured into position over the cartilage defect before injection of cells. A newer technique involves the growth of the chondrocytes directly onto the membrane, which is then glued onto the defect during an arthroscopic procedure.

Short- to medium-term results of ACI have been good; however, whether or not the long-term chances of developing OA are reduced, remains uncertain.

OSTEOARTHRITIS

OA is a very common disorder, and it is likely that it will appear in the exams. It is a degenerative joint disorder in which there is progressive loss of articular cartilage. OA can be *primary*, where there is no obvious underlying cause, or *secondary*, when it follows a pre-existing abnormality of the joint (e.g. fracture, rheumatoid disease, haemarthrosis, meniscal tear, etc).

All normal articular surfaces are lined by a thin layer of hyaline cartilage (in the knee there is an additional 'shock absorber' — the menisci, which are made of fibrocartilage). Initially, there is softening of the articular cartilage and the normally smooth surface becomes frayed (or fibrillated) and fissured, and eventually is worn away to expose the underlying bone. The subchondral bone, which is now under greater stresses, becomes thickened and sclerotic, and cysts may form (due to microfractures). As the disease progresses the cartilage left in unstressed areas proliferates and ossifies to form bony outgrowths called osteophytes (which some would say are an attempt by the body to restabilise the joint). Capsular fibrosis may occur secondarily, leading to a stiff joint. All synovial joints may be affected, although the weight-bearing joints, such as the knee and the hip, tend to be the most common. If the spine is affected, then this is known as spondylosis (which may have complications, such as nerve root compression by osteophytes).

The exact aetiology of the disease is unknown and a lot of work is being done in this area. However, it is known that the frequency increases with age.

We tend to think of OA as wear and tear, and this is how we explain it to our patients. There is indeed a significantly higher incidence of osteoarthritis in older people with a radiographic incidence of more than 80% of people more than 75 years old compared to 5% in those less than 25. However, if it were simply wear and tear then everyone should suffer from symptomatic arthritis as they get older, but they do not.

Repetitive joint motion in the presence of normal anatomy and joint function is likely to be beneficial for articular cartilage but the reality is that we often subject our joints to excessive stresses and forces that are likely to be harmful especially in those individuals who have some genetic or environmental predisposition to OA.

The aetiology is, therefore, multifactorial and involves not only the stresses that the cartilage is put under but also the ability of the cartilage to withstand those stresses.

Tip for medical students: Do not confuse OA with osteoporosis or osteomalacia, which are completely different conditions. Osteoporosis is where the amount of bone stock is less than you should have and osteomalacia is where there is failure of mineralisation (not enough calcification of the bone).

Symptoms of Osteoarthritis

1. *Pain.* This is the predominant symptom, usually aggravated by exercise and relieved by rest. It is progressive over months to years and

there are periods of remission and flare-ups, often due to trauma (the capsule may be stretched and inflamed). As the disease progresses and its severity worsens, the patient may have pain at night interfering with sleep.

2. *Stiffness.* This occurs especially after long periods of rest, and hence the patient can be very stiff in the morning, but this tends to improve as the day goes on.
3. *Deformity.* This is a feature of advanced disease and may result from muscular spasm, capsular and ligamentous contracture and distortion of the joint surfaces.

In your history it is important to focus on activities of daily living and social circumstances (e.g. mobility, ability to wash, cook and clean, home circumstances, social services, family backup, etc.). On examination movement is restricted, usually with accompanied crepitus, and in later stages of the disease there may be fixed flexion deformities.

A top tip, when examining a patient, is to look at their hands. If you notice swellings in the fingers (Heberden's nodes at the distal interphalangeal joints and Bouchard's nodes at the PIPJs), then this points to primary OA as the diagnosis.

X-Ray Changes

OA has the following X-ray changes (Figure 15.11):

1. Narrowing of the joint space (as the cartilage is worn away) is the most important sign. The Xrays should be taken in a weight bearing position to assess the narrowing correctly.
2. Osteophytes — bits of bone overgrowth, usually near the edge of the joint.
3. Subchondral sclerosis.
4. Subchondral bone cysts.
5. There may be evidence of previous disorders, such as old fractures, rheumatoid or congenital defects.
6. Structural damage — bony destruction and deformity is a late sign.

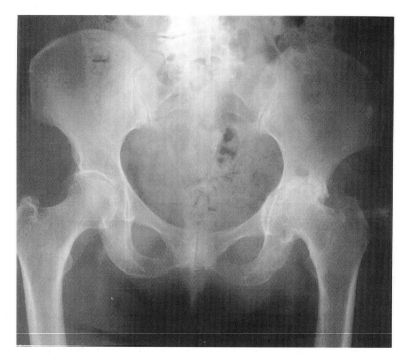

Figure 15.11. X-ray changes in osteoarthritis — the right hip has some osteoarthritic changes, although compared to the left hip it has relatively well-preserved joint space. On the left the joint space is completely obliterated; there are bone cysts, subchondral sclerosis and osteophytes. See Figure 15.12 for the postop film.

Management

In the early stages of the disease, treatment is conservative, using analgesics, weight loss, advice on altering load-bearing activities such as increased periods of rest, use of walking sticks or avoidance of activities that exacerbate the condition (in the younger patient this may mean giving up sports or changing their job). Physiotherapy to help increase the joint mobility and strengthen the muscles is often of great help. Injection of steroids and local anaesthetic into the joint space during acute flare-ups may be of some symptomatic benefit. More recently the use of intra-articular hyaluronic acid and dietary supplements such as glucosamine have been recommended. The data to support their use is conflicting but they certainly could be considered where arthroplasty is contraindicated or a long way off.

Patients often cope with their symptoms for many years. If, however, symptoms progress despite all of the above measures, then the following surgical options are available:

1. *Arthroscopic washout.* The commonest site for this is the knee, and the severity of the disease is assessed directly (and graded I–IV). The frayed cartilage is trimmed and any loose bodies are removed (pieces of cartilage or broken-off osteophytes). The joint is washed out to remove any remaining debris, and local anaesthetic is injected (sometimes a partial synovectomy is performed).
2. *Osteotomy.* This means the bone is divided ('osteo' = bone and 'tome' = cut), and sometimes a small area of the bone is removed to correct the deformity. Once divided the bone is left to unite either by external plaster or by internal fixation. Osteotomy can help relieve the pain but why it works is unknown (it is thought that it may be due to adjustment of the weight-bearing surfaces and changes in blood flow to the bone).
3. *Arthrodesis.* This means the joint is fused and will therefore restrict mobility. It is mainly used as a last resort for joints where the loss of movement is not too disabling (for example in the toes). For the hip and the knee, fusion is rarely performed nowadays as the results of arthroplasty are so good. If infection is a high risk then arthrodesis might be preferred over arthroplasty.
4. *Arthroplasty.* This can be replacement or excisional arthroplasty. In some joints, such as the metartarsophalangeal joints of the foot, it is better to excise the arthritic joint, allowing a fibrous and pain-free joint to form in its place. The hip and the knee have received the most attention for replacement arthroplasty, although there are many other prostheses available for the shoulder, the elbow and almost any other joint (although results have been poor in many joints, such as the ankle). We try to avoid joint replacement in the young (less than age 65), as it may last only 10–20 years before needing revision and the results of revision surgery are not as good as those of primary surgery. Nowadays, however, some joint replacements are lasting longer and longer and are being used in younger age groups.

Total Hip Replacement

Total hip replacement (THR) was pioneered by Sir John Charnley in the 1960s and is now a very successful procedure for arthritis of the hip (with a good result in about 95% of cases). The worn acetabulum is replaced by a high-density polyethylene cup into which a ceramic or metal head (part of the femoral stem) articulates. The components are usually cemented in place using an antibiotic-containing bone cement (methylmethacrylate). Uncemented prostheses are also available which are coated or 'sintered' and allow bone to grow into them.

You certainly do not need to know how to carry out a hip replacement, but for those of you who are interested, a small overview is given here.

There are several operative approaches to the hip joint although the commonest are the anterolateral or posterior approaches. In the anterolateral approach, an incision is made over the greater trochanter and the fascia is divided. The abductors (gluteus medius and minimis) are lifted off the greater trochanter to gain access to the capsule of the joint. The capsule is incised and removed. The head of the femur is dislocated and then the wear or damage to the acetabulum and femur can be assessed. The head of the femur is removed and the acetabulum is prepared using reamers to remove any cartilage and debris. The acetabular cup is cemented in (although uncemented prostheses are available). A hole is reamed (drilled) down the femoral shaft and, after a few trial stems are used, the correct prosthesis is cemented in (again, uncemented prostheses are available). Many prostheses nowadays are modular, meaning that different size neck lengths and different types of heads can be trialled for a best fit. The head is relocated into the acetabulum and the function of the joint is tested to see if it is stable. The soft tissues are closed in layers (a drain may or may not be used). The leg is placed in slight abduction using a triangular pillow, to maintain good stable position of the joint.

Rehabilitation begins about a day or so after the operation, initially with leg exercises, and once the X-rays have been checked the patient is allowed to fully bear weight. The usual hospital stay is about 7 days, although some patients go home sooner. If an uncemented prosthesis is used, then the patient may be asked to remain partially weight bearing with crutches for

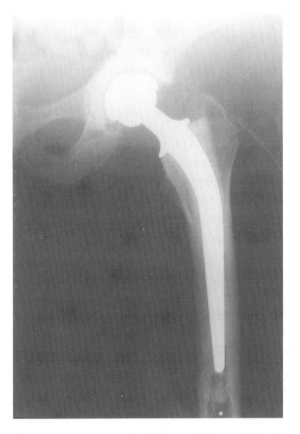

Figure 15.12. Total hip replacement — both the acetabulum and the femoral head have been replaced (note the cement around the femoral stem).

about 6 weeks (to allow the tissues to heal and bone to form around the prosthesis), after which time full weight bearing is encouraged.

There are many hip replacements on the market (over 100) but only a smaller number have long-term published results. As surgeons we are responsible for keeping up to date with the literature and deciding which prosthesis to use based on published data in the literature, our own experiences and information we learn by attending international meetings.

For those with long-term results, the data suggest that about 85% of THRs last over 10 years. After about 10 years, up to 10% can loosen and may need revision. However, the success rate of revision hips is not as good as the primary operation.

The main complications of THR include

Dislocation. About 3% of primary THRs dislocate. Patients are advised of the positions that can be risky including squatting or sitting on low chairs or movements that adduct the hip (i.e. sitting with crossed legs). There have been studies suggesting that the posterior approach to the hip carries a higher rate of dislocation.

Deep Ven Thrombosis (DVT). Studies have shown that up to 50% of THRs suffer a DVT and the risk is approximately halved with heparin prophylaxis. The risk of a pulmonary embolus (PE) is about 1–2% (although fatal PE is much lower). Nowadays we tend to encourage early mobilisation together with TED stockings and possibly some form of chemical prophylaxis. Practice will differ in different hospitals because of the lack of convincing evidence in the literature.

Deep infection (about 1–2%). This is disastrous and usually will require revision [in many cases this is performed as a two-stage procedure where the metalwork is removed in order to clear the infection (a Girdlestone's procedure) and traction is applied for several weeks before a definitive revision can be performed].

Nerve damage. The sciatic nerve is just behind the hip joint and can be stretched during the procedure (especially posterior approaches). This can lead to foot drop, which usually recovers but can take up to 18 months to do so. Also in the anterolateral approach the superior gluteal nerve can be injured leading to weakness of the abductors and a Trendelenburg gait.

Leg length discrepancy. The key is stability of the hip and sometimes the neck length needs to be increased in order to tighten the soft tissues. This usually can be addressed when the contralateral limb is operated on. Leg length difference is usually less than 5 mm in the vast majority of cases, but can be up to 2.5 cm in unusual circumstances, requiring a shoe raise on the other side.

Hip Resurfacing

In hip resurfacing only the damaged articular surfaces are replaced, in contrast to THR where the whole femoral head is resected. Hip resurfacing has always been an attractive concept and the theoretical advantages of hip resurfacing include reduced bone resection, closer restoration of normal anatomy and lower risk of dislocation.

Sir John Charnley, pioneer of the THR, in fact carried out the first hip resurfacing in the 1950s using Teflon on Teflon bearings but unfortunately these Teflon bearings wore quickly. The failure of materials (including metal on metal) plagued surgeons for the next 50 years but recently, surgeons have developed new technologies that create perfect rounded bearing surfaces that have so far shown very good clinical results and have been advocated for younger patients who want to restore as much bone stock as possible.

In these resurfacings the cap of the femoral head is replaced by a metal cover as is the acetabulum, creating a metal on metal bearing surface. Short-to medium-term results have been very encouraging, although this is an emerging technology and long-term results are needed before it can become a mainstream procedure. There are also a few unanswered questions relating to this technology. The biggest one is the raised levels of cobalt and chromium ions in the blood after metal on metal surfaces are used. In the vast majority of patients with metal–metal hip resurfacing there is an early rise in serum metal ions over the first 2–3 years but the levels then gradually diminish over time. There is a theoretical risk of carcinogensis, although convincing data to support this risk is yet to be published.

Total Knee Replacement

Total knee replacement (TKR) followed after THR; however, the success rate of this operation is as good as that for THR. We still tend to inform patients that the life of the joint replacement is about 10–20 years; however, some surgeons believe that a good knee replacement in a compliant patient can last a lifetime.

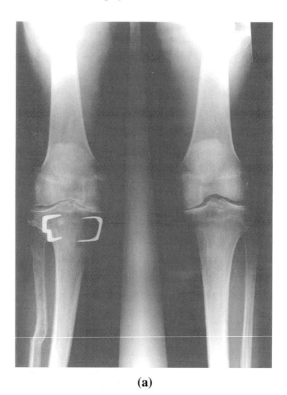

(a)

Figure 15.13. **(a)** Osteoarthritis of both knees — the medial compartment is more severely affected on both knees. Note that there are staples from an old right tibial osteotomy.

The joint is made of two metal prostheses with an intervening polyethylene articular disc between the distal femur and the tibial plateau and if only one compartment of the joint is damaged, this can be replaced by a unicompartmental prosthesis (results of this are excellent for the medial compartment but not so good for the lateral compartment). The whole joint is not replaced, just the articular surfaces (and hence joint resurfacing is perhaps a better name, as above). The materials used for the prostheses include titanium alloys, cobalt–chrome or stainless steel.

Again, for undergraduate exams you do not need to know the operative technique, but for those with an interest, an incision is made in front of the knee in the midline (about 25 cm long). The joint is accessed via the medial side of the patella as the patella is flipped back on itself (laterally) to get it out of the way. The distal femur and the tibial plateau are prepared by sawing off the irregular surfaces to allow the prostheses to fit on (using special jigs to ensure that all the angles are correct). Trial prostheses are used to attain the correct sizes to allow for optimal function and stability of the joint. The prostheses are cemented into place and a polyethylene disc is inserted between the tibia and the femur, acting like the articular cartilage, ensuring that there is no contact between the metal parts. The anterior cruciate ligament is divided and the posterior cruciate is sometimes kept (PCL retaining). If the patella surface is worn, then it can also be resurfaced using a polyethylene button. The knee is

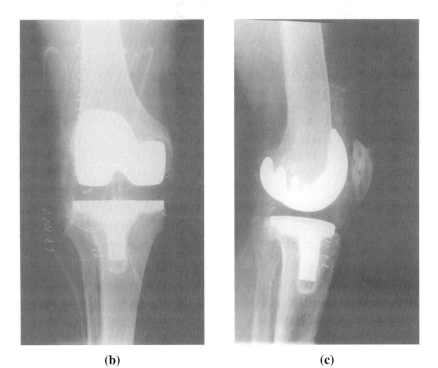

(b)   (c)

Figure 15.13. (*Continued*). **(b)** Right total knee replacement (TKR). AP view. **(c)** Lateral view (patellar surface has not been replaced).

washed out and the function is again tested, ensuring good flexion, patellar tracking and stability. Closure is again in layers, usually with two or three drains.

Postoperatively, the leg is placed in to a splint for support and protection. Bending of the knee is begun after one or two days, and a check X-ray is taken on day 2 or 3. Once active straight leg raising is achieved the patient can begin partial weight bearing, progressing to full weight bearing. The hospital stay is usually about 10 days and the patient should be mobilising independently, achieving flexion to 90° with a good active straight leg raise before discharge. Complications include DVT, which occurs in about 50–75% of TKRs (the incidence is halved if heparin prophylaxis is used), although many are asymptomatic. The risk of PE is about 1% (although fatal PE is said to be <0.1%). The infection rate is about 2–3% and is a disaster because the success of revision knees is again much lower than that of the primary procedure.

RHEUMATOID ARTHRITIS

Rheumatoid arthritis (RA) is a large subject that usually comes up in the medical section of exams; however, there are many operative procedures that can be performed to help the patients and so below are a few lines on this subject. Answers are best related in terms of treatment goals, and for RA these include:

1. *Prevention and treatment of the inflammatory synovitis.* Advice, exercises, joint protection and drugs such as the disease-modifying drugs — gold, penicillamine and immunosuppressants (methotrexate, pyrimidine synthesis inhibitors and anti-TNF therapies).
2. *Prevention of joint destruction and deformity.* Rest during acute exacerbations followed by rehabilitation and physiotherapy. RA patients are prone to tendon rupture, which may require operative repair.
3. *Joint reconstruction.* Joint replacements have a place in RA patients. The hip, knee, shoulder, elbow and MCPJs are examples of joints which can be replaced in advanced destruction, deformity or instability. You must, however, treat the symptoms and not the X-ray appearances.

Other operations that have a place are arthrodesis, osteotomy and synovectomy.

The X-ray changes of RA include soft tissue swelling, joint space narrowing and, later on, articular destruction and deformity.

AVASCULAR NECROSIS

This often comes up in multiple choice questions (MCQs). It is due to a disruption of the blood supply, either due to interruption of arterial inflow, such as after a fracture, or blockage of venous outflow, as in infiltrative disorders that block the venous sinusoids (e.g. Gaucher's disease). The causes include:

- Fracture/dislocation.
- Sickle cell disease (clumping of the RBCs leads to diminished capillary flow. There is a tendency for the infarcted areas of bone to become infected with unusual organisms such as salmonella).
- Decompression sickness (Caisson disease).
- Gaucher's disease (a rare familial disorder of lipid metabolism).
- Drug-induced (especially corticosteroids).
- Idiopathic.

AVN was classified by Ficat according to symptoms and the clinical and radiological findings. X-rays initially show no changes; however, after a few weeks reactive new bone forms in the adjacent living tissue, showing up as an increased area of density. Later on, the necrotic bone crumbles and the outline may be distorted. Bone scans show the region as an area of increased uptake due to the vascular reaction in the adjacent bone. The symptoms are usually pain and stiffness.

Idiopathic Avascular Necrosis (Osteochondritis)

In the above list the term 'idiopathic' appears really for want of a better term. There is a group of conditions called osteochondritides, which

are areas of patchy AVN of bone causing pain and limitation of movement, usually in adolescents. They are usually called by the names of
those who described them, and examples include AVN of the second
metatarsal head (Freiberg's disease), the navicular (Kohler's disease), the
lunate (Kienboch's disease) and the capitulum of the humerus (Panner's
disease).

The cause is unknown. There are two subgroups (traction aphophysitis
and osteochondritis dissecans), which still come under the heading 'osteochondritides', but because they have explainable causes they are listed
below separately. Note that they are not inflammatory conditions and so
the 'itis' is not strictly correct.

Traction Apophysitis

Repetitive pulling forces of a tendon may damage the apophysis to which
it is attached. The commonest example is the pull of the quadriceps on the
tibial tuberosity, called Osgood–Schlatter disease (two separate surgeons
who described the condition in the same year, 1903), which presents as
knee pain, usually in growing adolescents. It is typically a self-limited
condition that waxes and wanes, but which often takes months to years to
resolve entirely, through stopping sports and conservative measures. In a
small number of chronic cases where there is a bony ossicle in the patella
tendon, surgical excision is required and usually successful. Another
example of traction apophysitis is Sever's disease of the calcaneum, due to
the pull from the Achilles tendon.

Osteochondritis Dissecans

A piece of bone and its overlying articular cartilage may fall (dissect) off
and into the joint space due to repeated minor stresses. The commonest
site is the knee, with pain, swelling and limitation of movement. X-rays
may show a loose body or a crater on the articular surface of the medial
femoral condyle of the femur from which the fragment has fallen off.

Treatment depends on the size of the defect and the symptoms it causes. The options range from taking a 'wait and see' policy to surgery, which could include drilling, osteochondral autografting or autologous chondrocyte implantation. No good prospective randomised long-term trial results have been published to allow patients to make a really informed decision. A large defect will ultimately progress and lead to OA.

BONE TUMOURS

This is not a common topic in finals, although you may be asked to discuss this during a viva. Because there are so many types, students often learn them as a list and therefore do not know the relative importance of each type. In fact, all are incredibly rare, but you cannot be forgiven for not knowing two basic facts:

1. Secondaries to bone are much more common than primaries.
2. Primary bone tumours need to be managed by a specialist centre.

In order to help you learn about bone tumours it is helpful to have a basic understanding of the terms used to describe bones, which cannot be understood without a brief introduction to the development of long bones. A bone begins life as a cartilaginous model of approximately similar shape to the final product into which it will be converted. The primary centre of ossification appears at the centre of the shaft or diaphysis (Greek for 'in between') sometime during intrauterine life. The ossification spreads from here towards each end of the bone. Near the two ends of the bone there is a growth plate called the physis, from which longitudinal growth of the bone occurs initially as cartilage, which then undergoes ossification. At the outer end of the bone is the epiphysis (Greek for 'on top') and this is also cartilaginous. Sometime after birth a secondary centre of ossification appears at each epiphyseal end (Figure 15.14).

When you see an X-ray of a long bone of a child (depending on age), you see the ossified part of the epiphysis separated from the shaft by a gap, which is not actually a space but simply the unossified cartilaginous part of the bone which does not show up on the X-ray. From the physis,

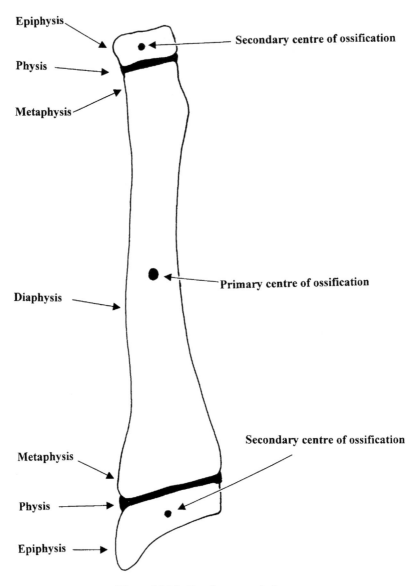

Figure 15.14. Development of a bone.

bone is laid down towards the diaphysis into an area of bone called the metaphysis (Greek for 'next to'). As the ossification from the primary centre and that from the secondary centre meet, fusion of the growth plate is said to occur, indicating skeletal maturity.

Primary bone tumours can develop in any of the tissues that make up the bone. They can be benign (given the ending '-oma') or malignant ('-sarcoma'). If derived from bone they are called osteoid tumours, such as an osteoma or osteosarcoma. Similarly, if they are derived from the cartilage they are called chondromas or chondrosarcomas, and if they are derived from the fibrous tissue they are called fibromas or fibrosarcomas. You can get combinations of the two, e.g. osteochondromas. There are also tumours derived from the marrow, including Ewing's sarcoma and myeloma. Some of the benign tumours can become malignant.

Symptoms from bone tumours usually include pain and swelling and certainly any such unexplained limb pain that lasts for more than a month (especially if pain occurs at night) should be investigated. Otherwise tumours may be picked up incidentally on X-ray or may be present as a pathological fracture.

Most of the tumours have characteristic X-ray appearances; however, there is a large amount of overlap and one X-ray appearance can have multiple differential diagnoses. The following X-ray appearances should be observed as forewarning signs of malignancy:

1. *Cortical destruction.* Is the cortical bone involved and eaten away?
2. *Periosteal reaction.* This looks like a fuzzy line outside of the cortex, indicating activity or irritation of the periosteum. This can be seen after a fracture or in infection, but can also be seen in the absence of the above in the presence of malignancy.
3. *Zone of transition.* The borders between the lesion and the normal bone. If the border can be drawn with a pencil (i.e. sclerotic margin) it is said to be a narrow zone of transition, which is less worrying than if the border is diffuse, which is associated with more aggressive tumours.

Other clinical indicators of malignancy include rapid growth of a lesion, tenderness and warmth (note that the latter two can also indicate infection).

344 Surgical Talk: Revision in Surgery

If a malignancy is suspected, thorough investigation is needed to establish the exact diagnosis and assess the size and spread. Other investigations include a chest X-ray, bone scans, CT and MRI. The ESR is usually raised, as is the alkaline phosphatase. A biopsy should really be performed by the surgeon who will ultimately operate on the lesion, and therefore patients should be referred to a specialist centre early.

Primary Tumours

These should be thought of as benign or malignant. There are many differential diagnoses of benign tumours. It is beyond the scope of this book to cover every differential diagnosis in detail. Other texts do that very well. So, below you will find some short notes that can be supplemented with further reading if you wish. For the purposes of exams it is fine that you have heard of the list below but it is less important that you learn it off by heart as it is mainly postgraduate stuff.

Aneurysmal bone cysts (ABCs). These are bone cysts that are expansile (hence their name). They usually affect those under the age of 30 and present with pain. On an MRI they display the pathognomonic sign of multiple fluid levels. Treatment of symptomatic bone cysts is usually to curette out the cyst and fill with bone graft.

Bone cysts (also called simple bone cysts or unicameral or solitary bone cysts). Most of these occur in the proximal humerus and femur, again in young patients. They are usually asymptomatic but if they take up a large amount of the width of the bone, they can fracture. If they do fracture, a bit of the cortex can fall into the cyst, which gives the classical 'fallen fragment sign'.

Chondroma (also known as enchondromas). These are benign tumours, which can be single or multiple (Ollier's disease). If multiple and associated with soft tissue haemangiomas, there is another syndrome called Maffucci's syndrome, which we only mention for MCQ purposes as you are unlikely to ever see one. Chondromas or enchondromas are the most common benign cystic lesions of the phalanges but can affect other long bones. In patients over 40 it is important to exclude a chondrosarcoma, into which a chondroma can (rarely) develop.

Fibrous cortical defect (also called nonossifying fibroma). These are common and have been reported to be seen incidentally on X-ray in up to 20% of children. They usually spontaneously regress, however, and so are rarely seen after the age of 30. They are nonpainful and benign defects of the cortex, as the name suggests, and usually affect the metaphasis of long bones. They should be left alone.

Fibrous dysplasia. This is a condition whereby bits of the bone (usually long bones) are replaced by fibrous tissue. It can be monostotic (localised) or polyostotic (generalised). Monostotic is more common (approximately 70–80%). In monostotic fibrous dysplasia a solitary segment is affected and the cause is unknown. It is usually picked up incidentally on X-ray, although it can present as a pathological fracture with pain.

In polyostotic fibrous dysplasia (20–30%) several bones are affected and it usually presents with progressive deformity (where the bones bend or enlarge), pain and pathological fracture. The classical X-ray appearance is described as a ground glass or smokey appearance. It has been questioned whether the Elephant Man had fibrous dysplasia, although most believe he had neurofibromatosis or Proteus syndrome.

There is a rare condition, worth a mention for a multiple choice exam and that is McCune–Albright syndrome, where polyostotic fibrous dysplasia occurs in association with pigmentation of the skin (café au lait spots) and, in females, precocious puberty.

Giant cell tumour (GCT). These are sometimes called osteoclastomas and are of unknown origin, although there are multinuclear giant cells under the microscope, giving them their name. They occur in young adults, but always after fusion of the growth plate. If the growth plate is still open, discard this diagnosis. They are usually around the knee (in the lower end of the femur or upper tibia) and always abut the articular surface. They are usually considered benign neoplasms, although some can be locally aggressive and some metastasise.

Osteochondromas. These are the commonest tumours of the bone. They are cartilage-capped exostoses that continue to grow as the bone grows (if multiple they may be part of a condition known as hereditary multiple exostoses). They usually present as a bony lump and appear on an X-ray as an abnormal outgrowth of bone — either finger-like or cauliflower-shaped projections (often they look smaller on an X-ray than the size to touch, because the cartilage does not show up). If there are symptoms they should be excised, and if they change in size after skeletal maturity, then this suggests possible malignancy (chondrosarcoma).

Osteoid Osteoma. These are benign tumours that do not become malignant. They are small and usually occur in those under 30, most commonly in the tibia or femur. They appear on the X-ray as a small radiolucent area (the nidus) surrounded by dense sclerosis and are hot spots on a bone scan. The main symptom is pain which characteristically responds to aspirin (but then again so do a lot of things). If left alone they may disappear spontaneously, but if the pain persists excision of the nidus should be undertaken, usually with instant resolution of symptoms. Large osteoid osteomas have been referred to as osteoblastomas although they behave much like ABCs and if seen usually relate to the spine. We will not say any more as it is simply too rare for us to worry about.

A mnemonic to remember the list is ABC FFG OO, if you are so inclined.

Malignant Tumours

Osteosarcomas. These occur in males more than in females, and usually in adolescents (although there is a second peak in those over 50, due to malignant change in Paget's disease). The commonest sites are around the knee or proximal humerus. Osteosarcomas usually occur in the metaphysis and are locally invasive, spreading distally via the blood (often to the lung). The main symptom is pain, especially at night, and there may be local tenderness. X-rays show a metaphyseal, translucent and destructive lesion. The tumour expands through the cortex, causing it to be raised, and a triangle of new bone is produced in the angle where the periosteum separates from the shaft called Codman's triangle. Eventually, it breaks through the cortex into the surrounding soft tissues, causing streaks of calcification within them (the 'sun-ray' appearance). Treatment usually involves chemotherapy and resection, which may mean amputation or wide local excision using an allograft or prostheses. About 60% survive 5 years.

Ewing's sarcomas. These are rare malignant tumours arising from the bone marrow, usually in young patients. Most of them occur in the diaphysis of long bones (in contrast to osteosarcomas which tend to be metaphyseal). Again, they present with a painful swelling, although because the lump is usually warm and tender they are occasionally diagnosed as having osteomyelitis. X-rays show a destructive lesion, sometimes with several layers of periosteal new bone around the lesion (called an 'onion skin' appearance). Treatment is usually chemotherapy, followed by surgical excision if possible.

Chondrosarcomas. These usually affect the middle-aged to elderly age group and are found in the pelvis or the proximal end of the long bones. There are two types: one arises from the surface of the bone (sometimes in the cartilage-covered cap of an osteochondroma) and the other arises within the medulla of the bone, often as a chondroma that either becomes malignant or has in fact been a slow-growing malignancy all the time. X-rays show an expanding radiolucent lesion with characteristic flecks of calcification. Treatment is by excision or, if necessary, amputation, since chondrosarcomas tend to metastasise late. Five-year survival is about 50%.

To summarise, if the patient is young (less than 30) always consider osteosarcoma or Ewing's sarcoma in your differential. In older patients (i.e. 40+) think of chondrosarcoma, myeloma and mets.

Secondary Tumours

Cancers that commonly metastasise to bone include breast, thyroid, renal, bronchus and prostate (not necessarily in this order, but it often helps to remember them by the mnemonic 'Bone Tumours are Rarely Bony Primaries'). The majority of metastases are lytic lesions, with the exception of prostate, which is usually osteosclerotic (however, breast and thyroid are sometimes osteosclerotic). They metastasise to bone that contains red marrow, otherwise known as the axial skeleton (spine, pelvis, ribs and the proximal end of the long bones). Secondary tumours may cause local pain or present as a pathological fracture. Pathological fractures are best treated by internal fixation, as they tend not to heal. By the time there are multiple bony secondaries the prognosis is poor and treatment is likely to be palliative. Radiotherapy is often used to treat local bone pain.

BONE INFECTION

Infection of bone (osteomyelitis) can be disastrous and extremely difficult to treat, and this is why such meticulous asepsis is undertaken in orthopaedic theatres and why antibiotic prophylaxis is always used when metalwork is involved. Acute osteomyelitis occurs either as a result of haematogenous spread or following trauma/operation. Infection of bones or joints acquired via the blood is common in children but rare in adults, who usually acquire the infection as a result of trauma or operation; the exception to this is in adults who are immunocompromised (including diabetics and those on steroids) or are intravenous drug abusers.

In acute haematogenous osteomyelitis, the usual organisms are *Staphylococcus aureus*, but occasionally *streptococci* or *coliforms* are responsible. They enter the blood in many ways, such as via a small skin abrasion or from an infected throat, and settle randomly on the bone. The symptoms usually include pain and fever, often with a preceding history of a sore throat or a superficial cut, etc. The limb is painful to move, and there is tenderness and possibly localised inflammation. Diagnosis can be difficult in a young child, who may simply look unwell and have a temperature. X-rays are normal at first, but later may show a hazy edge to the bone, indicating a periosteal reaction and new bone formation. A bone scan will show up increased activity while the X-rays are still normal.

Bloods should be sent for culture and white cell count, ESR and C-reactive protein (CRP), which should all be raised. Treatment is by intravenous antibiotics, analgesia and rest of the affected limb. The antibiotics are usually changed to oral after a few days and then given for up to 6 weeks.

Postoperative osteomyelitis where metalwork is *in situ* can be a disaster. Intravenous antibiotics are given and the metalwork may need to be removed and perhaps an external fixator applied if the fracture has not healed.

Chronic osteomyelitis can result if a sequestrum forms. This is an area of pus that is walled off by new bone, often discharging through a sinus. The infection can remain for many years, with recurrent acute flare-ups. Surgery to remove the sequestrum is indicated if healing is to ensue.

Acute Septic Arthritis

This usually affects large joints such as the hip in children and the knee in adults. The patient will feel unwell, often with a fever and rigors. The joint is painful, inflamed and swollen, and all movements are restricted.

X-rays may be normal initially and an ultrasound may show a joint effusion. Diagnosis is based on clinical presentation but can only be confirmed by aspirating the affected joint under aseptic conditions and sending the aspirate to bacteriology for microscopy and culture. Blood tests should include an FBC, ESR, CRP and cultures (do not forget that TB can be a cause).

If your index of suspicion is high or the aspirate confirms sepsis, treatment involves joint washout under general anaesthetic and IV antibiotics. If there is a prosthesis *in situ*, then the infection may settle only if the metalwork is removed.

Sometimes it is difficult to make a diagnosis, for example, when the patient has an acute monoarthritis and the aspirate shows a lot of white cells but no organisms. The differential diagnosis includes an acute monoarthritis (rheumatoid), gout, pseudogout, etc. However, clues from the history should help. Does the patient feel generally well or unwell, are they diabetic or on steroids, have they had any previous episodes, etc.?

If the blood markers are all normal and the patient is apyrexial and looks well, septic arthritis is unlikely. They can be treated with splintage, rest and nonsteroidal, anti-inflammatory drugs. If there is any doubt in your mind as to the diagnosis, the safe option is to admit the patient for observation.

NERVE INJURIES

These are common in finals and can appear both in medical and in surgical exams. When assessing power of a particular muscle group, try to use the MRC classification, which scores power from 0 to 5; 5 is normal power, 4 is weakness, 3 is ability to use muscle against gravity, 2 is movement with gravity eliminated (for example, able to move in a horizontal direction but not vertically), 1 is just a flicker of the muscle, and 0 means no movement detectable. It seems nonsensical to use plus or minus grades to a subjective scoring system, but no doubt you will see some people doing this.

Brachial plexus lesions can be of the upper or lower roots. The closer the lesion is to the spinal cord, the worse the prognosis will be.

Lesions of the upper brachial plexus (Erbs palsy, C5/C6) can occur at birth. Here, the abductors and external rotators are paralysed, so the arm is held close to the body, internally rotated ('waiter's tip' position), with loss of sensation to the C5/6 dermatomes.

Lesions to the lower brachial plexus (Klumpke paralysis, C8/T1) are rare and result in loss of intrinsic muscles of the hand, leading to a claw hand with loss of sensation in C8/T1 dermatomes.

Injuries to the individual nerves of the arm can occur anywhere along the course of the nerve, and the deficit will depend on the level.

Radial Nerve

The radial nerve is essentially the nerve which extends the fingers, the wrist and the elbow, and therefore testing the extension of each of these will give a clue as to the level. Sensation is not very accurate in helping to elicit the level, as it is predominantly a motor nerve.

Low lesions can occur with fractures around the elbow or forearm, and there is loss of extension of the carpophalangeal joints.

High lesions are more common and usually follow a fracture of the humerus or after a prolonged tourniquet time (the nerve is squashed or stretched but rarely severed). Damage usually occurs where the nerve travels around the shaft of the humerus (in the radial groove). The patient has a wrist drop, due to paralysis of wrist extensors and loss of sensation along the radial nerve distribution (this is a common case in exams). Because the nerve to triceps comes off proximal to the lesion, the triceps still functions normally.

Very high lesions can be caused by pressure in the axilla, such as through the incorrect use of crutches, or Saturday night palsy (the arm is hung over a chair when drunk). This leads to paralysis of triceps as well.

Ulnar Nerve

Damage to the ulnar nerve usually occurs at the elbow or the wrist. The usual picture is a 'claw-like hand'. The reason for this is that the ulnar nerve supplies all of the interossei, half of the flexor digitorum profundus (FDP) and the lumbricals to the ring and little fingers. A lesion at the wrist causes unopposed action of the extensors and the FDP, especially of the little and ring fingers, causing them to claw (the FDP is supplied just below the elbow and so a cut at the level of the wrist will not paralyse this).

Lesions at the elbow often have less clawing, since the ulnar half of FDP is now paralysed and the fingers are therefore straighter (a true claw hand is only seen in Volkman's contracture and proximal lesions of the brachial plexus).

Another test for the ulnar nerve is to ask the patient to grip a piece of paper between the thumb and the proximal phalanx of the index finger of a closed fist. In an ulnar nerve lesion the patient is unable to use adductor pollicis, and to cheat they flex the DIPJ using the flexor pollicis (supplied by the median nerve) to grip the paper. If they flex the DIPJ, then this is called a positive Froment's sign.

The sensation in the ulnar distribution of the hand is usually affected. There may be wasting of the interossei on the dorsum of the hand, and there is weakness of finger abduction and adduction.

In an exam, if you see a wrist drop think of the radial nerve, and if you see a claw hand think of the ulnar nerve. Median nerve palsy is usually seen at the wrist, as in carpal tunnel syndrome.

Carpal Tunnel Syndrome

The median nerve supplies the first two lumbricals and the thenar eminence muscles. The muscles are often referred to as the LOAF muscles, which stands for Lumbricals (first two), Opponens pollicis, Abductor and Flexor pollicis brevis.

The median nerve can be compressed as it passes under the flexor retinaculum (in the carpal tunnel). It is much more common in females than in males and the associations are pregnancy, rheumatoid arthritis, hypothyroidism, acromegaly and trauma, although most often it is idiopathic in menopausal women.

The classic symptoms are pain and paraesthesia in the distribution of the median nerve (see Figure 15.15). A small patch of skin over the thenar eminence is spared, because this is supplied by the superficial branch of the median nerve, which does not go under the flexor retinaculum.

The symptoms of pain and numbness are classically worse at night and might be relieved by shaking the hands. During the day symptoms may be brought on by activities that compress the nerve further, such as prolonged flexion of the wrist (e.g. typing or knitting). In advanced cases the muscles supplied by the median nerve may be weak and wasted. Ideally, diagnosis should be made early from the history, before any physical signs are present since once the muscle is wasted it invariably will not return even after surgical treatment. A test that can sometimes reproduce the symptoms is Tinel's test (tapping over the median nerve at the wrist to reproduce the symptoms). Always keep in mind a cervical rib or cervical spondylosis involving the C6 & C7 roots, which can cause similar symptoms. If a case is suspected, diagnosis can be confirmed by electromyographic studies across the wrist showing delayed conduction of the nerve impulses. Treatment of mild cases can be conservative, by using splints across the wrist or local steroid injections. Symptomatic cases where the nerve conduction is reduced require surgical decompression by division of the flexor retinaculum. The pain symptoms will improve; however, the numbness and wasting may not.

RADIAL NERVE   ULNAR NERVE   MEDIAN NERVE

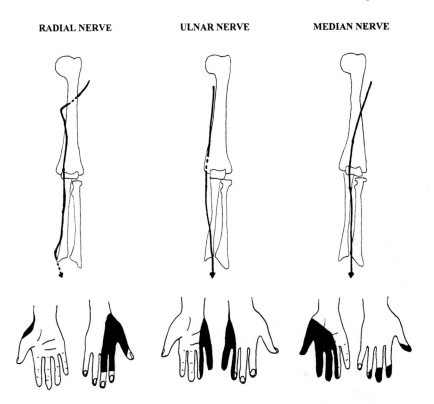

Figure 15.15. Distribution of the peripheral nerves to the arms. The shaded areas on the hands correspond to the sensory distribution of each nerve.

Dupuytren's Contracture

This is a common examination question. Named after the Frenchman who described it in 1931, Guillaine Dupuytren, it is a disorder where there is fibrosis and thickening of the palmar fascia (not the tendons!). It is commoner in men, usually of middle to elderly age. The aetiology is not known, although it can be inherited as an autosomal dominant gene. The associations include alcohol, drugs (such as phenytoin), cirrhosis and diabetes.

The condition often begins as a single nodule (which may or may not be painful). Later, bands of thickened tissue form on the palmar fascia which may adhere to the skin and there is progressive contracture of the fingers, usually the ring finger first, followed by the little finger, eventually to the point where the fingers are fully flexed. The condition can be bilateral and the feet can sometimes be affected. Operation is considered for progressive lesions some surgeons say they operate when the hand can no longer be placed flat on a table, although this is perhaps too simplistic an approach. It usually involves a fasciectomy, where the palmar fascia is divided. If the disease is advanced there may not be enough skin, necessitating a skin graft. The condition often recurs.

If you see this as a short case, the diagnosis is usually obvious although the differential diagnosis could include a skin contracture (an old laceration, scar or burn is, however, usually visible).

Ganglion

This is a common short case. A ganglion is a cystic swelling, most commonly seen on the dorsum of the wrist. Its exact origin is debated but is probably a cystic mucoid degeneration of the joint capsule or tendon sheath. It usually presents as a painless lump (but it can be painful) that may interfere with wearing a watch or may catch on clothes. A ganglion can disappear spontaneously, although a bash with a Bible was the traditional treatment. It is smooth and fluctuant and those at the wrist are usually fixed to deeper structures but not to skin. It can be aspirated (thick, gel-like material) and injected with hydrocortisone, although it commonly recurs, in which case it can be surgically excised.

Again, the diagnosis is usually obvious, but the differential could be a lipoma, fibroma or sebaceous cyst.

THE LIMPING CHILD

Paediatric orthopaedics is a postgraduate subject and is not really considered fair game for surgical finals. The limping child is, however, an important subject and you should know a little about the following.

There is a diagnostic calendar of conditions that affect the hip and this table illustrates the conditions and the rough age groups they tend to affect:

Age (years)	Diagnosis	Rough Incidence
0 (birth)	Congenital dislocation (CDH)	1 in 1000
0–5	Infections	
5–10	Perthes' disease (Legg–Cálve–Perthes)	1 in 10,000
10–15	Slipped femoral epiphyses	1 in 100,000
Adults	Avascular necrosis, rheumatoid arthritis and osteoarthritis	

The commonest cause of the painful hip in a young child is a transient synovitis secondary to a viral illness, often called the irritable hip, but this is a diagnosis of exclusion.

Congenital Dislocation of the Hip

At birth most hips are stable; however, a small number are dislocated or dislocatable. Most become stable within the first few weeks of life and can be considered to be physiological laxity of the joint capsule. The term congenital dislocation of the hip (CDH) is used in many books to describe what is perhaps better classified as developmental dysplasia of the hip (DDH), because the problem is not always a dislocation and it is not always present at birth but can develop and progress during the first few months of life. Regardless of the name, it can be defined as a congenitally determined developmental deformation of the hip joint in which the head of the femur is or may be completely or partially displaced from the acetabulum.

The incidence of DDH is about 2 per 1000 live births although somewhere between 5–20 per 1000 hips are lax at birth. Females are affected more than males and one-third are bilateral. The exact aetiology is unknown but there is a familial tendency and there is a high incidence of both joint laxity and a shallow acetabulum in first-order relatives of DDH patients. The position of the foetus in the uterus may play a part as there is a higher incidence in breech presentation, first-borns and those with oligohydramnios, all of which point to decreased intrauterine space.

It is also interesting to note that the incidence is much higher in North American Indians, who wrap their babies tight to the mother's body with the hips extended and the legs together, compared to the racially identical Eskimos, who carry their babies on the back with the hips widely abducted and flexed.

The best time to screen for DDH is at birth, during the routine post-natal examination. It is important for the screener to take a careful history looking for risk factors for DDH and obtain consent from the parents to carry out screening. On examination if there are any physical abnormalities (e.g. syndromic facies or scoliosis) this should be an additional warning sign. The buttock (gluteal) skin folds should be inspected and asymmetry should also set off your alarm bells (asymmetry of inguinal skin folds is less helpful in the new born although is significant in a 3–4-month-old baby).

Several tests have been described of which the commonest used in the textbooks are the Ortolani and Barlow tests.

In *Ortolani's test* the hips and knees are flexed to 90° and the thighs are grasped in each hand, the thumb over the inner thigh and the fingers resting over the greater trochanters. The hips are abducted gently and a resistance to abduction will be noted if the hip is dislocated, otherwise they abduct easily to 90°. When gentle pressure is applied to the greater trochanters by the fingers, a dislocated hip will relocate back into the joint and a click can be felt (positive Ortolani test). *Barlow's test* is a slight modification of this test. It is performed as above except that during the abduction phase, gentle but firm pressure is applied in the line of the femur so that a lax hip dislocates posteriorly. The hip pressure can then be reduced by performing the movement in Ortolani's test. Therefore, one could think of it as Ortolani's test detects a dislocated hip and Barlow's test detects a dislocatable hip.

If either test is positive, or your clinical index of suspicion is high, then the baby should have an ultrasound scan. This will show the shape of the cartilaginous socket and the position of the head of the femur. X-rays are not helpful as the femoral head does not start to calcify until about 10 weeks.

Treatment depends on the time of diagnosis, and generally the sooner the DDH is picked up the better the outcome. The actual treatments will vary from centre to centre but the principles of treatment are essentially the same, namely, to reduce the hip and hold the head of the femur in this position until the acetabular rim is sufficiently developed.

Reduction can be obtained by closed or open methods. The younger the patient the more likely that closed methods will be possible.

Closed Methods of Reduction

In the newborn this can be achieved initially with double nappies to abduct the hips, followed by a reassessment after 2–3 weeks with another ultrasound examination.

If the hip remains unstable it is possible to apply a special harness to hold the legs abducted. The most popular is called the Pavlik harness, which holds the legs in a position for a few months. It is imperative that the femoral head is shown to be in the right place using regular ultrasound.

If after another month the hip does not remain reduced using a spica, it will be necessary to perform an examination under anaesthesia. There are higher anaesthetic risks in babies and so it is better to plan this electively when an experienced paediatric anaesthetist is available.

In theatre under general anaesthetic, an arthrogram (dye injected into the joint) is usually carried out to look for concentricity of the hip and any anatomical abnormalities. Because the abductors are likely to be tight, some surgeons will perform a tenotomy (where the tendon is cut) to allow gentle reduction, without excessive force which can damage the delicate blood supply to the hip. This is performed under image intensifier control. A plaster hip spica is then applied to keep the hip in the reduced position.

If the hip cannot be easily concentrically reduced, then an open reduction will need to be carried out. In a very young child this is usually carried out at a later stage, when they are closer to a year old (because of the higher anaesthetic risks) and in the interim the hip is usually left untreated.

Open Reduction

The commonest open stabilising procedure is a derotation varus osteotomy of the femur. The leg is rotated to a position where the head has maximum covering in the acetabulum; the femur is then sawed just below the trochanters and the shaft allowed to rotate back to a neutral position, and the two ends are then fixed using a plate (e.g. Coventry screw plate). Once in a good position the hip is held there using a plaster spica for a few weeks.

Once the toddler is walking the hip is checked out regularly both clinically and radiologically and an assessment is made of the acetabular development. If unsatisfactory, then further surgery may be required such as a pelvic osteotomy (the commonest is called a Salter osteotomy) to reposition the acetabulum to better cover the femoral head. This type of surgery is usually delayed until the child is about 2 years old.

If the diagnosis is not picked up at birth but picked up in the next few months, then the same principles apply. After about 6 months, X-rays can be used to assess the acetabulum.

If the CDH is 'missed', then diagnosis may not be made until the age of 12–18 months, when the child begins to walk with an abnormal gait. There may be limb shortening, external rotation of the foot, asymmetrical skin creases and a positive Trendelenburg's test. Reduction of the hip in this age group can be achieved by either open or closed methods as above (although a lip of labrum or loose capsule often impedes reduction and so closed reduction is usually unsuccessful).

The prognosis is good if the dislocation is picked up early, although if left untreated it can lead to progressive deformity and disability. Genetic testing can be discussed with the parents due to the familial tendencies.

With bilateral dislocations the deformity and waddling gait are symmetrical and not so noticeable; in fact, such patients often carry on with their lives without much complaint. If you interfere with both sides you run the risk of one side failing and hence converting them to a unilateral asymmetrical deformity, and so most surgeons would not operate on such patients above the age of 6 years.

Perthe's Disease

This is a type of osteochondritis, since it is an AVN of the femoral head. The patient is usually a male, between 4 and 10 years of age, with a limp. Pain is dependent on the stage of the disease and although initially it may be painful, after a while it may become painless. If there is pain it is in the groin and may radiate down to the knee.

Early on, all movements are painful, making it difficult to differentiate the condition from infection or a transient synovitis, which is by far the commonest cause of the irritable hip.

Initially, X-rays are normal, although a bone scan may show an abnormality. The earliest change to be seen on an X-ray is increased density of the bony part of the epiphysis, which later on flattens and fragments. A bone scan is useful especially in early stages of the disease.

There are 'at risk' signs (both clinical and radiological) that point to a poorer prognosis, although the details of these are perhaps more than you need to know for surgical finals.

Treatment is initially bed rest until the pain subsides, and further operative treatment will depend on the X-rays but essentially involves trying to contain the head in the acetabulum to enable it to retain as good a shape as possible.

Slipped Capital/Upper Femoral Epiphysis

Slipped capital femoral epiphysis (SCFE) in the past was referred to as SUFE. It is an uncommon condition, usually found in children of pubertal age. It tends to affect two contrasting groups, one being the fat and sexually underdeveloped group and the other being the tall and thin group — boys more than girls.

Endocrine and mechanical factors might play a part, since fat children have a higher incidence. It has been proposed that SCFE is due to a hormonal imbalance at the time of a growth spurt.

The epiphysis slips posteriorly either as an acute event (acute slip — 20%) or over a period of time (chronic slip — 60%) or as a combination of the two (acute on chronic slip — 20%).

In an acute slip the patient usually presents with groin pain or pain referred to the thigh or knee. The leg may be slightly short, externally rotated, and initially all movements are painful. Treatment depends on the acuteness of presentation and the degree of displacement but usually involves surgery to reduce the epiphysis and hold it in place with a pin. In a chronic slip, reduction should not be attempted (as AVN may result) and the epiphysis is usually pinned where it is to prevent further slippage (*in situ* pinning).

One of the risks of SCFE you should know about is chondrolysis, where the articular cartilage breaks down. Although this can occur without surgery, the risk is higher if the guide wire or pin penetrates the articular cartilage.

Longer term all the hip disorders mentioned above can potentially increase the risk of disability, deformity and OA.

Irritable Hip

This is a diagnosis of exclusion commonly made in children between the ages of 1 and 10, and presents with a limp and pain in the hip. The cause is unknown but may be a viral synovitis as the patient often has a preceding upper respiratory tract infection. It is important to rule out septic arthritis, and so screening blood tests, including a full blood count, CRP and ESR, must be sent off. An ultrasound examination may be helpful.

Infection in a joint can lead to destruction of the articular cartilage and permanent damage within a short space of time, and therefore a child in whom you suspect infection needs urgent aspiration of the joint to obtain microbiological samples for microscopy and culture. If there is no bacterial infection and an irritable hip is diagnosed, then it usually settles with rest and analgesia over 2 or 3 days.

16

EAR, NOSE AND THROAT

Michael Oko

Ear, Nose and Throat (ENT) is an important subject and examination questions relating to it are common, although they tend to be at a reasonably basic level in the finals. Topics such as thyroid disease, dysphagia and lumps in the neck are important but are covered elsewhere in this book (Chapters 6 and 11). In this chapter we aim to summarise some key facts in the other important areas of ENT.

EXAMINATION OF THE EAR

Introduce yourself to the patient and pick up your auroscope. Chose an appropriately sized speculum to attach to the scope (make sure you are familiar with this instrument and can hold it as if you are used to doing so). Ask the patient if they have a better hearing ear (unless directed to examine a specific ear by the examiner) and proceed to examine the better hearing ear first. Look at the pinna (external ear) and the surrounding skin. Anteriorly look for preauricular sinuses and any other congenital abnormalities. Also, look for endaural and postauricular incisions using the light from the auroscope. An endaural incision is a surgical scar running from superior to inferior just above the tragus (the bit of skin-covered cartilage in front of the external auditory meatus). A postauricular incision runs in the hidden groove between the back of the pinna and the skull. These are often very subtle and only seen if you look closely. It is useful to keep talking and explain to the examiner what you are doing as you go along. Once you have examined the external ear, insert the auroscope into the external auditory canal, looking at the canal skin for any sign of infection. If you look posteriorly and the posterior canal appears defective, the patient has almost certainly had a mastoid operation. These are quite common in ENT exams as there are many patients who have had surgery many years ago and are still seen in the clinic for aural toileting of accumulated wax. As an undergraduate you will not be expected to answer anything too tasking. Perhaps it would suffice to know that it is a mastoid cavity and the reason people have this operation is either because of chronic infection within the mastoid cavity or a cholesteatoma, which is a benign, slow-growing epithelial tumour that causes progressive destruction of the ossicles, labyrinth, facial nerve and, hence, loss of hearing. It can sometimes lead to brain abscesses, meningitis or thrombosis of the sigmoid sinus.

As you finish looking around the external auditory canal wall, look toward the tympanic membrane and look for the light reflex (this is due to light bouncing off the angled tympanic membrane) antero-inferiorly and travel clockwise towards the attic region and look at the pars flaccida (the bit at the top of the tympanic membrane above the maleus) and see if it looks retracted or if there is any debris within it as it may have a cholesteatoma present. Continue examination of the pars tensa segment of the tympanic membrane in a clockwise fashion and note whether it is intact or not. If it is not intact what percentage of the drum is perforated? In exams you would probably see a stable tympanic membrane perforation which is on a waiting list for elective surgery.

Do not forget to examine the opposite ear. Free field hearing tests are a useful conclusion to your inspection of the ear, so make sure your technique for this is good (see below). You would also be expected to examine the function of the facial nerve.

Hearing Tests

Tuning Fork Tests

A common question is to ask you to perform the Weber's and Rinne's test. Classically, a 512 Hz tuning fork is used because if you use a higher-frequency tuning fork the sound decays too quickly and if you use a lower-frequency tuning fork you get a lot of vibrational sensation.

Rinne's Test

Always make sure you explain to the patient before you do anything. Explain that (1) you will be tapping the tuning fork and placing it in front of their ear and then (2) you will move it to their mastoid tip.

You then ask the patient to tell you which one was the loudest, (1) or (2), and repeat this on the opposite side. It is normal that air conduction or (1) should be better than bone conduction or (2) and this is a Rinne positive. You can get a Rinne negative if bone conduction is better than air conduction and this suggests a conductive loss. You can also get a false negative Rinne when the patient has a 'dead' or nonfunctioning ear on the side being tested and they actually hear the tuning fork test in the opposite ear. It is said that Rinne can pick up a 15–20 dB hearing loss.

Weber's Test

Gently strike the fork and place it on the forehead, asking the patient to which side the sound lateralises. The normal response is midline. In general, the patient perceives the sound in the ear with the better-conductive component. With a pure conductive hearing loss, the sound will be perceived louder in the poorer hearing ear ('towards the bad hearing ear'). With a pure sensorineural hearing loss, the sound will be perceived in the better hearing ear ('towards the good hearing ear'). Ambiguity develops when one ear has both conductive and sensorineural hearing loss. You can remember this test by doing it on yourself, whilst one ear is plugged with your finger to simulate a conductive loss.

It is thought that the Weber test is a more sensitive test than the Rinne and will pick up anything from a 5 dB conductive loss.

Free Field Hearing Tests

These are useful to know and should be carried out if you do not have ready access to an audiology laboratory. Done with confidence they look impressive in exams. Start with a whispered voice at 2 ft with tragal rubbing of the opposite ear. If you use both words and numbers (e.g. 66 BW) at this distance, they should normally be heard equally in both ears. If there is no response, then try a whispered voice at 6 in., then a conversational voice at 2 ft (40–60 db loss), 6 in. and up to a loud voice at 2 ft and finally 6 in. (>60 db loss). The test is aborted when 50% of responses are correct.

Pure Tone Audiometry

You may be expected to know what this is and possibly interpret some of the most common results. An audiometer produces pure tones and the test is carried out in a soundproofed room. The patient wears headphones connected to the audiometer. The patient listens until the sound first appears and then until it just disappears. A small vibrator can also be used applied to the mastoid process to assess bone conduction.

The threshold of hearing at different frequencies is plotted and this is the audiogram.

Evoked Response Audiometry

Essentially, the technique involves an auditory stimulus (a brief click or tone transmitted via a earphone or headphones) with measurement of the elicited resulting brain waveform response by surface electrodes. Brain stem evoked responses can be used to detect acoustic neuromas or determine hearing thresholds in children. Cortical responses can detect malingerers who may be seeking compensation for work-related hearing loss.

ENT SYMPTOMS

The common ENT symptoms include deafness, tinnitus and vertigo. A few brief notes follow.

Tinnitus

This is the auditory sensation of noise without external sound stimulation (i.e. a sound heard when there is no sound). It is extremely common and is associated with ageing and noise-induced hearing loss. It can be unilateral, bilateral or central and the patients often complain of a mechanical noise which appears louder when in bed trying to sleep (when there is no masking background noise). It can be disabling in some cases and may herald the appearance of an acoustic neuroma (see below) when unilateral (hence all unilateral cases should be referred to ENT for assessment). Treatment consists of positive reassurance, using background noise at bedtime (put the TV or radio on a timer) or a tinnitus masker (which produces white noise). Relaxation techniques have also been found helpful by many patients.

Vertigo

This is the illusion of movement experienced by the patient often with a rotatory component (dizziness) and should be distinguished from lightheadedness. The history often points to the diagnosis.

- Trauma + positional vertigo + nystagmus + short duration + fatiguability = benign paroxysmal positional vertigo (BPPV). This is due to a degenerative condition of the utricular neuroepithelium and may occur spontaneously or following head injury.
- URTI + severe vertigo + vomiting + lasting days = labrynthitis.
- Fluctuating hearing loss + vertigo lasting days + tinnitus + aural fullness = Menière's (see below), but rule out acoustic neuroma with MRI.

Remember that balance is dependent on sight (70%), proprioreception (15%) and the vestibular system (15%). Management of vertigo includes a detailed history and physical exam, appropriate investigations (PTA, MRI) and treatment (labyrinthine sedatives and physiotherapy, or surgical intervention in appropriate cases).

Causes of Deafness

Conductive deafness is due to interference with the conduction of sound at any point from the auricle to the oval window. Sensorineural deafness is the result of disease of the cochlea, auditory nerve or brain. The causes of deafness can be classified into these two categories or as congenital or acquired.

Congenital

1. Hereditary — autosomal recessive or autosomal dominant
2. Intrauterine insult
   Infections (e.g. CMV, rubella, etc.)
   Hypoxia (due to any cause, e.g. difficult delivery)

Acquired

Adults

1. *Ageing.* Presbyacussis (deafness of old age) is the most common. Patients are usually over 65 years of age with bilateral hearing loss of slow onset over many years with or without tinnitus. It is usually noticed by the family. There is a progressive symmetrical slope on PTA and if there is >40 db loss at 2 kHz then a hearing aid might help.
2. *Noise-induced hearing loss.* A history of long-term noise exposure at work is usual and may be associated with tinnitus.
3. *Otosclerosis.* This is an autosomal dominant inheritance with variable penetration. It presents more commonly in women with conductive hearing loss in adulthood with a classic dip (carharts notch) at 2 kHz on PTA. It is due to fixation of the stapes at the oval window and treatments are a hearing aid or stapedotomy.
4. *Meniere's disease.* This presents with a classical triad history of deafness, vertigo and tinnitus (DVT) in association with aural fullness (a sense of pressure in the middle ear, as if descending in an aeroplane) in a percentage of cases. The cause is unknown but one theory relates to excessive endolymphatic fluid. During acute episodes the patients feel very unwell and may suffer from nausea and vomiting. Audiometry shows low-frequency sensorineural loss which fluctuates

(you have to do an MRI of the cerebropontine angle and internal auditory meatus to rule out an acoustic neuroma). It runs a chronic history which burns out over time. The mainstay treatment is predominately conservative management with avoidance of caffeine, salt and other associated trigger factors. Surgical remedies for this condition include insertion of a grommet, saccus decompression, cortical mastoid and insertion of Gentamicin into the middle ear cleft. In extreme circumstances labarynthectomy and vestibular nerve section may be required.

5. *Acoustic neuroma.* This usually presents with slow onset of unilateral symptoms of hearing loss and tinnitus with or without vertigo. As it enlarges, it will cause headaches, other cranial nerve palsies (VI, VII, VIII) and intracranial hypertension. In rare cases it presents with bilateral symptoms. You should suspect an association of MENII (multiple endocrine neoplasia type 2). Investigation includes a full clinical exam, PTA (unilateral sensorineural hearing loss) and MRI. Treatment consists of observation with annual MRI for monitoring growth, radiotherapy with the gamma knife or surgery through a translabrynthine or middle fossa approach.

Paediatric Conditions

1. *Acute otitis media.* This is very common in general practice but you are less likely to see a case in an examination due to the pain of the condition. However, this may not stop the examiners from showing you a picture of an acutely inflamed eardrum.

   A history of a child who is febrile with an upper respiratory tract infection, rubbing their ear(s) and crying in pain should make you suspicious of this common condition. When you look at the tympanic membrane it is red and acutely inflamed, bulging or slightly retracted. Treatment consists of analgesia (usually paracetamol) and antibiotics (amoxicillin) and the condition usually improves after a few days. However, potential complications include glue ear (the middle ear is full of a sticky effusion), perforation of the tympanic membrane (these normally heal spontaneously after about 6 weeks) and mastoiditis (ostitis of the temporal bone with abscess formation, which can lead to meningitis and brain abscesses).

2. *Glue ear (otitis media with effusion = OME).* This is the most common complication of acute otitis media and may be associated with allergic rhinitis. The prevalence is high at 2 years of age and decreases towards the teenage years. Inattention at school, poor speech development and other abnormal milestones may be presenting features. There are a lot of conservative treatments available but none of definite proven benefit (Otovent nasal ballons, topical nasal steroids, decongestants) and the condition spontaneously resolves in the majority of cases. If there is persistent > 30 db bilateral hearing loss for > 3 months, then grommets may be considered. (These are small plastic ventilating tubes placed in the tympanic membrane under GA, which remain for 6–18 months). These are usually obvious on auroscopy.

COMMON CONDITIONS OF THE EAR PINNA

These can be divided into congenital and acquired.

Congenital

Microtia, accessory auricles, preauricular sinuses and various other malformations of the first branchial arch which may be associated with syndromes such as Treacher Collins.

Acquired Conditions (Can be Benign or Malignant)

Benign. Traumatic haematoma of pinna, sebaceous cyst, lipomas and pigmented navae.

Malignant. Squamous cell carcinoma (SCC) or, more commonly, basal cell carcinoma, the treatment of which is surgical resection which often in the pinna involves a wedge resection of the primary lesion itself and neck dissection if there has been regional spread to the deep cervical chain.

CONDITIONS OF THE EXTERNAL AUDITORY CANAL

These again can be divided into benign or malignant. The most common condition affecting the external auditory canal is chronic otitis externa, which is treated with aural toilet, a swab taken for microscopic cultures and sensitivity and usually only topical antibiotics in the form of Gentisone HC eardrops. Bony exostosis can also appear in the exam and this presents a smooth symmetrical narrowing of the external auditory canal in people who do a lot of swimming (the reason for this is not known). Treatment is conservative unless it is significantly problematic, then drilling away the bony exostosis can be done.

CONDITIONS OF THE TYMPANIC MEMBRANE (EARDRUM) — PERFORATION

Perforation of the eardrum is most commonly due to mucosal disease within the middle ear cleft which has resulted in an acute and subsequent chronic otitis media with perforation of the tympanic membrane. This is often referred to by otologists as chronic mucosal otitis media. Less commonly, you have squamous otitis media that presents as a perforation and can be associated with a cholesteatoma. These can progressively destroy the ossicles and hence impair hearing. You can think of this as a benign, 'onion-like' skin lesion (i.e. lots of layers) which grows in on itself and can progressively compromise all of the structures within the middle ear cleft and potentially spread superiorly through into the middle cranial fossa leading to an otogenic brain abscess.

DISORDERS OF THE FACIAL NERVE

To recap on the anatomy, the facial nerve runs from the cerebro-pontine angles into the internal auditory canal and then traverses the length of the temporal bone giving off three branches, which are the greater superficial petrosal, the nerve to stapedius and the chorda tympani before it exits the temporal bone through the stylomastoid foramen. It runs forward in to the substance of the parotid gland. Note that upper motor neuron lesions of the facial nerve spare the forehead (because of suprapontine crossover and sharing between the two sides) and lower motor neuron lesions do not. Do not forget that facial trauma and parotid lumps may also cause a facial paralysis but if you get one of these in the exam it will usually be obvious. Asking the patient to lift the eyebrows, close the eyes tight, purse the lips and 'blow and show me your teeth' will reveal function in the important branches.

Trauma to the temporal bone in the form of horizontal or transverse fractures can subsequently lead to a complete lower motor neuron lesion of the facial nerve. In about 5% of cases the facial nerve is exposed as it passes through the middle ear and hence acute otitis media, which puts pressure on the unprotected nerve, can lead to LMN facial nerve palsy.

Bell's Palsy

Bells palsy is an LMN lesion of the nerve of unknown cause, but possibly viral. This is a diagnosis of exclusion and a full clinical examination needs to be completed in addition to audiometry to make sure the facial nerve is not compromised within the substance of the temporal bone due to a cholesteatoma or other cause. It is controversial but many authors argue that these patients should be started off on high-dose steroids within 24 h of onset. In practice, full recovery may be expected in 85% of cases.

Vestibular Schwannoma (Acoustic Neuroma)

An acoustic neuroma is a benign lesion of the superior vestibular nerve, which is slow-growing and can be present with unilateral tinnitus, vertigo or a sensorineural hearing loss. Clearly this needs to be excluded in any patient who has any of the above symptoms and the diagnostic goal standard test of choice is MRI with gadolinium of the cerebro-pontine angle.

EXAMINATION OF THE NOSE

This is unlikely for finals, but simple to learn so we thought it was worth a brief mention. Introduce yourself to the patient. Look directly at the nose from in front, the side and on top as well as below. On examining the front determine which part of the external nose is bony and which part is cartilaginous. It is sometimes useful to hold your hand up in front of the nose to determine if there is any deviation due to the bony or cartilaginous portions of the nose.

In most examinations you will only be expected to use the auroscope to examine the nose, hence your view is limited to the first 1–2 cm within the nasal cavity. It is often helpful to ask the patient to breathe in through the nose and any obvious alar collapse can be identified. Use you thumb to lift the nasal tip and look for symmetry of the nasal cavity (think of it as being like a shotgun barrel!) and if it is not think of deviation of the nasal septum.

Only after doing this insert the auroscope into the nasal cavity and look at the septum in the midline to see if there is a septal perforation or any points of recent bleeding. Once you have identified the septum, identify the lateral nasal wall with the inferior turbinate being the most prominent and inferior. Make sure there is a gap between the septum and the lateral nasal wall and that this gap is roughly symmetrical. If it is not, it means the patient has a septal deviation and that could cause nasal obstruction and these patients are popular in ENT exams as they are often on routine waiting lists for a septoplasty.

On examining the lateral nasal wall look at the colour of the turbinate (it should normally be a healthy pinkish colour but is pale and boggy-looking in allergic rhinitis) and see if you can find any pale polypoidal lesions inside the nasal cavity as nasal polyposis is also another exam favourite.

To conclude your examination you should check for air flow by seeing if the patient can mist a mirror as they breathe out through their nose symmetrically on both sides and for absolute completeness test the sensation around the distribution of the maxillary division of the trigeminal nerve.

Common Conditions of the Nose for Exams

Epistaxis is a popular question as it is another way of asking a question about shock and haemorrhage. The most likely patient will be one with hereditary haemorrhagic telangectasia (Osler–Weber–Rendu syndrome) as they are frequent regular attendees to the ENT department with some of them needing over 100 units of blood per year. It is an autosomal dominant inherited condition which presents with facial telangectasia (look carefully at the lips and nose) and recurrent, sometimes torrential, epistaxis.

Management includes taking a full history, including any preceding trauma and current medication such as warfarin and aspirin, which some of these patients are on. If acutely bleeding, manage as per shock (see page 51). After you have donned the appropriate shielding apparatus to stop the patient aerosoling blood into your eyes and face, sometimes it is helpful to ask the patient to blow their nose to clear the old clots out and then you can use the light source to visualise the nasal cavity. As a house officer or A & E doctor you may need to insert a Mericel pack (this is a white tampon for the nose which is inserted after a local anaesthetic lignocaine 2% spray has had time to work and a lubricant such as KY jelly is applied to the tip of the tampon. Insert it straight back parallel to the hard palate, not upwards!). You should know that if this fails to control the bleeding then ENT should be contacted straight away and they will prob-ably insert a posterior pack using a Foley catheter balloon and repack the nose and, failing this, take the patient back to theatre for endoscopic control of the bleeding either through ligation of the sphenopalatine artery, maxil-lary or, in a worse case scenario, the external carotid artery. Beware also of patients who are packed who do not have the pack secured anteriorly. This may displace posteriorly and obstruct the airway.

The vast majority of the bleeds are from the front part of the nose in the Little's area (1 cm inside the nose and on the septum). However, in the elderly they tend to bleed slightly more posteriorly in the region of the sphenopalatine artery and tend to be more problematic.

Apart from admission and nasal packing, treatments range from laser to vessels, septodermoplasty, oestrogens and sealing up of the nasal cavity (Young's procedure).

Allergic Rhinitis

This is a type 1 hypersensitivity reaction to various inhaled or ingested allergens. Clinically, this presents with itching, sneezing, rhinorrhoea and nasal blockage. It costs the European Union approximately 22 billion a year in lost man-hours and treatments per year. About 60 to 70% of people with asthma also have rhinitis, which is not too surprising seeing that the same pseudostratified ciliated columnar epithelium exists in both areas. There are several different things patients may be allergic to and things that they cannot necessarily avoid in their environment. You have to think of the nose as an air conditioner which warms, filters and humidifies between 6 and 7 million liters of air per year. If you are allergic to something like house dust mite and you have a bed full of house dust mite, about a third of your life would be spent inhaling them. Management includes history taking of trigger factors, physical exam to check for polyps, skin prick tests for various antigens or RAST (radioallergosorbent test). The mainstay of treatment is actually allergy avoidance which requires allergy identification and then long-term use of antihistamines and/or topical nasal steroids. These should be prescribed with caution for children as they can cause growth retardation.

Sinusitis

Classic fronto-maxillary sinus (throbbing pain worse on bending forward) develops usually after an upper respiratory tract infection. There may be a foul smell and sometimes pus can be seen to exit from the nasal cavity. Treatment consists of nasal decongestants, antibiotics, analgesia and topical nasal steroids as indicated.

Indications for admission and CT paranasal sinuses. Systemically unwell, orbital or intracranial complications suspected (do neurobservations and check visual acuity or get an ophthalmologist to review).

EXAMINATION OF THE MOUTH

Look at the lips for telangectasia, ulcers, etc. Use your auroscope as a light source and a tongue depressor as a spatula to examine the upper teeth and parotid duct orifices (opposite second upper molars), hard palate, soft palate, uvula (if it is bifid then they could have an occult submucosal cleft palate, which is a contraindication to adenoidectomy), the anterior and posterior tonsil pillars, tonsils (look for asymmetry) and then the oropharynx behind the posterior tonsil pillars and uvula (at this point ask the patient to say 'Ahh' and look for asymmetry of movement of the soft palate).

Move onto the lower teeth and buccal sulcus all the way back to the retromolar trigone. Ask the patient to stick out the tongue and look for wasting, fasciculation, ulceration and deviation to one side (hypoglossal nerve paralysis causes the tongue to deviate to the same side as the paralysis). Then, ask the patient to point the tongue to the left and then the right as most cancers are on the lateral border of the tongue. Finally, ask the patient to lift the tongue to the roof of the mouth and inspect the floor of the mouth and the submandibular duct orifices just lateral to the frenulum. If you find something in the mouth, be prepared to examine the regional lymph nodes in the neck. You will not be expected to do indirect laryngoscopy but understand when referral to an ENT specialist is appropriate.

Tonsils/Adenoids

Tonsil and adenoid tissue normally are more prominent in children and the adenoids regress after about 13 years of age. They consist of lymphoid tissue, which is involved in immune processing of the substances we inhale and swallow. In some children there appears to be overproliferation or overactivity of these tissues and this leads to excessive infections or obstruction to the postnasal space or oropharynx, leading to obstructive sleep apnea. Most infections are dealt with by GPs with oral antibiotics and analgesia (penicillin ± metronidazole). Glandular fever is a viral cause of tonsillitis (Epstein–Barr virus) associated with contact (hence the term 'kissing disease') and marked cervical lymphadenopathy in young adults. It is also known as infectious mononucleosis.

A white cell count and a monospot test (detecting heterophil antibodies) are usually carried out and LFTs should be checked as occasionally patients can become jaundiced. Antibiotics, especially ampicillin, should be avoided (because they can cause a rash). Some patients feel tired and run down for up to a month or two. Some studies suggest that up to 10%

of patients develop symptoms of chronic fatigue syndrome. Splenic rupture is a rare but potentially fatal complication of acute glandular fever.

Complications of Tonsilitis

Peritonsillar abscess (Quinsy). This usually presents as marked trismus (difficulty in and limited mouth opening), intense sore throat, dysphagia and unilateral otalgia in a young febrile patient. Examination reveals unilateral tonsillar enlargement in addition to bilateral tonsillitis with or without cervical lympadenopathy. Treatment is admission, aspiration/incision and drainage, analgesia, IV antibiotics and fluids. If it fails to improve, suspect parapharyngeal abscess.

Parapharyngeal abscess. Suspect this if the patient appears to be unduly unwell, fails to improve after 24–36 h of high-dose IV antibiotics and has unilateral swelling of tonsil and neck. Get an urgent CT from skullbase to diaphragm and if an abscess is present it has to be drained through the neck.

Cancers of tonsils and adenoids. Squamous cell carcinomas and lymphomas are by far the commonest cancers that present with nasal blockage, unilateral glue ear, dysphagia, unilateral tonsil enlargement or ulceration with or without cervical lymphadenopathy. Diagnosis has to be confirmed histologically with fine needle aspiration (FNA) of neck nodes (or node excision biopsy for lymphoma) and staging with CT or MRI of neck and chest.

Obstructive Sleep Apnea/Snoring

This occurs both in children and adults and is common in males over the age of 40 who are overweight with sedentary occupations. It presents with marital disharmony due to loud snoring, multiple nocturnal waking and daytime somnolence. Examination usually reveals an overweight individual (BMI > 30) with a large neck (>17) who may have large tonsils, a long dependent uvula or a relatively small jaw. It is diagnosed with polysomnography showing more than 30 episodes of cessation of breathing for more than 10 sec over a 7 h period or apnea index > 5 (AI ⩾ 5 episodes of apnea >10 sec/h). It may be mild (AI = 5–20), moderate (AI = 20–40) or severe (AI ⩾ 40) and treatment includes weight loss, avoidance of alcohol and sedatives at night, dental positioning devices and CPAP. Surgery has a limited role in selected cases.

Larynx

Functions

Phonation. The ability to speak requires an intact larynx with functioning vocal cords, the respiratory bellows of the lungs and the mouth and tongue all working in unison.

Tumours and neurological injuries can cause paralysis of the recurrent laryngeal nerves and you should never forget to think of the neck and chest for an underlying pathology, particularly in smokers. To recap the anatomy, on the left the recurrent laryngeal dives into the chest and loops around the arch of aorta and ligamentum arteriosum before running up to the larynx, deep to the thyroid. On the right it loops round the subclavian artery before becoming recurrent.

Respiration. The larynx is a dynamic conduit between the trachea and the tongue base and has specialised epithelium and cartilage to line and support it. During swallowing respiration ceases, the epiglottis flips backwards and the cords are abducted to prevent aspiration.

Stertor. This is noisy respiration due to obstruction at the level of the tonsils and tongue base.

Stridor. This is noisy respiration due to obstruction at the level of the vocal cords and below and may be inspiratory, expiratory or biphasic.

Cancer of the Larynx

SCC is the commonest tumour of the upper aerodigestive tract and is intimately related to cigarette smoking, excessive alcohol consumption and social deprivation. In patients over 40 yrs who are long-term smokers, a persistent ulcer, lump, hoarse voice, dysphasia or any persistent (more than 2 weeks) ENT pain must be considered to have an SCC until proven otherwise. Clinical examination of the ENT including a flexible nasendoscopy of the larynx is mandatory; FNA of any neck nodes, panendoscopy and biopsy + CT skull-base to diaphragm are required to rule out occult tumors or stage positive biopsies. This applies to all ENT tumors including lymphomas. Treatment is based on histological type, TMN staging, comorbidity, patient suitability for surgery, radiotherapy or chemotherapy and patient preference. Generally, for T1–2 surgery or radiotherapy alone is used and T3–4 usually has both. Prognosis is dependent on the stage at the time of presentation with T1–2 having 80–90% 5-year survival while T4 can be as low as 10–15%. A big challenge to ENT practice is getting these patients in earlier when prognosis is better.

If needed, surgery may be minimally invasive (endoscopic resection) or open surgery. Open surgery may be conservative or radical depending on the the primary site and extent of lymph node involvement. Resection of the primary tumour site (e.g. laryngectomy) with or without neck dissection of lymph nodes and follow-on radiotherapy (5 days a week for 6 weeks) 6 weeks postop is a standard treatment option for advanced (T3–4) disease.

PAEDIATRIC AIRWAY ISSUES

Laryngomalacia

This is the commonest cause of stridor in children and is often mild and presents in the first week or two of life. The mother might report particular problems when feeding the child or laying it on its back and/or failure to thrive. Referral to an ENT surgeon is important if you suspect this. A flexible nasendoscopy under LA is usually carried out proceeding onto a microlaryngoscopy and bronchoscopy (MLB) to confirm the diagnosis. Treatment is usually conservative but laser epiglottoplasty is highly effective in appropriate cases.

Epiglottis

This is a true airway emergency and it classically presents with a drooling, acutely unwell febrile child. Get ENT and anaesthetic consultants involved early, Do not upset or try to examine the mouth in case you trigger acute airway obstruction. The airway is secured by intubating and then swabs can be taken of the epiglottis and IV antibiotics (usually third-generation cephalosporins) given.

Foreign Body

The sudden onset of stridor in a previously normal child must always be regarded as due to a foreign body until proven otherwise.

Always listen to the mother. If a mother is convinced that her child has inhaled and choked on something she probably is right even if your physical exam and CXR are normal. The only way to exclude a foreign body in the bronchus is by bronchoscopy.

Laryngeal Papillomatosis

This should be suspected in a child with progressive hoarseness or aphonia and airway obstruction. It is caused by human papilloma virus (HPV 6 and 11) and usually presents before the age of 5 years with a hoarse voice or, in some cases, stridor. Diagnosis is by direct laryngoscopy and treatment is usually laser resection. The papilloma virus has a strong tendency to recur and repeated treatments are often needed.

Subglottic Stenosis

Prolonged intubation and congenital abnormalities are the commonest causes and in children the subglottis is the narrowest part of the respiratory tract. Stridor and failure to thrive are presenting features. Treatment depends on severity and ranges from conservative observation if mild to tracheostomy and partial cricotracheal resection if severe.

17

THE EXAM

Ben Banerjee

Examinations are formidable even to the best prepared, for the greatest
fool may ask more than the wisest man can answer.

C. C. Colton

Most medical schools set a mixture of written, viva voce and clinical
examinations. Written papers may be essay questions, short answers, multiple choice questions (MCQs) or extended matching questions. Clinical
exams consist of either short case or long cases, or both. In some medical
schools, medical and surgical cases are examined together and this is
becoming more common. In some, surgical cases are examined in a separate section of the exam. It is important that you understand how the
exams run in your own medical school, as it will influence the way you
should prepare for them. You should speak to people who have done the
exams in previous years and look through as many past papers as possible. Each year at medical school the majority of students pass their finals.
Essentially, the aim of the examiners is to vet out anyone who clearly is
unsafe to be a houseman (foundation year 1). It is a bit like a game with
hard and fast rules. If you abide by the rules of the game you will pass,
and if you break them you could fail. The following list includes some of
the rules concerning how not to fail finals:

- Dress smartly and look respectable.
- Be polite to the patient and try to build up rapport, because if they do
  not like you they could land you in difficulty.
- Never hurt the patient.

380 Surgical Talk: Revision in Surgery

- Never make up anything, and never say anything dangerous. If you do not know something say that you will ask a senior for advice, or for a drug say that you would look it up in the *British National Formulary* (*BNF*).
- Wash hands before any physical examination and ensure your nails and hands are well groomed.
- The examiners are always right — do not answer back and do not argue.

If the examiners think that you would be unsafe as a junior doctor, then they will fail you. Know the management of emergency conditions well because if your viva is not going well the examiners will usually change the subject to one that you should know something about in order to be a safe doctor. For example, you should know the emergency management of a shocked patient. If you said you would do a CT scan before placing two large-bore venflons into the antecubital fossae and starting fluids, then you would deserve to fail.

WRITTEN PAPERS

It is important to deal with this part of the exam with care and a prepared approach. You should also aim to practise written answers before the exam. Except for clinical cases or objective structured clinical exams (OSCEs), marking is usually done anonymously by two examiners. Remember that many examiners attach great importance to legibility, accuracy and clearness of expression. In most universities answers have to be written in specific mark books and there are often requirements to write candidate numbers on each page, start each answer on a new sheet, etc. Try to follow these instructions in full. It may be advisable to use alternate lines in an answer book if this improves legibility, and it may also be a good idea to underline section headings, perhaps with a different colour. Use an appropriate pen for written answers and avoid unusual colours of ink. Resist the temptation to write so quickly that your writing becomes illegible.

Essay Questions

Many exams these days do not have essay questions. It would not harm for you to practice writing essays, however, in preparation for any exam as they are a great way to sort your thoughts out in a logical manner. Writing an essay to a time limit is a definite skill which can be enormously improved with practice. It is obvious that one should read the questions carefully before starting to answer the paper, but it is amazing how many students apparently fail to do this. The examiners will usually have decided in advance on an approximate allocation of marks for each point made and discussed. There may be some spare marks to award arbitrarily for excellence but they will be relatively few. What this means is that you will get most of the marks for simply mentioning or sketching out points and relatively few for elaboration. If you spend time answering things which have not been asked, no matter how good your answer is, there will be no marks. An example would be 'How might a peptic ulcer present?' and the candidate spends time discussing how it might be treated. Many medical schools (and postgraduate exams like MRCS) use 'close marking' schemes. The essence of these is that questions are all given marks close to the pass mark, i.e. 40 for a bad fail, 65 for a very good answer. This means that it is very difficult to make up for answers left completely unattempted. The only way to avoid simple types of error is to have a set plan of approach; since it is easy to make an error in the heat of battle, you must plan your strategy in advance. We would suggest the following:

- Read the instructions at the top of the paper carefully (i.e. how many questions should be answered, time allowed, etc.). Do not presume that they will be the same as for past papers you may have looked at during your revision. If you are not sure ask the invigilator, who is there for that purpose.
- Calculate exactly how much time should be spent on each question after allowing 5 min for reading the paper and 5 min for each essay plan.
- Slowly read each question in turn, until you are sure you understand what it is asking.
- Spend 5 min on each question thinking and writing a rough plan. Use the surgical sieve to prevent your forgetting anything. Do all the plans first.

- Only then start writing the essays themselves. Start with the one you feel you can answer best.
- Spend only the amount of time allowed on any one question.
- On no account fail to answer a question. If the worst happens and you run out of time, hand in your essay plan.

Multiple Choice Questions

The basic way most multiple choice exams are marked is that you get one mark for a correct answer, nothing for an answer not attempted and one mark is taken away for an incorrect answer.

This means that guesswork is unlikely to improve your marks and may in fact reduce them, since questions may be deliberately misleading. If possible, clarify what type of marking scheme is used in your medical school well in advance of the exam.

We suggest you approach MCQs in the following way:

- Calculate the time available and aim to go through the paper in 60% of that time.
- Go through answering only the questions you are fairly certain you know the answers to.
- Go back over the questions you have not answered and see if there are any that you can now answer with a fair degree of certainty.
- Questions using the words *always* and *never* are invariably false; likewise questions using the word *may* are usually true (for example, 'Vomiting is *always* present in bowel obstruction' — false).
- Make sure you spend a moment on each question considering the exact wording and sense of the question — this can make a big difference in the multiple choice. For example, 'Perforated peptic ulcer is always treated by operation' is not the same as 'Perforated peptic ulcer is usually treated by operation'.
- Leave questions unanswered when your answer would be complete guesswork.
- Some MCQs are not negatively marked and for these you should answer all the questions, even if you have to guess.

Extended Matching Questions

Extended matching questions are increasingly being used for medical students' exams. By using cases rather than just facts they can be used to test problem solving and the application of knowledge. Usually, a clinical scenario (a 'vignette') is described and candidates are offered a list of up to 20 possible responses. The candidate has to select the *single* best response for each vignette. Most commonly, several vignettes are grouped together within a clinical theme for a single set of responses. The 'best' response may be used more than once so do not be worried about this. Confusingly, it seems a common format is to list the responses before starting the vignettes. This type of question has the potential to be confusing (for examiners as well!), so make sure you understand the format and practice answering such questions well in advance of the exam (see examples at the end of this chapter).

Short Answer Questions

Even more than with essay questions the examiners will be awarding marks on the basis of individual points mentioned. Once again there will be few marks which can be flexibly awarded and no marks for points in the answer which do not address the question as actually asked. It is usually not necessary (or possible time-wise) to do a plan, but in many ways the answers should have the obvious structure of a plan anyway. As with essay questions you should first of all spend a few minutes reading the instructions and all the questions twice. Then, decide which questions you are going to answer and calculate the time to be spent on each question. Do not spend more time on any one question and make sure you finish all the questions.

Clinical Examination

You should be smartly dressed and arrive early. This is often the most worrying part of the exam for students. It can be quite difficult to think clearly in such a high-tension situation and it is important that you have prepared your basic history-taking and examining techniques in advance so that you can perform these on 'auto-pilot' and concentrate specifically on your answers to the examiners. One of the best ways to prepare yourself is with practice with your colleagues or with medical staff on the firms you are attached to. It is possible for you to work much longer periods when revising and practicing together.

Viva Voce Examination

This usually takes the form of the candidate sitting at a desk opposite two examiners. Topics can cover any area of surgery, and sometimes X-rays, specimens or surgical instruments may be shown. In some medical schools the viva is the last part of the exam and then commonly the examiners will know something of the candidates' performance to that point. In other medical schools the viva is only held for deciding who should get a distinction or for those with borderline marks who are in some danger of failing.

The examiners quickly develop an overall impression of you; therefore, it is important not to ponder far too long over the first question asked. If you do not understand a question, after a short period of reflection tell the examiners that you do not understand and ask them to rephrase the question. If you do this they will usually give some extra information or a hint to help you in the correct direction. This is much better than simply asking them to repeat the question when you will probably get no extra information and will still be unable to answer.

Always try to classify your answer in a logical way (e.g. the surgical sieve). Start with the simple and more common things and work to the more complex and rare elements. Remember, if the questions appear to be getting harder this usually means you are doing well, as the examiners need to assess how good you are, so that they can give you a grade. Most people leave the room remembering only the last question asked — which is, as explained, usually the most difficult. This is why you should never ask the candidate leaving the viva before you what they were asked.

Objective Structured Clinical Exams

Many medical schools now use OSCEs as part of their examinations. The principle of these is to provide uniformity in the exam for all students and not have the unpredictabilty that is inherent in the standard clinical exams. There is usually no negative marking in an OSCE. Since all candidates will be examined on the same material, it is possible to standardise marking across examiners in a way that would not otherwise be possible. Often actors are used instead of real patients. The usual approach for an OSCE exam is to have a number of 'stations' at which the candidate has to carry out tasks. For example, one station might be to carry out an abdominal exam, another to consent a patient for a colostomy, etc. Examiners may be present to mark the candidate, which can sometimes be off-putting; however, they would not normally speak or question the candidate directly. Some stations may also consist of X-rays with a list of questions or pictures of clinical signs, etc., in which the candidate completes an answer sheet which is marked afterwards. Where actors are used they are usually asked to give out only one piece of information at a time. For example the question 'Do you have abdominal pain?' would produce the answer 'Yes' and you would then have to ask 'Where is the pain', etc. as a separate question. There is nothing inherent in an OSCE examination which should trouble the well-prepared candidate. One problem can be completing the task within the time allowed at each station, and you should therefore find out the format of the exam well in advance and practise doing things to time.

Short Cases

These were traditionally used in most medical schools but are gradually being replaced by OSCEs. A large number of cases, usually with physical signs, are assembled together in one place. The candidate is taken from case to case by the examiners.

The examiners usually work in pairs, with one questioning and the other marking. Do not be put off by this. There is no truth in the commonly held belief that you have to get through a particular number of short cases to be able to pass. Remember to briefly introduce yourself to the patient, ask them if they mind your examining them and make sure you preserve their dignity but without compromising on exposure. Most marks will be awarded for using the correct technique of examination and not necessarily for reaching a diagnosis. Not all short cases will take the same length of time to deal with. If the case is very straightforward (for example a case of Dupuytren's), simply state the features and diagnosis so that the examiners can either move on or ask you extra questions about treatment, etc. Above all, be guided by the examiners as to what you should examine and how quickly.

Common short cases include:

- neck lumps (especially thyroid)
- groin lumps (especially hernias and testicular lumps)
- hands (Dupytren's, ganglions and nerve lesions)
- skin cancers and lumps (e.g. BCCs, lipomata and neufibromata)
- abdominal examinations (enlarged liver or stomas)
- lower limbs (varicose veins, ACL tears, knee osteoarthritis or chronic ulcers)
- feet (hammer toes, hallux rigidus or hallux valgus)

Long Cases

Most medical schools expect the candidate to be examined on a surgical long case, although the time available with the patient varies enormously (20–60 min). The principle of the long case is that the candidate is left alone with the patient to take a history and carry out an examination. Leave 5 min at the end to quickly gather your thoughts on how you are going to present the case to the examiners. The time allowed with the patient varies from 20 min to 1 h. In medical schools where 1 h is allowed, there is usually enough time for a full standard history and examination, and time itself should pose no problem. When the time is shorter, the candidate may have to limit the history and examination to the most important points. This will be understood by the examiners, and if asked about something you have not had time to do, you must state this clearly. It is a fatal error to waffle or, even worse, make something up. Remember also that the examiners may take you back to the case and go over the points in question with you. If you are found to have made something up, then usually you will automatically fail this part of the exam. If possible, present the case without looking at your notes continuously (sample presentations are given below). Eye contact with the examiners will help to make a good impression.

Common long cases include abdominal operations (e.g. postop bowel resection for cancer or inflammatory bowel disease), vascular cases (carotid disease, aortic aneurysm or peripheral vascular disease), orthopaedic cases (joint replacements for osteoarthritis) and breast lumps (usually elderly patients).

When you present your long case to your examiner, have a provisional diagnosis or differential in your mind. It is sometimes possible to predict what questions the examiner is going to ask you, and it will help if you have thought of the answers before the question is asked. Here are some sample presentations from real finals cases. Note that they are concise and contain only the relevant facts. Leave 5 min at the end of your clerking to get your ideas together and to write a quick summary.

SAMPLE LONG CASE CLERKINGS

Case 1

Mr. J S is a 67-year-old retired builder. He has attended today for the purpose of the exams. He presents with a year's history of progressive pain in his left hip. Over the last 3 months, however, the pain has worsened, and it now interferes with his sleep. He occasionally needs a stick and has particular difficulty in climbing stairs. Whereas in the past he could walk long distances, he can now only walk 200 yd before he is limited by pain in the groin and he also has difficulty in putting on his shoes and socks. His GP prescribed Ibuprofen, which despite some initial help is now of no use.

There has been no history of trauma and he denies any problems with his other joints. He is married and lives in a two-storey house with his wife.

In his past medical history he had an appendicectomy at age 12 but otherwise has been fit and well, with no cardiorespiratory disease. He has no relevant family history and his only medication is Ibuprofen. He denies any allergies and does not smoke or drink.

On systems review the only positive findings were those of prostatism, where he reports nocturia twice nightly, a poor stream and terminal dribbling of his urine.

On examination he is slightly overweight (weighing 110 kg, with a height of 5 ft 6 in. [If you could work out the body mass index, you certainly would impress the examiners. NB: BMI = weight^2 (kg)/height (cm) and is normally under 25.] But he looks generally well, with no signs of anaemia, jaundice or lymphadenopathy. Cardiorespiratory examination was unremarkable (have it written, in case they ask you about any particular point), and abdominal examination revealed an appendicectomy scar. I did not perform a rectal examination, but would normally do so, to feel the size and consistency of his prostate. On examination of his hips he has an antalgic gait with a positive Trendelenburg's test. There was no leg length discrepancy. He has a fixed flexion deformity of 10° on the left side and a decreased range of movement of the left hip (flexion 10–85°, abduction 35°, adduction 10°, internal rotation 10° and external rotation 15°). The movements were most painful in full flexion and internal rotation. Examination of the right hip and the back and both knees was normal. There was no neurovascular deficit and no signs of peripheral vascular or venous disease. In summary, this 67-year-old retired builder has a year's history of progressively worsening pain in his left hip which is now affecting his lifestyle and ability to sleep at night. My provisional diagnosis is that of osteoarthritis.

The examiners will then ask what investigations you would like to perform (plain X-rays) and will make you comment on them. They are likely to ask you about anything you have said. If your diagnosis is correct, then the questions they may ask you are as follows:

1. What is the treatment? (Conservative versus surgical — lose weight, physio, etc., although the patient is likely to need a hip replacement.)
2. You say in your history that he has prostatism — is that relevant? (Yes, he may go into postoperative retention.)

3. The examiners may talk to the patient and ask you about your positive findings. [Trendelenburg's test, leg length, fixed flexion (Thomas's test).]

Case 2

Mrs. J P is a 51-year-old housewife who is currently an in-patient at this hospital, awaiting surgery. She presents with a lump in her left breast. She first noticed the lump two weeks ago whilst showering and it has not changed since then. She has no symptoms from the lump and she had never noticed any breast lumps before. Her main concern is that this is a cancer.

Her menarche was at age 12 and her periods were always regular up until her menopause 2 years ago. She has been on hormone replacement therapy since. She has no family history of breast cancer. She went to her GP, who sent her to the breast clinic last week, where she underwent a needle test and a mammography. She says the results were suggestive of cancer and she has been admitted for surgery. She has no relevant past medical history and is on no medication, but is allergic to penicillin, which gives her a rash. She lives with her husband John, who is 57 and they elected to have no children. She smokes 10 cigarettes a day and drinks only occasionally.

Systems review was negative for any problems in the cardiovascular, respiratory, abdominal and neurological systems. On examination she looks well and is not pale or jaundiced. Examination of her breasts reveals that both nipples are inverted, although she says this has been present for as long as she can remember. She has a 3 cm hard lump in the upper outer quadrant of her left breast. The lump has an irregular outline but is mobile and not tethered to the chest wall or the skin. She has no lymphadenopathy and no evidence of metastatic spread on examination of her abdomen, chest and spine. Cardiorespiratory examination was unremarkable.

In summary, this 51-year-old postmenopausal lady has a suspicious 3 cm lump in her left breast. She has undergone triple assessment in the clinic and has been admitted for surgery tomorrow.

The examiners will ask questions like

1. What is your differential diagnosis? [Benign or malignant, etc. Cancer, fat necrosis, fibroadenoma (rare in this age group).]
2. If you saw this lady in the clinic what investigations would you perform? (Triple assessment.)
3. Are there any further investigations that can be performed? (Trucut and staging procedures.)
4. What treatments are available?

Sample OSCE Station (1)

'This patient has a lump in the left groin, please examine it and say what you think it is'. (The station consists of a male patient with a left inguinal hernia, on a couch.)

Example Marking Scheme	*Available Marks = 10*
Introduces themselves to patient and asks permission to examine them. Adequate exposure, preserves patient's dignity	0/1
Asks patient to point to site of lump	0/1
Stands patient up	0/1
Asks patient to cough and inspects for lump	0/1/2
Palpates anatomical landmarks	0/1/2
Defines position of lump in relation to testicle	0/1/2
Identifies it as an inguinal hernia	0/1

Example OSCE Station 2

A 25-year-old man presents to A & E with an 18 h history of acute abdominal pain. Please carry out an appropriate examination of his abdomen. (The station consists of an actor in a gown and underpants on a couch.)

Example Marking Scheme	*Available Marks = 20*
Introduces themselves and asks permission to examine patient	0/1/2
Washes hands	0/1/2
Arranges adequate exposure whilst preserving patient's dignity	0/1/2
Inspects abdomen	0/1/2
Palpates lightly all quadrants	0/1/2
Palpates deeply all quadrants	0/1/2
Feels for liver, spleen, kidneys	0/1/2
Examines hernial orifices	0/1/2
Percussion	0/1/2
Listens to bowel sounds	0/1/2

Example Extended Matching Question 1

A. Perforated peptic ulcer
B. Appendicitis
C. Kidney stone
D. Bowel obstruction
E. Strangulated hernia
F. Ruptured ectopic pregnancy
G. Abdominal aneurysm
H. Mesenteric adenitis
I. Carcinoma of the colon
J. Endometriosis
K. Pancreatitis
L. Diverticulitis

For each patient presenting with abdominal pain select the correct diagnosis. Answers may be used more than once.

1. A 24-year-old man presents with right lower abdominal pain. The pain comes on gradually over 24 h and was initially left in the centre of his

abdomen. He has nausea but has not vomited. He has not opened his bowels for 24 h. Examination shows a temperature of 37.6°C and a right lower abdominal tender mass.

Correct answer = B

2. An 80-year-old man has developed poorly localised lower abdominal pain over 5 days. There is no nausea or vomiting. He has not had a bowel movement for 2 days and before this he has had loose stools. Examination shows him to be apyrexial and to have a soft abdomen with a palpable, slightly tender left lower abdominal mass.

Correct answer = I

Example Extended Matching Question 2

A. Paget's disease
B. Galactocele
C. Gynaecomastia
D. Fat necrosis
E. Carcinoma of the breast
F. Fibroadenoma
G. Mastalgia
H. Breast abscess

For the following case descriptions please select the most likely diagnosis. Answers can be used more than once.

1. A 45-year-old woman presents with an inflamed itchy nipple. Mammography is normal. Clinical examination reveals no breast lump or lymphadenopathy.

Correct answer = A

2. A 60-year-old man presents with a hard mass in the right breast which is fixed to the chest wall.

Correct answer = E

INDEX

abdomen, examination   167
abdominal pain   165
abscess   34, 37, 38
achalasia   106, 115
acoustic neuroma   367, 370
acute abdomen   170
acute diverticulitis   151
acute otitis media   367
acute pancreatitis   85
acute respiratory distress syndrome
  (ARDS)   322
adhesions   3
airway   47, 72
aldosterone   18
alkaline phosphatase   22
allergic rhinitis   372
amnesia   69
anaesthetic   33
anaesthetist   27, 73
aneurysm   5, 238, 242
aneurysmal bone cyst (ABC)   344
angiodysplasia   154
angioplasty   237
ankle brachial pressure index (ABPI)   233
anorectal abscess   161
anterior cruciate ligament rupture   325
anterior draw test   285
anterior resection   26, 141
antibiotics   30, 31, 34, 37
anticoagulant   26

aortic aneurysm   231, 239
appendicitis   127, 130–132, 172
arthrodesis   331
arthroplasty   331
arthroscopy   324
articular cartilage   326
ATLS®   65, 294
autologous chondrocyte implantation
  (ACI)   327
avascular necrosis   303, 339
axillary nerve   320

Badger's sign   63
Baker's cyst   284
Bankart lesion   320
Barlow's test   356
Barrett's oesophagus   107
Barton's fracture   317
basal cell carcinoma   214
Battle sign   62
benign breast disease   180, 193
benign prostatic hyperplasia (BPH)   6,
  39, 259, 260
Bier's block   315
biliary colic   84
bilirubin   80, 99
bladder
    cancer   257
    diverticulae   259

393

blood   15, 40
blood gas analysis   37
body water   13
Boerhaave's syndrome   113
bone
     cyst   344
     graft   302
     tumour   341
Bouchard's nodes   288, 329
bowel obstruction   3
Bowen's disease   215
brain injury   64
branchial cyst   198
branchial sinus   200
breast
     abscess   195
     clinic   179
     examination   175
     lump   9, 10
     triple assessment   180
     reconstruction   193
breast cancer   9, 11, 177–179, 183–185,
185, 187, 190, 191
     screening   192
     staging   182
Buerger's test   233
burns   70–77

Caisson disease   339
cancer
     bladder   264
     gallbladder   91
     larynx   376
     pancreas   91, 98
     prostate   259, 263
capillary refill time   55
carbon monoxide   73
cardiac tamponade   49
carotid body tumour   200
carotid disease   242

carotid endarterectomy   243
carpal tunnel syndrome   316, 352
cast bracing (*see* functional bracing)
catheter   40, 255
central line   57, 58
central venous pressure (CVP)   22
     line   22
cerebral perfusion pressure (CPP)   61
cerebrospinal fluid (CSF)   60, 62, 63
cervical spine   45
Charcot's triad   103
chemotherapy   189
chest drain   39, 50
chin lift   47
cholangitis   32, 81, 90, 103
cholecystectomy   86, 89
cholecystitis   85
     acute   7, 84
     chronic   83
chondrolysis   360
chondroma   344
chondromalacia patella   283
chondrosarcoma   347
claudication   236
coagulopathy   101
Codman's triangle   346
colicky pain   9, 10, 166
Colles fracture   315
colloid   15, 40
colorectal cancer   140, 147
colostomy   26, 143
compartment syndrome   300, 319
complex regional pain syndrome   303
complication   36, 119
computerised tomography (CT)   80
concussion   63
congenital dislocation of the hip
     (*see* DDH)
contre coup injury   64
contusion   64
core biopsy   181

Courvoisier's rule   99
craniocleidodysostosis   287
crepitus   283
cricothyroidotomy   48
Crohn's disease   134, 136–140
cruciate ligament   284
crystalloid   14, 15
cubitus varus   319
Cushing response   67
cystic hygroma   200
cystoscopy   258

deafness   365
deep vein thrombosis (DVT)   30, 33,
    35–38, 251
delayed union   302
dermoid   200
developmental dysplasia of the hip
    (DDH)   355
diabetes   26–28
diagnostic peritoneal lavage
    (DPL)   51
dislocation   291
    shoulder   319
diverticular disease   151, 154
diverticulitis   152, 153
drain   19, 38, 39
ductal carcinoma *in situ* (DCIS)   180, 187
Dukes staging   141
duodenal ulcer   123
Dupuytren's contracture   288, 353
dynamic hip screw (DHS)   311
dysphagia   105, 106

ear, examination   361
embolism   234
empyema of the gallbladder   85
enchondroma   344
ERCP   81, 82, 89

endoscopic ultrasound   81
endotracheal tube   49
enteral feeding   21, 22
epididymo-orchitis   272
epiglottis   378
epistaxis   371
Erbs palsy   350
escharotomies   74, 76
Ewing's sarcoma   347
external fixator   298
extracellular fluid   13
extracorporeal shock wave lithotripsy
    276
extradural haemorrhage   64

facial nerve   197, 209
fasciotomy   235, 301
fibroadenoma   180
fibrocystic disease   180
fibroma   5
fibrous cortical defect   345
fibrous dysplasia   345
fine needle aspiration   180
fissure *in Ano*   158
fistula   19
fistula *in Ano*   159
fixed flexion deformity   283
flail chest   45, 49
fluid balance   15, 20, 40
follicular carcinoma   205
fracture   62, 69, 70
    basal   62, 70
    classification   289
    complications   299
    depressed   62
    distal radius   314
    femoral   322
    healing   292
    malunion   303
    management   294

fracture (*Continued*)
  neck of femur   305
  nonunion   302
  open   62, 295
  radius and ulna   312
  reduction   295
  rehabilitation   299
  scaphoid   317
  skull   62, 69, 70
  supracondylar humerus   318
  tibial   322
free field hearing test   363
Freiberg's disease   340
Froment's sign   351
functional bracing   297

gait   281
  antalgic   281
  short-legged   282
Galleazzi fracture   314
gallstone   25, 82–84
gallstone ileus   90
ganglion   354
Garden classification   308, 309
Gardeners' syndrome   149
gastrectomy   35
gastric cancer   109, 110
gastric ulcer   123
gastrointestinal stromal tumour   111
Gaucher's disease   339
giant cell tumour   345
Girdlestone's procedure   334
Glasgow Coma Score (GCS)   46, 66,
  67, 70
glue ear   368
goitre   202
Goodsall's rule   160
Greenstick fracture   290
Guedel airway   48
gunstock deformity   319

haemarthrosis   326
haematuria   4, 5, 257, 274
haemorrhage   34, 51
haemorrhagic shock   55
haemorrhoid   154, 157
haemothorax   49
haemotympanum   62
hand, examination   287
head injury   46, 59–61, 65–68
hearing test   362
Heberden's nodes   288, 329
heparin   30
hernia   217
  epigastric   227
  femoral   5, 221
  groin   220
  hiatus   106, 113, 114
  incisional   226
  inguinal   5, 221, 222
  obturator   227
  sliding   218
  strangulated   3
  umbilical   220, 226
Hickman line   22
Hill Sachs lesion   320
hip resurfacing   335
hip, examination   280
Hutchinson's pupil   64
hydrocoele   270
hyperglycaemia   22
hypertrophic pyloric stenosis   125
hypospadia   277
hypovolaemia   45, 63
hypoxia   46, 63

ileostomy   19, 26, 142
ileus   18, 35
infection   21, 30, 35
  chest   29, 33, 35, 36
  wound   34, 36

insensible loss 16, 20
insulin 22, 28
insulinoma 29
internal fixation 298
interspinous ligament 54
interstitial fluid 13
intracellular fluid 13
intracranial haemorrhage 64
intracranial pressure (ICP) 60, 61, 64
intravenous (IV) fluid 13, 17
intubation 48
intussusception 3, 129, 133
irritable hip 360
ischaemia
    critical 236
ischaemic leg 233

jaundice, complications 101

Kaposi's sarcoma 215
Kienboch's disease 340
Klumpke paralysis 350
knee, examination 282
knock knees 282
Kocher's method 320
Kohler's disease 340

Lachman test 285
laparascopic cholecystectomy 25, 31,
    86–88
laparoscopy 88
laparotomy 40, 51
large bowel obstruction 136
laryngomalacia 377
leg length discrepancy 280
leg ulceration 249, 250
'light bulb' sign 322
lipohaemarthrosis 324

lipoma 5, 210
liver function tests 79, 80
LOAF muscles 288
lobular carcinoma *in situ* 188
log roll 46, 52, 53
lymph node 5
lymphoedema 252

Maffucci's syndrome 344
magnetic resonance imaging (MRI) 81
Mallory–Weiss tear 123
mammography 181
mastectomy 184, 185
McBurney's point 131
McCune–Albright syndrome 345
McMurray's test 284
Meckel's diverticulum 127, 128
melanoma 212, 213
Meniere's disease 366
mesenteric adenitis 133
metaplastic polyp 151
methicillin-resistant *Staphylococcus
    aureus* (MRSA) 31, 34
middle meningeal artery 64
Monroe–Kellie Doctrine 60
Monteggia fracture 312
mouth, examination 373
MRC grading system 281, 350
mucocoele 89
Muir and Barclay formula 74
multiorgan failure 44
Multiple Endocrine Neoplasia (MEN) 122
Murphy's sign 84
Murphy's test 168
myoglobinuria 235
myositis ossificans 304

naevi 211
nasogastric tube 19, 47, 135

nasopharyngeal tube   48
nerve palsy   301
neurofibroma   211
nipple, discharge   196
normal saline   15, 17, 19
nose, examination   370
nutrition   21, 23

objective structured clinical examination
   385
obstructive jaundice   97, 98, 100, 101
oesophagus
      cancer   107, 108
      perforation   113
      varices   123
Ollier's disease   344
oncotic pressure   13
open reduction and internal fixation
   (ORIF)   297
oral contraceptive pill   30
Ortolani's test   356
Osgood–Schlatter disease   340
osmotic pressure   13, 14
osteoarthritis   327
osteochondral injury   326
osteochondritis   339
osteochondritis dissecans   340
osteochondroma   345
osteoid osteoma   346
osteomyelitis   348
osteophyte   328
osteosarcoma   346
osteotomy   331
otorrhoea   62

Paget's disease   188
pancreatitis   19
pancreatitis, acute   81, 94–97
Panner's disease   340

papillary carcinoma (*see* thyroid)
papilloma   212
parathyroid gland   208
parenteral nutrition   21, 22
parotid gland   197, 208–210
patella apprehension test   284
patella tap   283
pathological fracture   291
Pavlik harness   357
pearl ganglion   289
pelvic abscess   37
peptic ulceration   115, 124
perforation of the eardrum   369
peripheral arterial system   230
peritonitis   131, 166
Perthe's disease   359
pes cavus   283
pes planus   283
Peutz–Jeghers syndrome   150
pharyngeal pouch   106, 112
physiotherapy   29, 30, 33, 36
pilonidal abscess/sinus   162
pivot shift test   285
plasma   13
pleiomorphic adenoma   210
Plummer Vinson syndrome   106
pneumothorax   49, 50, 58
Poiseuille's law   56
polyps   3, 133
      adenomatous   148
      colonic   148
      hamartomatous   150
popliteal aneurysm   231, 241, 284
popliteal cyst   284
posterior draw test   285
postoperative complication   4, 11, 33
potassium   14, 18–20
primary survey   44
prophylaxis   31, 32
prostate specific antigen (PSA)   260
pulmonary embolism   251

pulmonary embolus 30, 37
pure tone audiometry 364
pyloroplasty 118
pyrexia 19, 22, 36, 38

quinsy 375

radial nerve 350
radical prostatectomy 264
raised intracranial pressure 68
Ranson's criteria 95
rectal cancer 142
rectal prolapse 160
reflex sympathetic dystrophy 303
renal cell carcinoma 257, 266
renal colic 273
renal failure 20, 102
renal tumour 266
resuscitation 44, 47, 51, 72
rhabdomyolysis 71
rheumatoid arthritis 338
rhinorrhoea 62
Richter's hernia 218, 227
Rinne's test 362
rotator cuff 286, 319
"rule of nines" 75

salivary calculi 209
salivary gland 208
salivary gland neoplasm 210
Salter–Harris classification 304, 305
saphena varix 5
scalp laceration 62
scaphoid fracture (*see* fracture)
sebaceous cyst 5, 211
secondary intention 35
secondary survey 44, 52, 53
Seddon classification 301

Seldinger technique 57
semimembranous bursa 284
seminoma 268
sentinel node biopsy 187
sepsis 44
septic arthritis 349
sequestrum 349
Sever's disease 340
shock 46, 51, 54–56, 68
shoulder instability 321
shoulder, examination 285
sickle cell disease 339
sieve, surgical 2, 3, 7
sinusitis 373
skull X-ray 70
sliding scale 28
slipped capital/upper femoral epiphysis 359
small bowel obstruction 133
Smith's fracture 316
smoking 30
sodium 14, 19
Spigelian hernia 227
squamous cell carcinoma 214
steroid 26, 29, 35
stoma 26, 142
strangulation 134, 218
stroke test 283
subarachnoid haemorrhage 65
subdural haemorrhage 65
subluxation 292
subphrenic abscess 37
Sudek's atrophy 303, 316
sulphasalizine 77
suprapubic catheter 256
surgical airway 48

tamoxifen 189
tension pneumothorax 44, 49, 55
teratoma 268

testicular torsion 273
testicular tumour 268
third space losses 18, 19
Thomas's test 281
thrombophlebitis 36
thyroglossal cyst 207
thyroid 201, 202
    cyst 204
    function test 204
    nodule 203
    papillary carcinoma 205
    surgery, complications 206
    tumour 205
thyroidectomy 11
Tinel's test 352
tinnitus 364
tonsilitis 374
total hip replacement 332
total knee replacement 335
tracheal deviation 45
tracheostomy 48, 49
traction 298
traction apophysitis 340
transurethral resection of the prostate
    (TURP) 261
trauma 43
"Trauma Series" 47
Trendelenburg gait 334
Trendelenburg's test 281
triangles of the neck 198
trigger finger 289
triple assessment (*see* breast)
trochanteric bursitis 280
tumour node metastases (TNM)
    system 182
TURP, complications 262

ulcerative colitis 136, 138, 154
ulnar nerve 351
ultrasound 25, 80, 181
undescended testes 5, 277
upper gastrointestinal bleeding 123
ureteric colic 274
urethral injury 47
urethral stricture 259
urinary retention 33
urine output 15, 18, 19, 36, 39, 40

vagotomy 118
valgus 282
varicose vein 244–248
varus 283
venous ulceration 249
vertigo 365
vitamin K 80, 101
viva voce examination 25, 384
Volkman's ischaemic contracture 301,
    319, 351
volvulus 3, 134

Weber's test 363
Whipple's operation 92
Wilm's tumour 268
winging of the scapulae 286
wound dehiscence 35
written paper 380

Zollinger–Ellison syndrome 117,
    119, 121